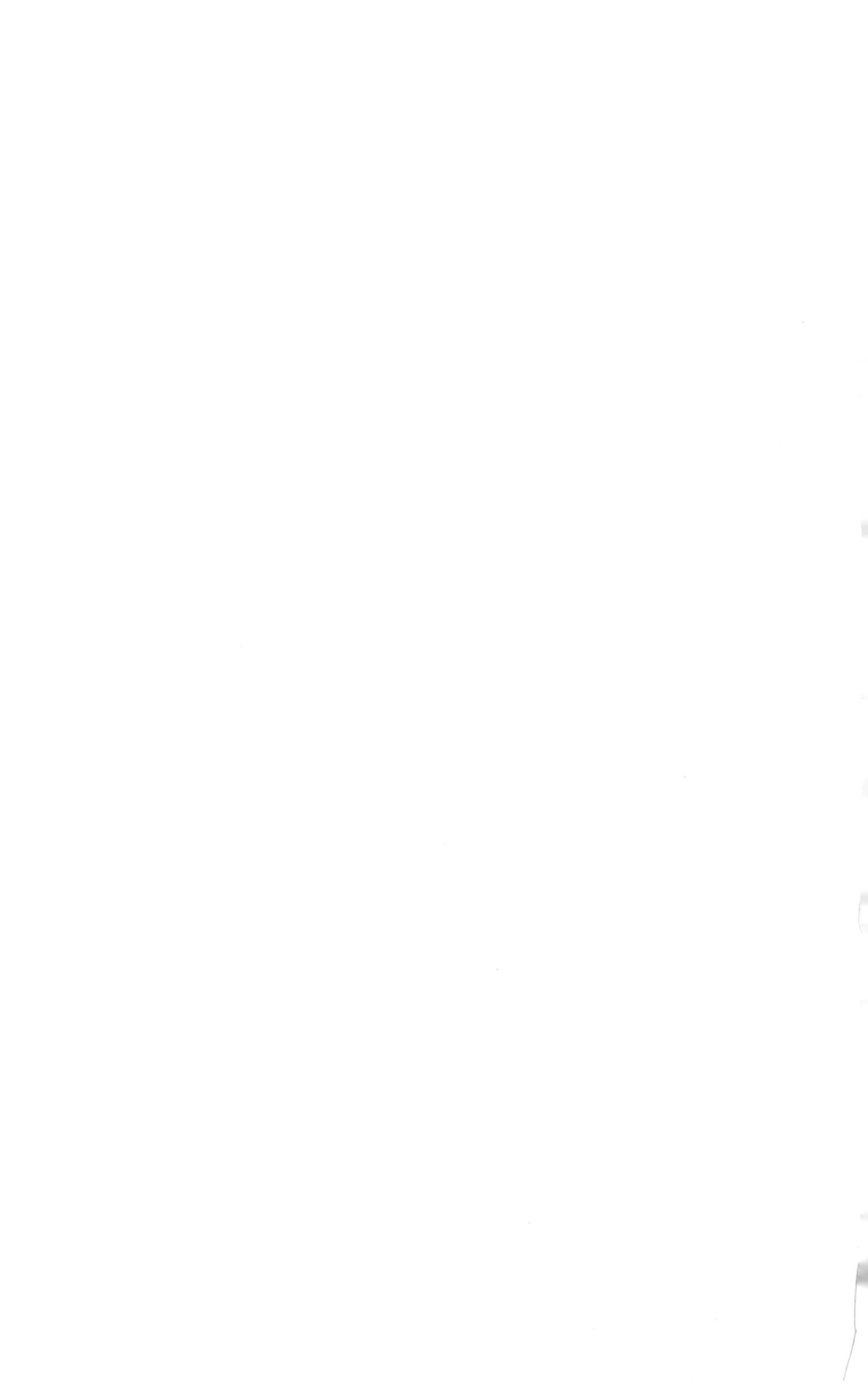

# CURRENT STATUS OF CLINICAL ORGAN TRANSPLANTATION

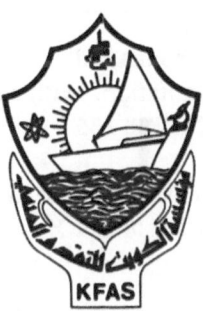

KFAS

# DEVELOPMENTS IN SURGERY

J.M. Greep, H.A.J. Lemmens, D.B. Roos, H.C. Urschel, eds., Pain in Shoulder and Arm: An Integrated View
ISBN 90 247 2146 6

B. Niederle, Surgery of the Biliary Tract
ISBN 90 247 2402 3

J.A. Nakhosteen & W. Maassen, eds., Bronchology: Research, Diagnostic and Therapeutic Aspects
ISBN 90 247 2449 X

R. van Schilfgaarde, J.C. Stanley, P. van Brummelen & E.H. Overbosch, eds., Clinical Aspects of Renovascular Hypertension
ISBN 0 89838 574 1

G.M. Abouna, ed. & A.G. White, ass. ed., Current Status of Clinical Organ Transplantation. With some Recent Developments in Renal Surgery
ISBN 0 89838 635 7

A. Cuschieri & G. Berci, Common Bile Duct Exploration
ISBN 0 89838 639 X

# CURRENT STATUS OF CLINICAL ORGAN TRANSPLANTATION

with some recent developments in renal surgery

*edited by*

GEORGE M. ABOUNA

ARTHUR G. WHITE (associate editor)

*Department of Organ Transplantation, Faculty of Medicine*
*Kuwait University and Mubarak Al-Kabeer Hospital*
*Kuwait City, Kuwait*

1984 **MARTINUS NIJHOFF PUBLISHERS**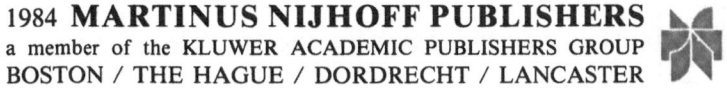
a member of the KLUWER ACADEMIC PUBLISHERS GROUP
BOSTON / THE HAGUE / DORDRECHT / LANCASTER

**Distributors**

*for the United States and Canada*: Kluwer Academic Publishers, 190 Old Derby Street, Hingham, MA 02043, USA
*for the UK and Ireland*: Kluwer Academic Publishers, MTP Press Limited, Falcon House, Queen Square, Lancaster LA1 1RN, England
*for all other countries*: Kluwer Academic Publishers Group, Distribution Center, P.O. Box 322, 3300 AH Dordrecht, The Netherlands


**Library of Congress Cataloging in Publication Data**

Main entry under title:

Current status of clinical organ transplantation with
    some recent developments in renal surgery.

    1. Kidneys--Transplantation--Congresses.  2. Trans-
plantation of organs, tissues, etc.--Congresses.
I. Abouna, George M.  II. White, Arthur G.  [DNLM:
1. Transplantation--Congresses.  2. Kidney--Transplanta-
tion--Congresses.  WO 660 C976]
RD575.C87  1984      617'.95      84-1553
ISBN 0-89838-635-7

ISBN 0-89838-635-7 (this volume)

*this book is dedicated to
Adam, Andrew, Benjamin,
Judith, Linda and Sarah*

# Foreword

MICHAEL F.A. WOODRUFF
*Emeritus Professor of Surgery,*
*University of Edinburgh*

This book grew out of a very successful conference on Organ Transplantation held in Kuwait in December 1982. The material presented at the conference has been expanded and brought up to date, and the result is a well written and authoritative account of many aspects of organ transplantation by a distinguished team of contributors drawn from many countries.

A unique feature of the book is the account it contains of the development of organ transplantation in the Middle East. Although, as yet, it has been virtually impossible in Islamic countries to take organs after death for use as transplants, it is beginning to look as if this situation may change. Meanwhile, using living volunteer donors and a small number of cadaveric organs sent from other countries, transplant teams in Kuwait and Turkey are obtaining results with kidney transplants which are as good, in terms of both transplant survival and patient survival, as those reported from acknowledged centres of excellence in the United States, Europe and other countries where organ transplantation has been established for many years.

Professor Abouna and his colleagues have shown that they not only can achieve astonishingly good results in clinical transplantation but can also produce a book that deserves to be read, and I am sure will be read, widely throughout the world.

# Preface

The idea to edit this book on 'Clinical organ transplantation' emerged shortly after a succesful First International Middle East Conference on Organ Transplantation which was held in Kuwait in December 1982. At that Conference several eminent experts and pioneers in the field of Organ Transplantation together with local transplant surgeons and scientists reviewed the current status of the art and the latest developments in Organ Transplantation, each in his own field. Subsequently it was agreed that these reviews and experiences be up-dated for publication in this book and this was achieved in December 1983. The book therefore contains up-to-date and authoritative reviews of the current status of transplantation of several vital organs including the kidney, liver, heart, heart-lung, pancreas and bone-marrow. In addition it covers several topical and controversial areas in the field of Clinical Organ Transplantation including histocompatibility matching and the role of DR and non-HLA antigens, immuno-modulation and recipient pre-treatment with blood and platelet transfusions, developments and future trends in clinical immunosuppression, the cellular diagnosis and treatment of allograft rejection and the procurement, preservation and sharing of organs.

There is also a Part on the Current Developments and Results of Renal Transplantation in the Middle East and another on some of the recent techniques in Renal Surgery including Work-Bench Surgery and Extracorporeal Lithotripsy.

The book is not intended to be a comprehensive volume on Organ Transplantation but rather as a brief review on Current practices and future trends in several aspects of clinical organ transplantation and it is hoped that it will serve as a guide to the surgeon and physician in training in Organ Transplantation, as well as to the established transplant clinician as a reference.

It is with great pleasure that we record our thanks to our colleagues and other contributors to this volume and we appreciate their help and prompt cooperation which was often given at very short notice. We are grateful to many of the staff of the Department of Organ Transplantation of Kuwait University for their dedicated support in the preparation of this book, particularly Dorothy Temudo, Ahmed Sayed Sobki, E.M. Philips, Susan Keddie, Francis Braganza and Jessy

George. We appreciate the cooperation and the patience of our publisher Martinus Nijhoff and particularly the valuable advice given by Mr. Commandeur of the Editorial staff at different stages in their preparation of the book.

Finally we acknowledge, with deep gratitude the generous financial grant given by the Kuwait Foundation for the Advancement of Science which made the publication of this book possible.

GEORGE M. ABOUNA

# Recent pronouncement by two major religions on organ transplantation

*A. Roman Catholic position as expressed by the message of Pope John Paul I to the Transplantation Society Congress in Rome, 6 September 1978.*

We owe a special greeting to members of the Seventh International Congress of the Organ Transplant Society. We are very touched by your visit, which is a homage to the Pope, and particularly by your desire to throw light on and to study more deeply the serious human and moral problems at stake in the researchers or in the surgical technique which are your lot. We encourage you, in this field, to request the help of Catholic friends, expert in theology and in morality and with a thorough knowledge of your problems, possessing a sound knowledge of Catholic doctrine and a deeply human understanding.

We are content today to express to you our congratulations and our trust, for the immense work that you put in the service of human life in order to prolong it in better conditions. The whole problem is to act with respect for the person and for one's neighbours, whether it is a question of donors of organs or beneficiaries, and never to transform man into an object of experiment. There is respect for his body, there is also respect for his spirit. We pray to God, the Author of life, to inspire you and assist you in these magnificent and formidable responsibilities. May he bless you, with all your dear ones!

*B. Muslim position as expressed by the Islamic Fatwa Committee (Religious Ruling) assembled by Ministry of Islamic Affairs in Kuwait, issued on 31 December 1979.*

If the donor is dead, it is permissible to take his organs whether or not he had so willed provided there is dire necessity, since the necessity to save a human life overrides the prohibition (of wounding the dead body). The priority is given to a recipient to whom a promise was made (by the deceased donor). It is preferred that organs be taken from a deceased who had already so willed, or whose family grants the donation.

If the donor is a living person, various possibilities are to be considered: If taking the organ would cause the donor's death, such as the heart or lungs, then the procedure is absolutely forbidden whether or not there is a consent; for if he consents it will be tantamount to suicide; If he does not consent then it will be murder: and both are prohibitted. If taking away the organ will not cause death, the donor being able to live without it, the ruling is based on the outcome: If by reason of losing that organ the donor becomes incapable of performing his duties (or conversely the recipient is enabled to commit evil deeds) ... such as follows donation of both hands and legs, rendering the person incapable of earning his living, or doing this only through illegitimate means, then the procedure will be prohibitted irrespective of consent. If this is not the case, as it is when the organ is a kidney, an eye, a tooth or blood, then the procedure is permissible provided that the donor gives consent and that the transplant operation is very likely to be successful. Without a consent it will be an assault subject to punishment by appropriate penalty or compensation as prescribed by the relevant sections of Islamic jurispudence.

# Contents

Foreword by M.F.A. Woodruff                                                    VII

Preface by G.M. Abouna                                                          IX

Pronouncements by major religions on organ transplantations                    XI

List of Contributors                                                          XVII


Part One: Histocompatibility matching and the blood transfusion effect

1. High and low responsiveness in renal transplantation and its impact on
   HLA matching,
   J.J. van Rood and G.F.J. Hendriks                                            1
2. HLA A and B matching, the mixed lymphocyte reaction and renal
   allograft survival in a single centre,
   A.G. White and G.M. Abouna                                                   7
3. The role of vascular endothelial cell antigens in renal transplantation,
   J. Cerilli and L. Brasile                                                   15
4. Blood transfusion(s) and cadaveric renal transplantation in the
   Netherlands,
   G.G. Persijn and J.J. van Rood                                             23


Part Two: Immunosuppression and immunological monitoring

5. The development of immunosuppression,
   T.E. Starzl, B.W. Shaw and S. Iwatsuki                                      39
6. Antilymphocyte globulin infusion in the treatment of acute allograft
   rejection: a prospective study,
   M.S.A. Kumar, A.G. White, P. John and G.M. Abouna                          49
7. Cyclosporin in renal transplantation: results of the Minnesota randomised trial,

D.E.R. Sutherland, J.S. Najarian, M. Strand, D.S. Fryd, R.M. Ferguson, R.L. Simmons and N.L. Ascher                                    57
8. Antilymphocyte globulin and thoracic duct drainage in renal transplantation,
J. Traeger, J.L. Touraine, J.M. Dubernard and M.C. Malik            61
9. Monitoring of organ allograft rejection by fine needle aspiration
cytology,
P. Häyry, J. Ahonen and E. von Willebrand                          79


Part Three: Donor procurement and organ preservation

10. Organ procurement and transportation,
F.K. Merkel and K.M. Sigardson                                     97
11. Procurement of kidneys from non heart beating donors,
T.J.M. Ruers, J.P.A.M. Vroemen, J.A. van der Vliet and
G. Kootstra                                                       107
12. Donor age in cadaveric renal transplantation,
J.A. van der Vliet, G.G. Persijn, B. Cohen and G. Kootstra        115
13. Prolonged preservation of imported cadaveric grafts by ice cooling
with Eurocollin's solution versus hypothermic pulsatile perfusion,
G.M. Abouna, M.S.A. Kumar, A.G. White, S.K. Dadah and
O.S.G. Silva                                                      123
14. A new approach to prolonged kidney preservation,
G. Kootstra, B.G. Rijkmans and W.A. Buurman                       131


Part Four: Vascular access surgery in renal transplantation

15. The upper arm A.V. fistula for chronic haemodialysis: long term
followup,
F.J. Dagher                                                       141
16. Permanent vascular access for haemodialysis: the Kuwait experience,
S.K. Dadah, M. Samhan, O.F. Omar and G.M. Abouna                  147


Part Five: Renal transplantation

17. Current status of renal transplantation,
J. Cerilli                                                        153
18. The living donor for kidney transplantation: a review of 100 consecutive donors,
P. John, M.S.A. Kumar, M. Samhan and G.M. Abouna                  163

19. Kidney transplantation in diabetic recipients: factors leading to improved results,
D.E.R. Sutherland, D.S. Fryd, C.E. Morrow, F.C. Goetz,
R.M. Ferguson, F.L. Simmons and J.S. Najarian     173
20. Fungal infections in 135 renal transplantations,
M. Haberal, Z. Oner, N. Yulag, H. Gulay and N. Bilgin     177
21. Bilateral renal transplantation: effect on pelvic hemodynamics and sexual function in male patients,
F.J. Dagher, A. Billet and L. Queral     183

Part Six: Renal transplantation and dialysis in the Middle East

22. Renal replacement therapy in Kuwait,
G. Kusma, N.A. Hilali and G.M. Abouna     187
23. The development of renal transplantation programme in Kuwait and the results in the first 142 grafts,
G.M. Abouna, A.G. White, M.S.A. Kumar, S.K. Dadah and
M. Samhan     193
24. Living related kidney transplantation in Turkey,
M. Haberal, N. Bilgin, N. Buyukpamukcu, U. Saatci, M. Karamehmetoglu, Z. Oner, A. Besim, H. Gulay, O. Dallar and Y. Sanac     209

Part Seven: Pancreas transplantation

25. Clinical pancreas and islet transplantation: registry statistics and an overview,
D.E.R. Sutherland     215
26. Pancreas transplantation in Lyon 1976–1983,
J.M. Dubernard, J. Traeger, G. Kamel, E. Bosi, A. Gelet, S. El-Yafi,
F. Canton, M.C. Malik, H. Codas and J.L. Touraine     225
27. Pancreas transplantation at the University of Minnesota: experience with 68 recent cases,
D.E.R. Sutherland, F.C. Goetz, P.L. Chinn, B.A. Elick, R.L. Simmons and J.S. Najarian     233

Part Eight: Heart and heart-lung transplantation

28. Cardiac transplantation,
S.W. Jamieson, P.E. Oyer, E.B. Stinson and N.E. Shumway     239
29. Heart-lung transplantation,

S.W. Jamieson, E.B. Stinson, P.E. Oyer, J. Theodore, S. Hunt and
N.E. Shumway                                                          247
30. Immunosuppressive therapy for cardiac transplantation,
S.W. Jamieson, P.E. Oyer, E.B. Stinson and N.E. Shumway              253


Part Nine: Liver transplantation

31. Current status of liver transplantation,
T.E. Starzl, S. Iwatsuki and B.W. Shaw                               261


Part Ten: Bone marrow transplantation

32. Current status of bone marrow transplantation,
E.D. Thomas                                                          269


Part Eleven: Recent advances in renal surgery

33. Renal autotransplantation and extracorporeal renal surgery,
G.M. Abouna                                                          285
34. Hypothermic *in situ* perfusion and surface cooling in renal surgery,
C. Chaussy, F.J. Marx, W. Sturm and A. Schilling                    297
35. Extracorporeal shock wave lithotripsy: a new aspect in the treatment
of kidney stones,
C. Chaussy, E. Schmiedt and D. Jocham                               305

Index                                                                319

# List of contributors

G.M. ABOUNA
Professor & Chairman
Department of Organ Transplantation
Kuwait University, Faculty of Medicine,
and Mubarak Al-Kabeer Hospital,
P.O. Box 24923, Kuwait

J. AHONEN
Docent of Surgery
University of Helsinki
Haartmaninkatu 3A
SF 00290 Helsinki 29,
Finland

N.L. ASCHER
Instructor in Surgery
Department of Surgery
University of Minnesota
Minneapolis, Minn, USA

A. BESIM
Hacettepe
University Hospital
Ankara, Turkey

N. BILGIN
Professor of Surgery
Hacettepe University Hospital
Ankara, Turkey

A. BILLET
Resident in Surgery
Department of Surgery
University of Maryland School of
Medicine & Hospital
Baltimore, MD 21201, USA

E. BOSI
Nephrologist
Claude Bernard University
Edouard Herriot Hospital
Pavillon V, Lyon, France

L. BRASILE
Research Associate
Department of Surgery
Albany Medical College
Albany, N.Y., USA

W.A. BUURMAN
University of Limburg
Hospital St. Annadal
Department of Surgery Annadal I
6214 PA Maastricht, The Netherlands

N. BUYUKPAMUKCU
Professor of Paediatric Surgery
Hacettepe University Hospital
Ankara, Turkey

F. CANTON
Edouard Herriot Hospital
Department of Urology and Transplantation
Pavion V, Lyon, France

J. CERILLI
Professor and Chairman
Department of Surgery
Albany Medical College
Albany, N.Y., USA

C. CHAUSSY
Professor of Urology
Ludwig-Maximilians-Universitat Munchen
Urologisch Klinik & Poliklinik

Klinikum GroBhadern
Marchioninistr 15
D. 8000 Munchen 700, FRG

P.L. CHINN
Pancreas Transplant Fellow
Department of Surgery
University of Minnesota
Minneapolis, Minn., USA

H. CODAS
Edouard Herriot Hospital
Department of Urology and Transplantation
Pavion V, Lyon, France

B. COHEN
Eurotransplant Foundation
University Hospital
Leiden, The Netherlands

S.K. DADAH
Registrar
Department of Organ Transplantation
Mubarak Al-Kabeer Hospital
P.O. Box 43787, Kuwait

F. DAGHER
Professor
Department of Surgery
University of Maryland School of
Medicine & Hospital,
Baltimore, MD 21201, USA

O. DALLAR
Resident in Surgery
Hacettepe University Hospital
Ankara, Turkey

J.M. DUBERNARD
Professor of Urology
Claude Bernard University
Lyon, France

B.A. ELICK
Chief Transplant Coordinator
Department of Surgery
University of Minnesota
Minneapolis, Minn., USA

R.M. FERGUSON
Assistant Professor of Surgery

University of Minnesota
Minneapolis, Minn., USA

D.S. FRYD
Assistant Professor of Surgery
University of Minnesota
Minneapolis, Minn., USA

A. GELET
Surgeon
Edouard Herriot Hospital
Dept. of Urology and Transplantation
Pavion V, Lyon, France

F.C. GOETZ
Professor of Medicine
University of Minnesota
Minneapolis, Minn., USA

H. GULAY
Resident In Surgery
Hacettepe University Hospital
Ankara, Turkey

M. HABERAL
Professor of Surgery
Hacettepe University Hospital
Ankara, Turkey

P. HAYRY
Professor of Transplantation Surgery
& Immunology
University of Helsinki
Haartmaninkatu 3A
SF 00290 Helsinki 29, Finland

G.F.J. HENDRIKS
University Hospital
Rijnsburgerweg 10
2333 AA, Leiden The Netherlands

N.A. HILALI
Assistant Registrar
Nephrology & Dialysis Unit
Amiri Hospital, Kuwait

S. HUNT
Clinical Assistant Professor
Department of Cardiology
Stanford University Hospital
Stanford, CA 94305, USA

S. IWATSUKI
Assistant Professor of Surgery
University of Pittsburgh
Medical School
1084 Scaife Hall
Pittsburgh PA 15261, USA

S.W. JAMIESON
Assistant Professor
Department of Cardiovascular Surgery
Stanford University School of Medicine
Stanford, CA 94305, USA

D. JOCHAM
Urologist
Ludwig-Maximilians-Universitat Munchen
Urologisch Klinik & Poliklinik
Klinikum Grobhadern
Marchioninistr 15
D. 8000 Munchen 700, FRG

P. JOHN
Registrar
Department of Organ Transplantation Surgery
Mubarak Al-Kabeer Hospital
P.O. Box No 43787 Kuwait

G. KAMEL
Surgeon
Edouard Herriot Hospital
Department of Urology and Transplantation
Pavion V, Lyon, France

M. KARAMEHMOTOGLU
Professor of Anaesthesiology
Hacettepe University Hospital
Ankara, Turkey

G. KOOTSTRA
Professor of Surgery
University of Limburg,
Hospital St. Annadal
Department of Surgery
Annadal I, 6214 PA Maastricht,
The Netherlands

M.S.A. KUMAR
Consultant Surgeon
Department of Organ Transplantation
Mubarak Al-Kabeer Hospital
P.O. Box 43787, Kuwait

G. KUSMA
Senior Registrar
Nephrology & Dialysis Unit
Amiri Hospital, Kuwait

M.C. MALIK
Claude Bernard University
Edouard Herriot Hospital
Pavillon V, Lyon, France

F.J. MARX
Professor of Urology
Ludwig-Maximilians-Universitat Munchen
Urologisch Klinik & Poliklinik
Klinikum GroBhadern
Marchioninistr 15
D.8000 Munchen 700, FRG

F. MERKEL
Associate Professor of Surgery, Immunology,
& Medicine
Rush-Presbyterian St. Luke's Medical Centre
Chicago, Ill., USA

C.E. MORROW
Medical Fellow
Department Of Surgery
University of Minnesota
Minneapolis, Minn., USA

J.S. NAJARIAN
Professor & Chairman of Surgery
University of Minnesota
Minneapolis, Minn., USA

O.F. OMAR
Registrar
Department of Organ Transplantation
Mubarak Al-Kabeer Hospital
P.O. Box 43787, Kuwait

Z. ONER
Associate Professor Transplantation Unit
Hacettepe University Hospital
Ankara, Turkey

D.E. OYER
Associate Professor
Department of Cardiovascular Surgery
Stanford University School of Medicine
Stanford, CA 94305, USA

G.G. PERSIJN
Eurotransplant Foundation
University Hospital, Leiden, The Netherlands

L. QUERAL
Associate Professor of Surgery
University of Maryland School of Medicine
& Hospital
Baltimore, MD 21201, USA

B.G. RIJKMANS
University of Limburg
Hospital St. Annadal
Department of Surgery
Annadal I, 6214 PA Maastricht The Netherlands

J.J. VAN ROOD
Department of Immunohaematology
and Bloodbank
University Hospital
Rijnsburgerweg 10
2333 AA Leiden, The Netherlands

T.J.M. RUERS
University of Limburg
Hospital St. Annadal
Department of Surgery
Annadal I, 6214 PA Maastricht The Netherlands

M. SAMHAN
Registrar
Department of Organ Transplantation
Mubarak Al-Kabeer Hospital
P.O. Box 43787, Kuwait

V. SAATCI
Professor of Pediatric Nephrology
Hacettepe university Hospital
Ankara, Turkey

Y. SANAC
Professor of Surgery
Hacattepe University Hospital
Ankara, Turkey

A. SCHILLING
Urologist
Ludwig-Maximilans-Universitat Munchen
Urologische Klinik & Poliklinik
Klinikum GroBhadern
Marchioninistr 15
D.8000 Munchen 700, FRG

E. SCHMIDT
Professor of Urology
Ludwig-Maximilians-Universitat Munchen
Urologische Klinik & Poliklinik
Klinikum GroBhadern
Marchioninistr 15
D.8000 Munchen 700, FRG

B.W. SHAW
Assistant Professor of Surgery
University of Pittsburgh
Medical School
1084 Scaife Hall
Pittsburgh PA 15261, USA

N.E. SHUMWAY
Professor
Department of Cardiovascular Surgery
Stanford University School of Medicine
Stanford, CA 94305, USA

K.M. SIGARDSON
Transplant Coordinator
Chicago Regional Organ & Tissue Bank
Chicago, IL 60612, USA

O.S.G. SILVA
Department of Anaesthesia, and
Transplantation
Mubarak Al Kabeer Hospital
Kuwait

R.L. SIMMONS
Professor of Surgery
University of Minnesota
Minneapolis, Minn., USA

T. STARZL
Professor of Surgery
University of Pittsburgh
Medical School
1084 Scaife Hall
Pittsburgh PA 15261, USA

E.B. STINSON
Professor
Department of Cardiovascular Surgery
Stanford University School of Medicine
Stanford, CA 94305, USA

M. STRAND
Transplant Coordinator
Department of Surgery
University of Minnesota
Minneapolis, Minn., USA

W. STURM
Urologist
Ludwig-Maximilians-Universitat Munchen
Urologische Klinik & Poliklinik
Klinikum GroBhadern
Marchioninistr 15
D.8000 Munchen 700, FRG

D.E.R. SUTHERLAND
Associate Professor of Surgery
University of Minnesota
Minneapolis, Minn., USA

J. THEODORE
Associate Professor of Medicine
Department of Medicine
Stanford University School of Medicine
Stanford, CA 94305, USA

E.D. THOMAS
Professor of Medicine
Associate Director for Clinical Research
Fed Hutchinson Cancer Research Centre
1124 Columbia Street
Seattle, WA 98104, USA

J.L. TOURAINE
Professor of Nephrology
Claude Bernard University
Edouard Herriot Hospital
pavillon V, Lyon, France

J. TRAEGER
Professor & Chairman of Nephrology

Claude Bernard University
Edouard Herriot Hospital
Pavillon V, Lyon, France

J.A. VAN DER VLIET
University of Limburg
Hospital St. Annadal
Department of Surgery
Annadal I, 6214 PA Maastricht,
The Netherlands

J.P.A.M. VROEMAN
University of Limburg
Hospital St. Annadal
Department of Surgery
Annadal I, 6214 PA Maastricht,
The Netherlands

A.G. WHITE
Associate Professor
Department of Organ Transplantation
Kuwait University, Faculty of Medicine
Mubarak Al-Kabeer Hospital,
P.O. Box 24923, Kuwait

E. VON WILLEBRAND
Docent of Clinical Immunology
University of Helsinki
Haartmaninkatu 3A
SF 0029o, Helsinki 29, Finland

S. EL YAFI
Claude Bernard University
Lyon, France

N. YULAG
Professor of Microbiology
Hacettepe University Hospital
Ankara, Turkey

# 1. High and low responsiveness in renal transplantation and its impact on HLA matching

J.J. VAN ROOD and G.F.J. HENDRIKS

The question whether or not HLA matching can modify the amount of immunosuppressive drugs needed for good graft survival can, of course, be answered in the affirmative. It is a well established fact that grafts exchanged between HLA-identical sibling donor-recipient combinations require less immunosuppression and survive better than grafts exchanged between mismatched living related combinations, and, of course, than grafts obtained from cadaveric donors.

The real challange lies with cadaveric donorgrafts. In this presentation, we will first discuss the influence of the immune status of recipients on graft survival. The central question here is 'how can high and low responders be detected?' Next we will discuss how good graft survival can be achieved in high responders. Finally, we will present some data on the interaction of HLA matching and the amount of immunosuppression needed.

As an introduction, let us summarize the different interacting factors which determine the graft outcome.

The most important single factor is the immune status of recipients, i.e., whether they are high or low responders. For the low responders neither pretransplant bloodtransfusion(s) nor HLA-A, -B or -DR matching are necessary. For the high responders, pretransplant bloodtransfusion and matching are prerequisites for good graft survival (1).

Consequently defining whether or not the recipient is a high responder before transplantation thus should be one of our first priorities. It is really amazing that so little progress has been made in that respect until quite recently.

Originally, functional tests were used, such as DNCB skin reactivity (2). That approach turns out to be poorly reproducable. Immunogenetic markers seem to be more promising.

We and others have shown that HLA-DRw6 positive individuals are high responders as far as the formation of antibodies against streptococcal non-MHC and HLA-DR antigens are concerned (3–5).

The observation that HLA-DRw6 positive recipients are high responders after renal transplantation has been confirmed by Ting (personal communication), Koene (personal communication), Soulillou (6) and UK transplant (Annual Report 1982). As is to be expected, matching for HLA-DR in DRw6 positive recipients dramatically improves graft survival.

Further support that HLA-DR matching is of great importance in DRw6 positive individuals is provided by the following analysis. Based on above results, we would expect that the results in DRw6 positive patients would have improved over the years in which HLA-DR matching was implemented while this would not be the case in DRw6 negative patients. The improvement would be gradual because, in the beginning, HLA-DR typing could only be performed retrospectively after transplantation. Only recently, has it become possible to reliably type donors and recipient before transplantation and to match them on the basis of HLA-DR. Our results have indeed shown that the 1 year graft survival in the HLA-DRw6 regative recipients remained the same over the years while there was a striking and quite significant improvement of graft survival in the DRw6 positive recipients.

This is thus again an argument that the improvement obtained with HLA-DR matching comes almost exclusively from matching in HLA-DRw6 positive individuals. Matching for HLA-DR may, therefore, compensate for the high responsiveness of HLA-DRw6 positive recipients.

DRw6 positive patients who receive kidneys from donors with no mismatches for HLA-DR can, of course, be divided in two groups: identical ones and compatible ones. The majority of the patients will have received a kidney which carried two HLA-DR antigens which were identical to those of their donors. Some of the patients will have received a donor kidney which was only compatible i.e. it carried only one of the two DR antigens present in the recipient. One of those antigens will be HLA-DRw6. If one compares the graft survival of the homozygous HLA-DRw6 donors versus that of the compatible homozygous DRw6-non-6 donors a striking difference is observed. When the donors are HLA-DRw6 positive, graft survival is excellent, i.e., 90% after one year, compared to only 70% in recipients of grafts from DRw-non-6 donors.

This is a most intriguiing finding. It is not only DRw6 in the recipient which is important, but also the presence of DRw6 in the donor. DRw6 positive recipients seem to be converted into low responders when confronted with DRw6 positive grafts. If the kidney is compatible for a non DRw6 antigen, the recipient remains a high responder. How important is the role of DRw6 in the graft? We can answer that question by studying the survival of grafts in DRw6 positive recipients which were mismatched for one DR antigen. Figure 1 shows the increase in graft survival at one year in grafts from DRw6 positive donors (85%) as compared to these from DRw6 negative donors (55%).

It appears that the positive effect of DRw6 in the donor may override the high responder effect of DRw6 in the recipient.

We should thus modify our previous conclusion: DRw6 positive recipients behave as high responders if the donor is DRw6 negative. However, donor selection i.e. the donor carries DRw6, improves graft survival in DRw6 positive recipients. In that situation mismatches for other HLA-DR antigens, and one or more HLA-A/B antigens do not seem to adversely effect graft survival.

Of course the above results raise the following logical question: how would DRw6 in the donor act in a DRw6 negative recipient?

Figure 2 shows that if a patient receives a kidney mismatched for *one* DR antigen it makes a significant difference whether this one mismatched DR antigen is DRw6 or any of the other DR antigens. When the one mismatched antigen is DRw6, graft survival was over 85%. However, when it was DR-non-6 antigen, graft survival was only about 62%. These results could be explained by assuming that DRw6 does not exist at all, i.e. that it may represent a 'null gene', so that if you had a mismatch for DRw6 you had in fact no mismatch at all. However, it is a bit difficult to see how the absence of an antigen could lead to such a good graft survival. Another possibility is that DRw6 does in fact exist, but that it can activate the suppressor circuit or to turn the recipient into low responders. To test this possibility Hendriks analysed a group of DRw6 negative patients who had received a kidney mismatched for *two* DR antigens (7).

Figure 3 shows that for the grafts which were mismatched for two DR antigens in which one of these two DR mismatched antigens was DRw6, graft survival was again 85% while in the other group it was as expected about 60%. These results are difficult to explain unless one assumes that DRw6 is able to activate a suppressor circuit or is able in some other way to block the homograft reaction in the recipient. Precisely the same findings were obtained in haplo-identical living related grafts. If the haploidentical donor provides a mismatch for DRw6, graft survival is excellent. From these findings we can conclude that if DRw6 is present in the donor it may not be necessary to match. Every recipient whether he is DRw6 positive or negative will have a good graft survival. They all will behave as if they were low responders. On the other hand if a DRw6 positive recipient gets a DRw6 negative kidney even if it is compatible for the non-DRw6 antigens in the

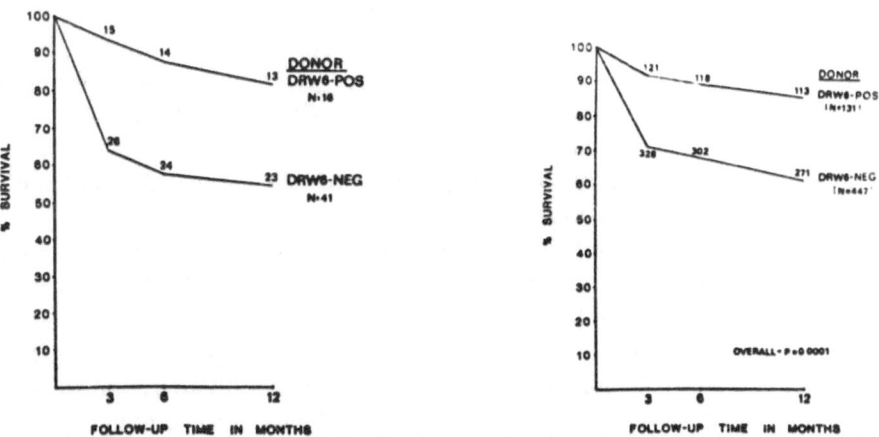

*Fig.1 (left)* DRw6-pos. recipients of 1-DR-MISM. First renal allografts (N=57).
*Fig.2 (right)* DRw6-neg. recipients of 1-DR-MISM. First renal allografts (N=578).

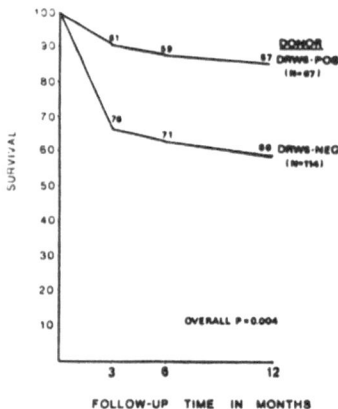

*Fig.3* DRw6-neg. recipients of 2-DR-MISM. First renal allografts (N=181).

recipient, graft prognosis will be relatively poor (60% or less). In such a situation the DRw6 positive recipient acts as a high responder.

These findings confront us with questions we have never asked before. The first one of course is: how are these two findings related? What is their mechanism? It is clear that we have to rethink our naive definitions of high and low responders. A DRw6 positive person can act as a high or as a low responder depending on what HLA antigens are present in the kidney donor.

The most intriguing question of all is: what is the biological meaning of all this, if any?

Could it be that an epitope on DRw6 resembles or crossreacts with epitopes which are carried by micro-organisms and or parasites against which one is better off if the immune response is rather weak? (7–9).

All the above data were collected from patients who had received pretransplant blood transfusions and were for the great majority treated with standard doses of imuran and prednison. Some of them were treated with ATG as well. On further analysis it became clear that ATG treatment for severe prednisone resistent rejection crises cancelled what we will call the 'DRw6 effect'. Thus, although DRw6 positive recipients had more rejection crises than DRw6 negative ones, if those rejections were treated by ATG instead of high doses of prednisolone the kidney was not lost (10).

Finally, the question whether HLA matching, graft function and the amount of immunosuppression are directly related should be addressed. Now that graft survival after 3 and 12 months is over 80% in many centers using many diffirent immunosuppression regimes, it will become increasingly difficult to determine the importance of matching. The overall results are simply too good to show much differences. In this situation, however, differences may be found by comparing graft *function* and HLA matching.

Table 1 shows that HLA-DR matched grafts function better than mismatched

Table 1. The beneficial effect of HLA-DR matching on the outcome of kidney graft function (3 months post-operatively).

| Nr. of DR mismatches | Creatinin clearance (ml/min) | |
|---|---|---|
| | $\leq 50$ | $> 50$ |
| 0 | 4 | 16 |
| 1 | 24 | 13 |
| 2 | 8 | 8 |

Fisher's exact $p = 0.006$.

grafts. Likewise van Hooff has shown previously that HLA-A/B matching diminishes the amount of immunosuppression needed (11).

In conclusion, it seems that we can identify at least some of the high responder recipients before transplantation by HLA-DR typing (HLA-DRw6). Such patients should preferentially receive an HLA-DRw6 positive kidney. If a rejection crisis occurs in these patients, it will often be prednisone-resistent but ATG sensitive. With these and other measures, graft survival will be enhanced and it will become increasingly difficult to show an effect of HLA matching on graft survival. However, the effect of HLA matching can be seen if not graft survival but graft function and/or the amount of immunosuppressive drugs (prednisone) given are used as point of reference.

**Acknowledgements**

This work was in part supported by the Dutch Foundation for Medical Research (FUNGO) which is subsidized by the Dutch Organization for the Advancement of Pure Research (ZWO), the J.A. Cohen Institute for Radiopathology and Radiation Protection (IRS), the Eurotransplant Foundation, the Dutch Kidney Foundation and the Kuratorium für Heimdialyse in Germany.

**References**

1. Van Rood JJ: Pretransplant blood transfusion. Sure but how and why! Transpl Proc XV: 915–916, 1983.
2. Diamondopoulos AA, Hamilton DNH, Briggs JD: A new predictive factor for the outcome of renal transplantation. In: Proceedings EDTA Congress, Robinson BHB, Hawkins JB (eds). Tunbridge Wells UK, Pitman Med Publ Co Ltd 1978 (vol 15) pp 283–288.
3. Lehner T: The relationship between human helper and suppressor factors to a streptococcal protein antigen. J Immunol 129: 1936–1940, 1982.
4. Baldwin FHJ, Claas EHJ, Van Es LA, Van Rood JJ, Paul LC, Persijn GG: Renal graft rejection and the antigenic anatomy of human kidneys. In: Transpl Clin Immunol (Touraine JL et al (eds). Amsterdam, Excerpta Medica, 1981 (vol XIII) pp 140–146.

5. Hendriks GFJ, Claas FHJ, Persijn GG, Witvliet MD, Baldwin W, van Rood JJ: HLA-DRw6-positive recipients are high responders in renal transplantation. Transpl Proc 15: 1136–1138, 1983.
6. Soulillou JP, Bignon JD: Poor kidney-graft survival in recipients with HLA-DRw6. N Engl J Med 308: 969–970, 1983.
7. Hendriks GFJ, D'Amaro J, Persijn GG, Schreuder GMTh, Lansbergen O, Cohen B, Van Rood JJ: Excellent renal allograft prognosis with DRw6 positive donors in the face of HLA-DR mismatches. The Lancet (In press) 1983.
8. Hendriks GFL, Schreuder GMTh, Claas FHJ, D'Amaro J, Persijn GG, Cohen B, Van Rood JJ: HLA-DRw6 and renal allograft rejection. Brit Med J 286: 85–87, 1983.
9. Woodruff M, Van Rood JJ: Possible implications of the effect of blood transfusion on allograft survival. The Lancet, May 28: 1201–1203, 1983.
10. Hoitsma HJ, Reekers P, Van Lier HJJ, Van Rens JG, Koene RAP: HLA-DRw6 and treatment of acute rejection with anti-thymocyte globulin in renal transplantation. Brit Med J (Submitted).
11. Van Hooff JP, Van Es A, Persijn GG, Van Hooff-Eykenboom IJEA, Kalff MW, Van Rood JJ, De Graeff J: Cadaveric graft survival, clinical course, blood transfusions, HLA-(A and B) match, and -DR match in adult patients transplanted in one centre. In: Proceedings EDTA Congress (Robinson BHB, Hawkins JB, Naik RB (eds). Tunbridge Wells UK, Pitman Med Publ Co Ltd, 1979 (vol 16) pp 359–365.

# 2. HLA A and B matching, the mixed lymphocyte reaction and renal allograft survival in a single centre

ARTHUR G. WHITE and GEORGE M. ABOUNA

## Introduction

Renal transplantation was started in Kuwait, Arabia, in 1979 and since that date 147 renal allografts have been performed. This article describes the results of matching for HLA A and B antigens and the mixed lymphocyte reaction (MLR) in 130 consecutive grafts conducted by the same team in a single centre. One hundred and two grafts were from living donors and 28 from imported cadavers. These patients are described in detal elsewhere (1). Although the contribution of HLA matching is already well established in the living related donor situation, no such information is available for the Arab population. This population is characterised by a high proportion of consanguinous marriage and large family size (2).

## Patients and methods

HLA A and B antigen typing was carried out by a conventional two stage microlymphocytotoxicity test (3) using mainly commercial antisera. Lymphocyte crossmatching was performed using an extended incubation period at room temperature on unfractionated lymphocytes and a detailed knowledge of the panel reactive antibody (PRA) was obtained by monthly screening of the patients whilst on the dialysis programme.

The mixed lymphocyte reaction (MLR) was performed by standardised procedures in microplates using 250 $\mu$l culture volumes with lymphocyte concentrations for responding cells of 1 x $10^6$ ml. and for the mitomycin treated stimulating cells 3 x $10^6$ ml. All recipients were tested against potential donors and unrelated controls in one way and two way cultures and also against pooled allogeneic cells.

Furthermore a transformation control using phytohaemagglutinin was incorporated. Incubation was for 5 days at 37°C in a humidified 5% carbon dioxide atmosphere, pulsing with 1 $\mu$c of tritiated thymidine per culture well for the last 24 h. Harvesting was performed using an automated cell harvester and counting of the incorporated radioactivity with a liquid scintillation spectrometer. The results were expressed in terms of a stimulation index, calculated by dividing the response of the recipient to the donor's mitomycin treated cells by the response of the recipient to his own mitomycin treated cells. Other ways of interpreting the results, such as relative response of the recipient to third party or pooled cells or the two way MLR, made no difference to the interpretation of the results. Donor/ recipient combinations with a one way stimulation index of less than 2 were considered to be MLR negative and an index of greater than 2, MLR positive.

HLA typing was carried out for all 130 allografts and the MLR performed in 72 of these. Breakdown of the patients into HLA match grade and the relationship to the donor is summarised in Table 1. Ninety eight patients had a living related donor, 4 received a living unrelated donor kidney and 28 an imported cadaver graft. The majority of patients were in the 1 or 2 HLA mismatch (MM) category. Grafts were considered failed if irreversible rejection occurred or if the patient was lost for any reason.

## Results

The percentage actuarial graft survival in the living donor group calculated over a follow up period of 3 to 48 months in relation to HLA match grade is shown in Figure 1. There were no significant differences in graft survival in relation to HLA match grade. Figure 1 also displays the results of graft survival in the cadaver kidney recipients which have been subdivided into those with less than 2 or greater than two mismatches. The difference between these two categories was not significant.

The MLR was performed in 72 donor/recipient combinations and the relationship of the HLA match to the MLR response is shown in Table 2. Of particular interest was the fact that 2 'full house' identical combinations were MLR positive and that in the HLA two mismatch group, 4 donor/recipient combinations were MLR negative, one of which was an unrelated 'wife' donor and 2 of which parental donors. The relationship of the MLR to actuarial graft survival is shown in Figure 2 and the relationship to the number of rejection episodes and graft function in Table 3. There were no significant differences between the strength of the MLR and graft survival in the living donors although there was a trend to better graft survival and function in those that were MLR negative $(p > .10)$. All the recipients of cadaver grafts were MLR positive with their donor and as would

*Table 1.* HLA A and B matching and donor/recipient relationship.

| Relationship | 'Full House' identical | 0MM | 1MM | 2MM | 3MM | Total |
|---|---|---|---|---|---|---|
| Living related donor | 17 | 19 | 31 | 28 | 3 | 98 |
| Living unrelated donor | 0 | 0 | 2 | 2 | 0 | 4 |
| Cadaver donor | 0 | 0 | 0  1 | 10 | 17 | 28 |

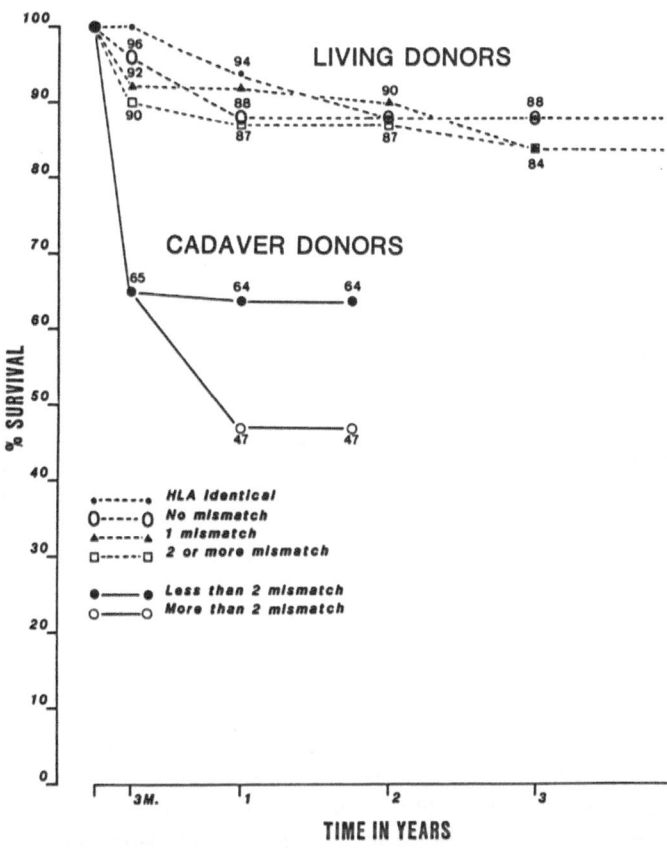

*Fig.1.* HLA A and B Matching and actuarial graft survival.

*Table 2.* HLA A and B matching and the MLR response.

| MLR response | 'Full House' identical | 0MM | 1MM | 2MM | 3+MM | Total |
|---|---|---|---|---|---|---|
| Living donors | | | | | | |
|   MLR negative SI < 2 | 8 | 5 | 1 | 4 | 0 | 18 |
|   MLR positive SI > 2 | 2 | 5 | 13 | 16 | 1 | 37 |
| Cadaver donors | | | | | | |
|   MLR positive SI > 2 | – | – | 1 | 5 | 11 | 17 |

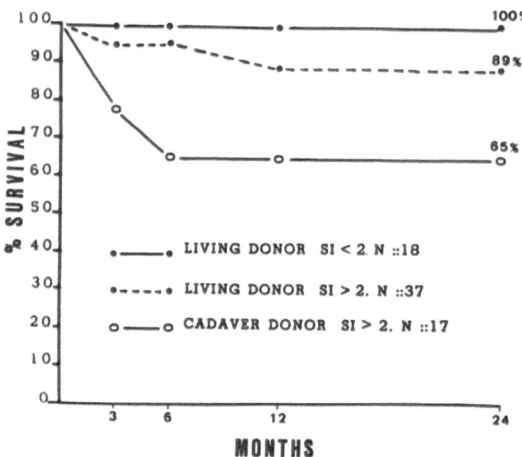

*Fig.2.* Actuarial graft survival in patient groups subdivided on the strength of the MLR.

be expected there was a significant difference between this group and the living donors that were MLR negative (p < .001).

### Discussion

The results obtained in this study showed no significant differences in the living related donor group between HLA identical and the 2MM grafts. This is somewhat at variance with earlier reports. Opelz, Mickey and Terasaki (4) report a 1 year graft survival in HLA identical siblings of 90% compared to 70% graft survival in HLA non identical siblings (p > .005). They also found that there was no difference in graft survival in those sibling transplants that were full house identical compared with those that had OMM. Our data would support this with a 1 year graft survival in both these groups of approximately 90%.

Morris (5) summarises the consensus view that HLA identical siblings have an approximate 80% graft survical compared with one haplotype sharing siblings or parent child grafts of about 65% at 3 years. However, Simmons *et al.* (6) found no differences in transplant function (if technical losses, diabetes or hyper acute rejection are excluded) between HLA identical siblings (79%), haplotype mismatched (75%) or child to parent or parent to child (79%) at 2 years. Dausset and Hors (7) also found no difference between HLA identical (96%) and haploidentical living related donor grafts (94%) at 2 years. Similarly our data presented here showed no significant contribution of matching for HLA A and B antigens to graft survival in the living donor group. However, the true relevance of these results could only be measured if we had large number of patients in a completely mismatched group. The vast majority of our living donor patients are 2MM or less. Additional factors that could influence our results are that this series is reported by a single centre and team and this may be an example of the 'centre

*Table 3.* The MLR response and graft outcome.

| | Living donors | | Cadaver donors |
|---|---|---|---|
| | MLR negative SI <2 SI >2 SI >2 N =18 | MLR positive N = 37 | MLR positive N =17 |
| *Actuarial graft* Survival at 2 years | 100% (18) | 89%(33) | 65%(11) |
| Number of rejections episodes and average per patient | 17(0,94) | 53(1.43) | 32(1.9) |
| Number of patients with no rejection | 6 (33%) | 6 (16%) | 1 (6%) |
| Average serum creatinine mgm/100 ml | 1.15 | 1.64 | 1.55 |

effect' whereby a multiplicity of other factors nullify the effect of HLA selection (8). Furthermore it is not unreasonable to suggest that in the population under study, where there is a degree of inbreeding (2), that many of the patients may well be matched for as yet undefined HLA or non HLA antigens. Certainly it might be anticipated that there would be less polymorphism in such a population.

There were 28 patients who received a cadaver kidney in this series and although the actuarial graft survival in the group with less than 2MM at 2 years was 64% compared with 47% in the greater than 2 MM category, the small numbers involved do not permit the calculation of a significant difference between the groups. In fact the evidence for a significant contribution of HLA A and B matching is still somewhat controversial even in much larger series (9).

The mixed lymphocyte reaction has been mainly used to assess donor recipient compatibility of living donor transplantation and it is the belief of some investigators that to perform living related donor transplantation without MLR analyses is clearly wrong (10). In the living donor situation there is considerable evidence that this approach is justified. Bach *et al.* (11) as early as 1970, sound a highly significant correlation between the results of the MLR and renal function and the timing of rejection episodes. Similarly Miller and Hattler (12), Cochrum *et al.* (13), Ringden and Berg (14), Walker *et al.* (15) and others have found a significant relationship between the MLR and graft function in the living related donor situation. In the living donor situation the distinction between those patients that are truly MLR negative with their donors is usually clear cut and can be confirmed by two way cultures. In the analysis of the data presented here we divided our patients into those that had a stimulation index of less than 2 (MLR negative) and greater than 2 (MLR positive). The results shown in Figure 2 indicate that there is no significant difference in graft survival between those patients that were MLR negative with their living donor and those that are MLR positive. This may be a consequence of the relatively small numbers studied and a significant difference might be obtained if there were more patients in the two categories. It is obvious that with an overall living donor graft survival approaching 90% at 2 years that very large numbers indeed would be necessary. The relationship of the MLR to cadaveric graft survival is not clear. Cochrum *et al.* (13), Walker *et al.* (15) and Berg and Ringden (17) have shown a significant relationship between the MLR and cadaver graft survival whereas Cullen *et al.* (16) found no relationship. In the cadaver situation the MLR results are reported in a variety of ways making interpretation difficult. If we consider a division into truly MLR negative and positive all our cadaver recipients were MLR positive with their donor and analysis of the MLR contribution is not possible.

There is a trend (Table 3) to fewer rejection episodes and better graft function in the MLR negative group although these differences do not approach significance for the reasons outlined earlier. Of perhaps greater importance is the data shown in Table 2, which describes the relationship of HLA to the MLR. Two HLA A&B 'identical' living donor recipient combinations were MLR positive and 4 patients who were 2 mismatches with their donors were MLR negative. This may indicate, for the population under study, a higher incidence of recombination between the HLA A&B loci and the D locus than that previously reported in other populations (18).

In conclusion, the study reported here, does not provide evidence for a significant contribution of either HLA A&B matching or the MLR to graft survival in the patients studied. The most acceptable explanation for this is the 'centre effect' although the genetic make up of the local population cannot be excluded.

### Acknowledgements

Our thanks are due to A.M. Al Hindi, A.R.M. Ahmed, H.Al Moussa and K.T. Raju, staff of the Immunology Laboratory, Organ Transplantation Department, for their excellent technical assistance in this work.

### References

1. Abouna GM, Kumar MSA, White AG, Daddah S, John P, Samhan M, Omar OF Kusma G: Experience with 130 consecutive renal transplants in the Middle East with special reference to histocompatibility matching, anti rejection therapy with ALG and prolonged preservation of imported cadaveric grafts. Transplant Proc (in press) 1983.
2. Al-Nassar KE, Conneally PM, Palmer CG, Pao-o Y: The genetic structure of the Kuwait populations: Distribution of 17 markers with genetic distance analysis. Human genetics 57:192–198, 1981.
3. Terasaki PI, McClelland JD, Park MS, McCurdy B: In: Manual of tissue typing techniques,

67–74. (Ray JG, Hare DB, Pederson PD, Kayhoe DE (eds.) DHEW Publication no (NIH) 75–545, 1974.

4. Opelz G, Mickey MR, Terasaki PI: HLA and Kidney Transplants: Reexamination. Transplantation 17:371–382, 1974.

5. Morris PJ: Histocompatibility antigens in Human Organ Transplantation. Surgical Clinics of North America 58:233–244, 1978.

6. Simmons RL, Kjellstrand CM, Condie RM, Buselmeier TJ, Thompson EJ, Yunis EJ, Mauer SM, Najarian JS: Parent-to-Child and Child-to-Parent Kidney Transplants. Experience with 101 transplants at one centre. Lancet (1): 321–324, 1976.

7. Dausset J, Hors J: HLA and Kidney Transplants. Nature New Biology 238: 150–152, 1972.

8. Opelz G, Mickey MR, Terasaki PI: Calculations on long term graft and patient survival in Human Kidney Transplantation. Transplant Proc IX: 27–30, 1977.

9. White AG: In: Organ Transplantation (Chatterjee SN (ed.)) Chapter 3, p 62. Wright PSG Inc, Bristol,1982.

10. Cerilli J: Presidential Address; Role of Kidney Transplantation and its Implementation. Transplantation 32 : 459–462, 1981.

11. Bach JF, Debray-Sachs M, Crosnier J, Kreis H, Dormont J: Correlation between Mixed Lymhocyte Culture performed before Renal Transplantation and Kidney Function. Clin Exp Immunol 6: 821–827, 1970.

12. Miller J, Hattler BG: Reactivity of Lymphocytes in Mixed Culture in response to Human Renal Transplantation. Surgery 72: 220–-228, 1972.

13. Cochrum KC, Perkins HA, Payne RO, Kountz SL, Belzer FO: The Correlation of MLC with Graft Survival. Transplantation Proceedings 5: 391–395, 1973.

14. Ringden O, Berg B: Correlation between Magnitude of MLC and Kidney Graft Survival in Intrafamilial Transplantation. Tissue Antigens 10: 364–372,1977.

15. Walker J, Opelz G, Terasaki PI: Correlation of MLC Response with Graft Survival in Cadaver and Related Donor Kidney Transplants. Transplantation Proceedings 10: 949–951, 1978.

16. Cullen PR, Lester S, Rouch J, Morris PJ: Mixed Lymphocyte Reaction and graft survival in 40 Cadaveric Renal Transplants. Clin Exp Immunol 28: 218–222, 1977.

17. Berg B, Ringden O: Correlation Between Relative Responses in Mixed Lymphocyte Culture, HLA-D and DR Typing, and Graft Survival in Renal Transplantation. Transplantation 33: 291–297, 1982.

18. Bradley BA, Festenstein H: Cellular Typing. British Medical Bulletin 34: 223–232, 1979.

# 3. The role of vascular endothelial cell antigens in renal transplantation

JAMES CERILLI and LAUREN BRASILE

## Introduction

The lymphocyte has traditionally been used as the target cell in evaluating histocompatibility in human renal transplantation. The rationale for the use of the lymphocyte is based on the assumption that the antigens expressed in the kidney which serves as transplantation antigens are equally expressed on the lymphocytes. It was assumed with better matching techniques graft survival would improve. In reviewing several studies evaluating the impact of HLA matching on graft survival, the effects of matching for HLA antigens have been disappointing. Reports from several centers indicate there is little difference (10–30%) in graft survival in cadaveric kidney transplants between four antigen matches and three, two, one or even zero antigen matches (1,2,3). Except in the cases of living-related HLA identical, mixed lymphocyte negative grafts, matching for HLA antigens has been disappointing. Even in the HLA identical, living-related group rejection occurs 5–10% of the time. These findings lead researchers to look outside the HLA system for alloantigens that could serve as transplantation antigens.

## Endothelial cells as a source of alloantigens

The endothelium lining the vasculature within the grafted kidney was a logical choice in the search for alloantigens since it is the first point of contact between donor tissue and recipient immunocompetent cells. It is also the site of lesions that lead to graft rejection. Morphological evidence supports blood vessels being the primary target in all types of rejection - early, intermediate or late rejection (4,5,6). The patterns of vascular damage in the grafted kidney included widespread endothelial damage such as that seen in hyperacute rejection and arteritis characterized by mononuclear cell infiltration and intimal proliferation or fibrosis. Early work by Vitto(7,8) had suggested that dog endothelium was rich in alloantigens. Vitto concluded from these early studies that vascular endothelium may provide the sensitizing milieu in a transplanted organ where the initial recognition occurs. Upon recognition of the significance of grafted endothelium serving as an early target and being immunologically important in all types of rejection, studies were begun to evaluate the clinical significance of vascular endothelial cell (VEC) alloantigens.

## Early clinical studies

Endothelial cells to be used as the targets in a cytotoxicity technique were isolated from umbilical cords, the lymphocytes, granulocytes, and monocytes were isolated from the cord blood. Work performed during the mid-70's by ourselves (9,10,11), Stastny (12,13), and Paul (14) indicated the presence of antibodies, in the serum from recipients who had rejected their renal allografts, that were cytotoxic to vascular endothelial cells and not cytotoxic to B or T lymphocytes. The presence of anti-vascular endothelial cell antobody correlated better with graft rejection than the presence of any other antibody. We (9) found that 95% of patients who had rejected their renal allografts developed cytotoxic antibody to VEC, and some of this antibody was found to be VEC specific. Absorption studies indicated that this cell specific, anti-VEC antibody could not be removed by absorbtion with pooled VEC from umbilical cords.

The VEC antigen system demonstrated a high correlation with the clinical courses of patients undergoing a renal transplant in that essentially all patients who exhibited anti-vascular endothelial cell antibody pretransplant or who developed it post-transplant, lost their grafts from rejection.

In 1979 Paul (15) reported a case study where a recipient exhibited IgG directed against the endothelium of the graft's peritubular capillaries and venules pretransplant. The antibody was not detected post-transplant until the graft was removed, whereupon antibody directed against VEC was again detected in the circulation. The onset of rejection became clear 26 h post-transplant, and the graft was removed 7 days post-transplant. Since a renal transplant may induce a polyclonal antibody response displaying a wide range of classes and specificities, of which only a small part may actually cause graft damage, eluates from rejected grafts were studied (16,17). By studying those antibodies deposited in rejected grafts it was thought that information about the specificity of the antibodies participating in graft rejection could be found. These studies confirmed the detrimental impact of anti-VEC antibody upon graft survival. In no case was antibody directed against VEC deposited in kidneys not transplanted or in grafts with good function (16). While 40% of the eluates from rejected kidneys contained antibody directed against VEC only 10% of the eluates exhibited antibody directed against T cells (16,18). These studies may have underestimated the incidence of antibody directed against VEC since the eluates were collected after the grafts were removed.

## Studies on the antigenicity of the kidney

Since a plethora of antibody is produced at the time of graft rejection, studies were performed to evaluate the antigenicity within the kidney (19,20). While it has been acknowledged for some time that antibody deposition and cellular infiltration can be limited to either the arterial of the venous portion of the renal vasculature (4), some surprising results were found. The developing picture of the antigen expression on kidney endothelium is the opposite of the antigen expression found on the lymphocyte which is used for prospective matching. ABO antigens were found to be localized along the endothelium of blood vessels. VEC specific antigens are abundantly expressed throughout the renal vasculature and are found in particularly high concentration along the peritubular capillaries and veins. The high concentration of VEC specific antigens expressed along renal vessels is in agreement with previous work by Stastny (21) and Cerilli (11) where the highest frequency of antibody found in circulation and in the kidney at the time of rejection is antibody directed against VEC antigens. HLA - A and B locus antigens were found to be in the lowest concentration along renal vessels, while the DR antigens were found to be concentrated along the vasculature (22).

## VEC specific antigen expression on monocytes

By the late seventies the significance of VEC antigen system had become apparent. Unfortunately, a standard VEC crossmatch could not be performed prospectively due to the unavailability of donor VEC until the time of the transplant. Since some of the patients exhibited anti-VEC antibody prior to transplantation and the recipient's immune system could not possibly have become sensitized to VEC pretransplant, work began to identify another cell type that could express these antigens and afford a mode of sensitization (13,23,21). A logical mode for sensitization was through transfusions, therefore cells isolated from peripheral blood were tested for the presence of VEC specific antigens. The peripheral blood monocyte was found to also express VEC specific antigens. In screening studies utilizing T and B lymphocytes, monocytes and VEC from the same umbilical cords, it was found that when the lymphocytes were negative there was 92% concordance of positive reactions with transplant serum between monocytes and VEC (11). With this finding, work began to develop a monocyte crossmatch to be used prospectively. It was proposed that if a prospective crossmatch identifying performed anti-VEC/monocyte antibody could be developed, it would be possible to detect VEC antibody thereby eliminating much of the accelerated rejection seen in this group of patients would be characterized and phenotypes established by sera screening protocols and family studies, it would be potentially possible to type and match for VEC antigens prospectively. With the identification of VEC specific antigens being expressed in the peripheral blood monocyte, the nomenclature for these antigens has now evolved to be identified as the E - M of sometimes VEM antigen system.

## The E - M antigen system in HLA identical, living-related transplants

A multicentered retrospective study was instituted to study recipients of HLA identical living related grafts who had experienced irreversible rejection (23,24). This approach was undertaken to minimize the role of the HLA antigens in studying the organ specific VEC antigen system. Twenty-five recipients fit the criteria of this protocol and were entered into the study. Of the twenty-five recipients of HLA identical living-related grafts who experienced total graft rejection, nineteen (76%) exhibited antibody in their sera cytotoxic to their respective donor's monocytes. The VEC/monocyte antibody was detected in the patients pretransplant sera in fifteen of these nineteen recipients. The remaining four patients with a positive donor monocyte crossmatch were found to have this antibody in their post-transplant sera available for testing. In no instance was cytotoxic antibody directed against donor T or B lymphocytes found. The onset of rejection in patients with a positive pretransplant monocyte crossmatch was calculated to be a mean of thirteen days post-transplant, while in the patients who developed this antibody post-transplant we were able to detect the presence of cytotoxic donor antimonocyte antibody in their serum prior to the onset of rejection (25). In contrast, in a control group of sixteen recipients of HLA identical living-related grafts experiencing good clinical courses, the antibody was never detected.

The results from this retrospective study points towards a correlation between the development of donor specific anti-VEC/monocyte antibody and the onset of rejection. These results also indicate the importance of detecting sensitization to donor VEC/monocyte antigens pretransplant. It is currently becoming a recognized policy to avoid transplantation in patients exhibiting donor specific monocyte/VEC antibody regardless of the HLA matchgrade.

## E - M antigen expression of granulocytes

Cells that are derived from common lineage tend to express similar antigens. It has been hypothesized by Lalezari (26,27) that granylocytes, VEC and peripheral blood monocytes are derived from common percursor cells and therefore the granulocyte would be expected to express the E-M antigens. Controversy still surrounds this issue, in addition to the recognized E - M antigen system, monocyte specific antigens have been reported, and additional antigens shared by granulocytes, VEC and peripheral blood monocytes (26).

An enlightening study utilizing post-transplant sera from recipients who had rejected their HLA identical living-related grafts was screened to determine the specificity of antibody developed post-transplant. The sera was screened against T and B lymphocytes, monocytes and granulocytes from the same donor (25).

Results from this study indicate that the VEM antigens are distinct from granulocyte antigens. Only one serum had concordant results with monocytes. Absorbing this serum with granulocytes, removed the cytotoxicity directed against granulocytes but did not effect the cytotoxicity directed against the monocytes.

**Clarification of the specificity of the VEM antigen system**

The VEM antigens are slowly becoming recognized as transplantation antigens. Patients who develop anti-VEM antibody directed against their donor's vasculature either pre or post-transplant have a high incidence of graft rejection regardless of HLA matching or MLC reactivity. Sera from recipients of HLA identical living-related grafts exhibiting positive monocyte crossmatches with their donors, were screened against T and B lymphocytes, granulocytes, monocytes and VEC from the same umbilical cord donors (28). Included in the study were recipients who exhibited antibody in their sera, cytotoxic to their respective donors monocytes and yet, who never experienced a severe rejection episode.

The recipients who rejected their HLA identical living-related grafts exhibited antibody cytotoxic to both endothelial cells and monocytes. The recipients who did not reject their grafts although their sera contained antibody cytotoxic to monocytes exclusively; no cytotoxicity directed against concordant, VEC was detected. This study confirmed the existence of monocyte specific antigens in addition to the VEM antigens system. The use of the VEC panel is one simple method to separate monocyte specific antibody from VEM reactivity. Therefore, a positive monocyte crossmatch remains a contraindication to transplantation regardless of HLA matching unless a VEC panel indicated the antibody to be monocyte specific.

**Summary**

Blood vessels are the primary target in all types of rejection. Since the endothelium is rich in alloantigens, the VEC may be the sensitizing milieu in a transplanted organ. In addition to ABO and HLA antigens, VEC express a tissue specific antigen system. Antobody cytotoxic to VEC and not cytotoxic to T or B lymphocytes has been found in sera from recipients who have rejected their renal allografts. The presence of anti-VEC antibody correlated better with graft rejection than the presence of any other antibody in the patient who exhibits anti-VEC antibody pretransplant or who develops it post-transplant usually lose their grafts from rejection. The VEC specific antigens are abundantly expressed throughout the renal vasculature, this high concentration of VEC antigen may explain the correlation between the presence of anti-VEC in patient sera and a poor clinical course. The peripheral blood monocyte was found to also express VEC specific antigen. This finding provided an explanation for a mode of sensitization to VEC antigens prior to transplantation through transfusion. A clinical assay to screen for preformed anti-VEC/monocyte antibody was developed in the hope of eliminating much of the accelerated rejection seen in patients exhibiting this antibody. The currently accepted nomenclature for the VEC/monocyte antigens is the VEM antigen system. The VEM antigens are slowly becoming recognized as transplantation antigen. Endothelial cell panels can be utilized to identify highly sensitized patients. Therefore, a positive monocyte crossmatch may be considered as a contraindication to transplantation regardless of the HLA matchgrade in patients exhibiting cytotoxic antibody to VEC.

# References

1. Ting A, Morris PS: Powerful Effect of HL-DR Matching on Survival of Cadaveric Renal Allografts. Lancet 2: 282–285, 1980.
2. Opelz G, Terasaki PI: International Histocompatibility Workshop Study on Renal Transplantation. Histocompatibility Testing: 592–624, 1980.
3. Opelz G, Terasaki PI: International Study of Histocompatibility in Renal Transplantation. Transplantation 33, 1: 87–95, 1982.
4. Busch GJ, Garovoy MR, Tilney NL: Variant Forms of Arteritis in Human Renal Allografts. Transplantation Proceedings II: 100–103, 1979.
5. Anderson ND, Wyllie RG, Shaker LJ: Pathogenesis of Vascular Injury in Rejecting Rat Renal Allografts. Johns Hopkins Medical Journal 141: 135–147, 1977.
6. Bucsh GJ, Reynolds ES, Galvaneck EG et al: Human Renal Allografts. Medicine 50: 29–83, 1971.
7. Vetto RM, Burger DR: The Identification and Comparison of Transplantation Antigens on Canine Vascular Endothelium and Lymphocytes. Transplantation 11, 4: 374–377, 1971.
8. Vetto RM, Burger DR, Endothelial Cell Stimulation of Allogenic Lymphocytes. Transplantation 14, 5: 652–653, 1972.
9. Cerilli J, Holliday JE, Koolemans-Beynen A: An Analysis of the Cell Specificity of the Antibody Response Accompanying Human Renal Allograft Rejection. Surgery 83: 6, 1978.
10. Cerilli J, Holliday JE, Fesperman DP: Role of Antivascular Endothelial Antibody in Predicting Renal Allograft Rejection. Transplantation Proceedings IX, 1, 1977.
11. Cerilli J, Brasile L: Endothelial Cell Alloantigens: Transplantation Proceedings, VII, 3, 1980.
12. Moraes JR, Stastny P: A New Antigen System Expressed in Human Endothelial Cells. The Journal of Clinical Investigation (60): 449–454, 1977.
13. Moraes JR, Stastny P: Human Endothelial Cell Antigen: Molecular Independence from HLA and Expressed in Blood Monocytes. Transplant Proceeding IX (1), 605–607, 1977.
14. Paul LC, van Es LA, Kalff MW, de Graeff J: Intrarenal Distribution of Endothelial Antigens Recognized by Antibodies from Renal Allograft Recipients. Transplantation Proceedings XI, 1: 427–430, 1979.
15. Paul LC, Claas Frans HJ, van Es LA, Kalff MW, Graeff JD: Accelerated Rejection of a Renal Allograft Allograft Associated with Pretransplantation Antibodies Directed Against Donor

Antigens on Endothelium and Monocytes. The New England Journal of Medicine, 1258–1260, May 1979.

16. Baldwin III WM, Soulilou J-P, Claas FHJ, Peyrat MA, van Es LA, van Rood JJ: Antibodies to Endothelial Antigens in Eluates of 88 Human Kidneys: Correlation with Graft Survival and Presence of T- and B-Cell Antibodies. Transplantation Proceedings XIII, 3: 1547–1550, 1981.

17. Lee HM, Waldrep JC, Mendez-Picon G, Mohanakumar T: Antibodies Eluted from Rejected Human Renal Allografts: Specificity to B Lymphocytes, Monocytes, Primary Kidney Cells and Endothelial Cells. Transplantation Proceedings XIII, 1: 108–110, 1981.

18. Claas FHJ, Paul LC, van Es LA, Van Rood JJ: Antibodies Against Donor Antigens on Endothelial Cells and Monocytes in Eluates of Rejected Kidney Allografts. Tissue Antigens 15: 19–24, 1980.

19. Baldwin III WM, Claas FHJ, van Es LA, van Rood JJ: HLA A, B, DR and Endothelial-Specific Antigens in Kidney-graft Rejection. Immunology Today: 110–111, December, 1980.

20. Baldwin III WM, Claas FHJ, van Es LA, Van Rood JJ: Distribution of Endothelial-Monocyte and HLA Antigens on Renal Vascular Endothelium. Transplantation Proceedings XIII, 1: 103–107, 1981.

21. Moraes JR, Stastny P: A new Antigen System Selectively Expressed in Endothelial Cells. Journal of Clinical Investigation 60: 449–454, 1977.

22. Hirschberg H, Evensen SA, Henriksen T, Thorsby E: Stimulation of Human Lymphocytes by Allogeneic Endothelial Cells in Vitro. Tissue Antigens 4: 257–261, 1974.

23. Cerilli J, Brasile L, DeFrancis MB: Clinical Significance of Anti-monocyte Antibody in Kidney Transplant Recipients. Transplantation 32: 495–497, 1981.

24. Cerilli J, Bay W, Brasile L: Human Immunology. Human Immunology 7: 45–50, 1983.

25. Cerilli J, Brasile L, Clarke J: Specificity of Antibody Developed in Recipients who Reject Their HLA Identical Living-Related Grafts. Non-HLA Antigens in Health, Aging and Malignancy: 251–256, 1983.

26. Thompson JS, Oberlin V, Severson CD, Parsons T, Herbick J, Claas FJA: Demonstration of Granulocyte, Monocyte and Endothelial Cell Antigens Detected by Double Fluorochromatic Testing. Transplantation Proceedings VII, 3: 26–31, 1981.

27. Lalezari P: Organ-specific and Systemic Alloantigens: Interrelationships and Biologic Implications. Transplantation Proceedings VII, 3, 1980.

28. Cerilli J, Brasile L, Clarke J et al: Clarification of the Specificity of the Monocyte/Vascular Endothelial Cell System (In press).

# 4. Blood transfusion(s) and cadaveric renal transplantation in the Netherlands

G.G. PERSIJN and J.J. VAN ROOD

## Introduction

In the early days of regular haemodialysis renal patients were liberally transfused. Since the end of the sixties this policy has changed which is shown by a decrease in the median number of blood transfusions administered to the dialysis patients awaiting kidney transplantation (1). This change resulted from the realization that dialysis patients could be well maintained without regular blood transfusions by using the more sophisticated smaller artifical kidneys and without pretransplant bilateral nephrectomy. Furthermore, the restricted blood transfusion policy would reduce the risk of hepatitis and the induction of anti-HLA antibody production. Increased immunization of the potential transplant recipient was associated with lower kidney graft survival (2). Besides these aspects, sensitized kidney patients have a longer waiting time for a cadaver kidney transplant, and in some cases may not be able to receive a transplant at all due to cytotoxic antibodies.

Consequently, many dialysis centers avoided transfusing their potential kidney transplant candidates. This policy led to discomfort in some patients who had to live with very low haematocrit levels which handicapped them, in particular the bilaterally nephrectomized.patients, in many ways. In this way a group of never transfused patients awaiting a cadaveric renal transplant was 'created'. Paradoxically, kidney graft survival in this particular group of patients was not improved by avoiding blood transfusion and thus immunization. On the contrary, kidney graft survival times were worse if compared to graft survival in the transfused group of recipients. Opelz and Terasaki (3) were the first investigators who drew attention to this particular fact.

From a historical point of view it is interesting that others already had suggested that blood transfusions did not detrimentally influence kidney graft survival (4,5). Since that initial report many centers were able to demonstrate retrospectively a beneficial influence of pretransplant blood transfusions on kidney allograft survival in man. Prospective studies in monkeys (6) and dogs (7,8) had provided unequivocal evidence that pretransplant third party blood transfusions improve the fate of kidney allografts from unrelated donors.

## Acceptance of the blood transfusion effect

Since Opelz and Terasaki (3) originally reported on the beneficial effect of pretransplant blood transfusion on cadaveric kidney allograft survival, numerous additional reports have been published. The majority of them agree that blood transfusions do have a beneficial effect on cadaveric renal allograft survival. The Oxford group initially did not see a beneficial influence of pretransplant blood transfusion on kidney allograft survival (9). However, recent studies could demonstrate that there was a beneficial effect. It has to be stressed that the graft survival in their non-transfused group is rather high as compared to other centers (10). Experimental studies in animal models, like the rhesus monkey, clearly have demonstrated a positive influence of pretransplant blood transfusion on kidney allograft survival (6,11). The overall conclusion is that pretransplant transfusions have a beneficial effect on cadaveric kidney graft survival. However, no general agreement has been reached on the influence of different variables such as the exact number of transfusions; the composition of the transfusate and the risk of sensitization; the time interval between transfusion and transplantation; the use of HLA-matched blood transfusions; the use of blood transfusions in recipients of a related transplant; the effect of transfusions on subsequent transplants and finally, the influence of blood transfusions given to the kidney donor.

In addition the mechanisms, underlying the beneficial effect of blood transfusion on kidney graft survival, remain unknown and speculative. The current state of affairs of some of the above mentioned parameters will be described.

## Number of transfusions

Survey of the world literature. There is no unanimity concerning a beneficial dose-related transfusion effect. Sometimes, studies from the same center disagreed with their own previous reports (12,13,14,15,16). Some reports showed that even a single blood transfusion was as effective as many transfusions (17, 18,19). Other investigators observed that the best graft survival was obtained with 2 or 3 units of blood (10,20,21,22) while others demonstrated the maximum effect on graft survival with up to 5 units of blood (23,24,25). Also the results, obtained during the 8th International Histocompatibility Workshop, did not give a definite answer on this point (26). In this international multicenter study there seemed to be dose-effect of transfusions. Indeed, all the different subgroups of patients according to the number of transfusions had significantly better graft survival compared to the graft survival in non-transfused recipients. However, graft survival in the transfused groups was not statistically different from each other. This observation was confirmed in the prospective study too (15,16). Nevertheless, the best survival was achieved in the group of recipients who had received more than 20 blood transfusions.

## Prospective study

In the Netherlands it was decided that never-transfused and/or nulliparous kidney patients awaiting a cadaveric kidney transplant should prospectively be transfused with one unit of washed ABO-identical blood. Another group of never-transfused and/or nulliparous patients was given 1 or 3 units of cotton-wool filtered blood (see next section). Blood was not stored longer than 3 days and considered to be fresh.

It was found unethical to continue transplanting non-transfused kidney patients. Consequently, a prospective non-transfused control group was not available for this study. The aims of this protocol were to investigate the influence of different variables such as the number of transfusions, the composition of the transfusate, the time interval between transfusion and transplantation and the HLA-type of the blood transfusion and kidney donor. The choice to use washed erythrocytes was based on the results in the retrospective study. Besides this, the risk of immunization against HLA-antigens was low, especially when 1 unit was given. By washing the blood and removing the buffy-coat about 40–60% of the leukocytes are removed.

Table 1 shows the relevant data of the recipients in this prospective study. All patients, who were transfused according to this protocol but who later required additional transfusions prior to transplantation for medical reasons wer excluded from this study.

Most of the serum samples tested after the transfusion of these patients showed no detectable lymphocytotoxic antibody activity. In 2 cases very weak activity amounting to approximately 5% kill above background developed. This activity had disappeared in subsequent serum samples. All patients received 1–6 blood

*Table 1.* Profile of the prospective study (1977–1980).

| Number of Transfusions | Compo-sition of Transfusate | Number of patients male | female | Age in years | Haemo-dialysis period in months | Average HLA-mismatch kidney donor-recipient |
|---|---|---|---|---|---|---|
| 1 | Leukocyte poor | 31 | 9 | 16-56 (36)[a] | 3-68 (19)[b] | 1.6 |
| 1 | Leukocyte free | 6 | – | 31–56 (36.5)[a] | | 1.7 |
| | | | | | 3–21 (10)[b] | |
| 3 | Leukocyte free | 3 | 3 | 16–50 (37.5)[a] | | |

[a] The mean age in years.
[b] The mean haemodialysis period in months.

transfusions, mostly leukocyte-free blood (cotton-wool filtration method) during transplantation (27).

Figure 1 shows that kidney graft survival in these 40 patients is 78% after 5 years. This is significantly better than 28% graft survival in our retrospective non-transfused group (N=74) (p 0.001) (This curve is not shown).

Other authors have shown in single-center studies also an improvement in kidney graft survival in patients who had received one or very few blood transfusions before transplantation (9,17,28,29). Opelz observed only 10% better graft survival following one transfusion compared to kidney graft survival in non-transfused recipients after 6 months. Best graft survival in this multicenter study was obtained in patients with more than 20 transfusions (15).

## The composition of the transfusate

Considerable disagreement exists concerning the composition of the transfusate. Most clinicians attempt to avoid possible sensitization by blood transfusions because of the poorer graft survival obtained in recipients with lymphocytotoxic antibodies. However, the beneficial transfusion effect on kidney allograft survival was mostly noticed when the patients had received whole blood or leuko-

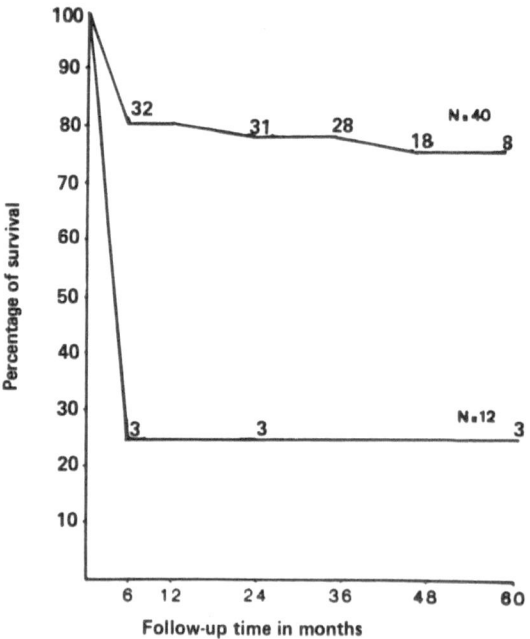

Fig. 1. Five-year graft survival results of a prospective blood transfusion study in the Netherlands. The upper curve represents 40 patients who received prospectively 1 unit of leukocyte-poor blood. The lower curve represents 12 patients who received 1 or 3 units of leukocyte-free blood (overall p = 0.001).

cytepoor blood transfusions (3,10,17,20,22,29,30,31).

The literature shows no general agreement on the effect of frozen blood on kidney allograft survival. Opelz (32) and Safwenberg (33) have reported that frozen blood is ineffective in improving cadaveric kidney graft survival. Contrarily, other investigators could demonstrate that frozen blood was as effective as other blood products such as whole blood, packed cells or leukocyte-poor blood (28,34,35,36,37). This beneficial effect of frozen blood was dependent on the method used for freezing, as mentioned by Fuller *et al.* (38). The deglycerolization method by agglomeration should be preferred to the deglycerolization method by centrifugal washing.

To avoid the detrimental effect of sensitizing the potential kidney transplant recipient and to save the beneficial influence of pretransplant blood transfusion, several prospective blood transfusion protocols have been designed. One special approach is worth mentioning here, namely the protocol introduced by Nube *et al.* (39) (see further) and later followed by Albert *et al.* (40). Nube (39) proposed to transfuse the potential kidney graft recipient with 2 or 3 units of HLA-A and -B compatible leukocyte poor blood transfusions. Albert (40) had a similar approach, although here, the recipients were transfused with HLA-A and -B matched leukocyte-poor blood. In this study it was impossible to transfuse all patients with HLA-A and -B compatible blood. Thus, there remained differences for the HLA-A and -B antigens between blood transfusion donor and kidney recipient.

Very recently, Borleffs *et al.* (41) have observed a beneficial effect of pure platelet transfusion on kidney graft survival in the Rhesus monkey. This elegant approach might be of clinical advantage because pure platelet transfusions do not induce leukocyte antibody formation.


*Dutch data*


The blood transfusion protocol introduced in the Netherlands in 1977 included also a group of previously non-transfused patients who were transfused with 1 or 3 units of cotton-wool filtered blood. With this technique the fresh blood is almost totally depleted from leukocytes and is called leukocyte-free blood (27). Most of the dialysis specialists, who discussed the transfusion protocol with their patients, favoured the donation of only one transfusion. Table 1 gives the relevant information of this group. All patients received transfusions of leukocyte-free blood varying from 1 to 4 units, during the operation. Figure 1 shows that kidney graft survival in this group of recipients is 25% after 5 years. This is significantly different from the survival in the group prospectively given 1 unit of leukocyte-poor (p=0.01). The survival in the group pretreated prospectively with 1 or 3 units of leukocyte-free blood does not differ significantly from the survival in our retrospective non-transfused group. A few remarks should be made. Firstly, none of the patients in this prospective study needed a blood transfusion. Secondly, during this protocol, it turned out, quite quickly, that patients transfused with 1 or 3 leukocyte-free blood transfusions rejected their kidney very rapidly. This observation prompted the nephrologists to switch to the 'leukocyte-poor' protocol. This explains why only 12 patients are in the leukocyte-free group. Thirdly, the 3 patients with a functioning graft are all from the same transplant centre. Interestingly, it was later learnt that the blood used for preparation of leukocyte-free blood in this centre was already one week old which is against the protocol. It is known that dead leukocytes, fragments etc. are not removed from one week old blood by cotton-wool filtered filtration. This might explain the 'transfusion effect' in these 3 patients.

### HLA-A and -B matching of the blood transfusion donor and recipient

Blood transfusions given to potential kidney recipients are in fact a two-edged sword: the benefit in renal allograft survival and the detrimental effects such as anti-HLA antibody production or the risk of transmitting infections. These latter two risks increase with the number of blood transfusions. Therefore, it is very clear that one should be very reluctant to transfuse indiscriminately. Furthermore, it is known that the beneficial blood transfusion effect is dependent on the presence of small amounts of leukocytes. Consequently, to obtain a beneficial effect of blood transfusions on renal allograft survival and to avoid the detrimental effect of presensitizing the potential recipient, one could choose the following transfusion protocol. Transfuse the never-transfused patients awaiting a cadaveric kidney transplant with a small number, i.e. 2 or 3, units of HLA-A and -B compatible or identical blood.

Such a suggestion was already made by Dr.J.Sachs at the British Transplantation Society meeting in Newcastle in 1978 (42). The only disadvantage to this approach, however, is that patients with a common HLA-A and -B phenotype are in favor, because for them one can find always HLA-A and -B identical or compatible blood donors. The first investigators who introduced and used this blood transfusion policy in man were Nube et al. (39). Later, Albert et al. (40) reported their results using a similar transfusion scheme. However, in this study blood transfusion donors and potential kidney recipients were not always HLA-A and -B identical or compatible. They were well matched, i.e. the average HLA-A and -B mismatch was 0.86. Cytotoxic antibodies were found in 25% of the patients who received well-matched washed red blood cells. Furthermore, their data did not show a beneficial transfusion effect on graft survival if blood transfusions are matched for HLA-A and -B. Very recently the Leuven group published a Letter in the New England Journal of Medicine that they were unable to demonstrate a beneficial effect of HLA-A and -B compatible blood transfusions on renal allograft survival. However, this statement was based on only 4 patients of which 2 lost their grafts. Another 26 patients, who had received previously random blood transfusion and later HLA-A and -B compatible blood transfusions, had all functioning grafts at 1 year.

*Dutch data*

Nineteen Dutch dialysis patients, who had never been transfused or pregnant, prospectively received two or three HLA-A and -B compatible blood transfusions at three weekly intervals. One additional patient received only one transfusion. Blood was made leukocyte poor by removal of the buffy coat after centrifugation (1800 r.p.m. for 20 min). Blood samples were collected at various intervals after each transfusion to screen for the presence of lymphocytotoxic antibodies against a panel of 50 selected HLA-A and -B typed donors. Before each transfusion one unit of autologous blood was withdrawn, frozen by the glycerol method and stored at −70°C. Thus, autologous blood was available during procedures such as pretransplant nephrectomy. Up until now, 15 patients have received primary cadaveric graft under the auspices of Eurotransplant.

During the transplantation prodecure all patients received leukocyte-free random blood transfusions. Standard immuno-suppressive therapy consisted of azathioprine and prednisone. The relevant data of these 15 patients are summarized in Table 2 (after Nube *et al.* (39)). Thirteen patients were transplanted in one centre and two, due to unforeseen circumstances, in another center. From the retrospectively performed HLA-DR typings, it appeared that all patients had received at least one HLA-DR mismatched blood transfusion. Thus, no patient received blood transfusions identical or compatible for the HLA-A and -B and -DR antigens. The mean number of HLA-DR mismatches between blood transfusion donor and kidney recipient is 1.4. Serum samples of two patients, showed on one occasion very weak lymphocytotoxic activity without specificity after a transfusion. A third patient showed a very strong antibody activity 6 weeks after his last blood transfusion (reached against 54% of the panel cells), with unknown specificity. Subsequent screenings showed no lymphocytotoxic activity. Two weeks before this serum sample was taken, this particular patient received an

*Table 2.* Profile of the HLA-A and -B matched blood transfusion group.

| Number of blood-transfusions | Number of male | female | Age in years | Haemodialysis period in months | Average mismatch kidney donor-recipient HLA-A and -B | HLA-DR |
|---|---|---|---|---|---|---|
| 1–3 | 14 | 1 | 19–52 (35.4)[a] | 7–59 (25.2)[b] | 1.3 | 1.2 |

[a] The mean age in years.
[b] The mean haemodialysis period in months.

anti-influenza vaccination. Finally, one patient showed strong lymphocytotoxic activity in subsequent screenings after receiving HLA-A and -B matched blood transfusions. No other blood transfusions were given to this patient in the period between his last HLA-A and -B matched transfusion and the transplantation.

Figure 2 shows that kidney graft survival in this group of pre-transfused patients is 86% at 2 years. Two out of 15 patients lost their grafts due to irreversible rejection and haemodialysis treatment was reinstituted. The remaining 13 patients have a functioning graft of at least 18 months. None of the patients has died in this protocol group. Graft survival in a historically non-transfused group (N=14) from the same center was extremely low namely 7% at 2 years.

### Timing of the transfusion

The role of the duration of the interval between blood transfusion and transplantation is still uncertain. Buy-Quang et al. (17) have reported that a better graft survival was achieved when transfusions had occurred within 6 months before grafting. More recently, Hourmant et al. (20) from the same group have stated that the transfusion effect was strongest if the last unit was given within 3 months of transplantation. Werner-Favre et al.(43) and Fauchet et al. (44) have also found the same effect. However, the latter (44) showed also that all 8 patients who had received the last transfusion more than 12 months before transplantation

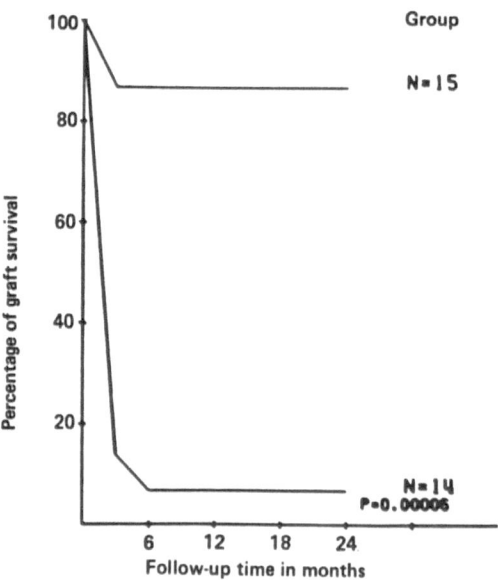

*Fig. 2.* Two-year kidney graft survival in 15 patients who received prospectively 2–3 units of HLA-A and -B compatible blood transfusions. The lower curve represents a historical non-transfused group of 14 patients (overall p = 0.0006). (From Nubé *et al.* 1982).

had a functioning graft. Yet, many other clinical data including those of the International Workshop study did not support these findings (19,22,26,45,46). One of the main problems in cadaveric renal transplantation is that one never knows when the patient will be transplanted. This consideration has led to prospective protocols in which the patient will receive peri or preoperative blood transfusion. Thus, blood transfusion given within 6 h before (peri) or during (per) transplantation.

Stiller *et al.* (47), Williams *et al.* (10), Hunsicker *et al.* (34) and the NIH-Registry Report (1977) demonstrated that transfusions given to non-transfused recipients at the time of transplantation have a beneficial effect on kidney graft survival. Again, others, including ourselves, have not been able to confirm this (44,48,49,50). Recently, Fassbinder *et al.* (51) showed that 2 units of buffy-coat rich erythrocytes, one given 4 h and the other one given 1 h before transplantation, gave a 74% kidney graft survival at 2 years in a group of never transfused patients. A similar transfusion protocol in previously transfused patients resulted in a 72% graft survival at 2 years. Therefore, they concluded that blood transfusions with sufficient leukocytes given peri-operatively have a beneficial effect on kidney graft survival too. The different protocols used in the different centers make it very difficult to draw firm conclusions on the effect of per or peri-operative blood transfusions (52).

**Prospective study**

The time between transfusion and transplantation in the group of 40 patients who received prospectively 1 unit of leukocyte-poor blood varied from 21 days to 1108 days (mean: 251 days). A clearcut correlation between the time of transfusion and kidney graft outcome was not observed (Table 3). However, the impression exists that patients had a much easier clinical course after grafting when they had received 1 leukocyte-poor blood transfusion within 200 days prior to their transplantation rather than longer than 200 days before transplantation. On the other

*Table 3.* Time interval between blood transfusion and kidney transplantation in the different prospectively transfused groups.

| Time interval (days) | Function/Total at 1 year | |
|---|---|---|
| | Leukocyte-poor | Leukocyte-free |
| 0–100 | 10/12 | 1/5 |
| 101–200 | 8/11 | 2/6 |
| 201–300 | 4/4 | – |
| 301–400 | 5/6 | 1/1 |
| 401–500 | 2/3 | – |
| 501 | 3/4 | – |

hand, 6 out of 8 transplants into patients receiving leukocyte-free blood within 200 days before transplantation failed within 3 months.


## Other factors

Besides the already described parameters which seem to play an important role in the effect of pretransplant blood transfusions on kidney allograft survival many other factors seems to be relevant too. Reviewing the literature provides an enormous amount of such, sometimes conflicting, factors. Joysey *et al.* (53) found that the beneficial effect of transfusions was restricted to patients of blood group O. This finding has been confirmed by Bore *et al.* (54). However, others did not find such an association with blood group 0 (13,30).

Festenstein *et al.* (55) showed that a beneficial effect of pretransplant blood transfusion was only apparent in patients with well HLA-A and -B matched kidneys. No difference was found in graft survival in recipients who received a poorly HLA-A and -B matched kidney whether they were transfused or not. Also Spees *et al.* (36) found that the better the HLA-A and -B match between donor and transfused recipient, the better the transplant survival. The International Workshop Study showed a consistent correlation of HLA-A and -B matching and graft survival in non-transfused patients (26). The correlation was weaker in patients who had received only a few blood transfusions, whereas there was no correlation in patients with more than 10 transfusions. The effect of matching is largely outweighed by multiple blood transfusions.

Uldall *et al.* (46) reported that the best kidney graft survival was obtained in transfused patients who received an HLA-B locus identical kidney. Williams *et al.* (10) did not find any interaction between the transfusion effect and the degree of donor-recipient matching for the HLA-A and -B antigens. However, when HLA-DR matching was taken into account, he stated that a safe procedure to overcome the risk of transfusions is to ensure that the non-transfused recipient receives a well HLA-DR matched kidney. Fehrman *et al.* (56) only noticed a transfusion effect in male recipients, while no such an effect was seen in female recipients. Solheim *et al.* (49) also found a more pronounced effect of transfusions in males than in females. William *et al.* (10) could not demonstrate such a correlation.

Guttmann *et al.* (57) showed a highly significant correlation between the length of dialysis and the number of transfusions. Fehrman *et al.* (56) revealed that graft survival was positively correlated with pretransplant dialysis, more strongly than with transfusions. However, Buy-Quang *et al.* (17) stated that duration of dialysis was less important than blood transfusions and pregnancies, which was also observed by Solheim *et al.* (49).

Alexandre *et al.* (25) reported that very superior graft survival was obtained in transfused recipients who were treated with ALS or ATG. This observation was confirmed by Spees *et al.* (36). The transfusion effect was most optimal in patients who did not develop lymphocytotoxic antibodies, as found by Sirchia *et al.* (29). Also, others have reported the same findings (3), while Werner-Favre *et al.* (43) could not show any influence of antilymphocytotoxic or anti-B cell antibodies on kidney graft survival. Significantly better graft survival was observed by Andrus *et al.* (58) in multi-transfused recipients who remained free of CMV infection. No effect of autologous blood transfusions on kidney allograft survival was seen by Safwenberg *et al.* (33). A reduced transfusion effect was noticed in black recipients of a cadaveric kidney graft, by Spees *et al.* (36). Finally, the role of previous pregnancies on kidney allograft survival. Fauchet *et al.* (44) have suggested an additive effect of transfusions and previous pregnancies. Also, other investigators have stated that a pregnancy had much the same effect on kidney graft survival as blood transfusion (17,20,59). Analysis of the Dutch data showed that 15 never-transfused female recipients who had been previously pregnant had a 50 % graft survival at 1 year. This is a 20% improvement as compared to graft survival in patients who never had received blood transfusions nor had been pregnant.

Solheim *et al.* (44) demonstrated that identical graft survival was obtained in non-transfused women with previous pregnancies as non-transfused women without pregnancies.

## Mechanisms

The mechanism by which blood transfusions improve renal allograft survival is still unknown and remains speculative. Several hypotheses have been proposed such as a selection hypothesis and a protection hypothesis.

According to the first, patients who respond with high levels of cytotoxic antibodies, the so-called 'high responders' are selected out by the cross-match. They will be never transplanted unless a fully-matched, i.e., HLA-A, -B and -C identical donor-kidney becomes available. Patients who do not produce antibodies after many blood transfusions are the so-called 'non' or 'low responders' (32). Probably, they can be transplanted with any donor kidney. Against this hypothesis is that 1 single blood transfusion gives an improvement of graft survival (45). After administration of 1 single blood transfusion, no good division can be made into low and high responders. Besides this, graft survival is enhanced by blood transfusions in patients with all levels of cytotoxic antibodies (24). However, the selection hypothesis does not explain the reported beneficial effect of per-operative blood transfusions either (10,34,47).

Recently, a new approach has been developed to distinguigh haemodialysis patients as responders or non-responders, i.e., the use of the quantitative dinitrochlorobenzene (DNCB) skin test (35). Studies, in which blood transfusions given to such patients, interact with the DNCB- reactivity are under way. The second possibility is the protection hypothesis, which is based on the idea that antigens present in the donor blood induce enhancing antibody formation. Ferrara et al. (60) have shown that repeated stimulation with small doses of HLA-antigen induces a state of unresponsiveness in man. This phenomenon has been reported by other investigators in experimental animal models after multiple blood transfusions (61). The nature of these enhancing antibodies is still speculative. MLC-blocking antibodies, cold B-cell antibodies, anti Ia-like or anti HLA-DR antibodies and anti-idiotypic antibodies have been suggested as enhancing antibodies (16,19,43,62,63,64).

Another explanation for this protection mechanism might be the induction of suppressor cells after blood transfusions. Increased suppressor cell function has been reported 3 weeks after the administration of 2 units of packed red cells in chronic haemodialysis patients (66). Also, marked suppression of cellular immunity in never-transfused haemodialysis patients have been observed after transfusion of washed erythrocytes (67). This phenomenon was not observed when autologous blood was given.

Evidence has been demonstrated, in an experimental dog model, that blood transfusions led to a macrophage blockade which leads to improved renal allograft survival as suggested by Keown and Descamps (68). Finally, Goulmy et al. (69) have demonstrated that donor cell specific mediated lympholysis (CML) did not occur in 70% of the patients who did not reject their unrelated donor kidneys. All patients who have rejected their graft were CML-reactive. In only 1 case out of 7 studied, suppressor cells were shown to be present. All patients in this study had received 1 or more blood transfusions. A possible explanation for this specific CML-non reactivity could be that the specific anti-donor cytotoxic clones of the effector cells are eliminated by anti-idiotypic antibodies or by absorption in the graft.

In conclusion, most of the work done in animals as well as in humans suggest that nonspecific suppressor cells are responsible for the graft prolongation effect of pre-transplant blood transfusion.

However, the possibility remains that there might be different phases and steps caused by blood transfusions which results in the acceptance of a donor organ. Maybe, the use of monoclonal antibodies, such as the OKT-sera, in monitoring renal patients after the administration of blood transfusions will give a definite answer in the near future.

## Conclusions

Pre-transplant blood transfusions have a beneficial effect on cadaveric kidney graft survival. Some evidence exists for a similar 'transfusion effect' on living related transplants, especially in the group of patients who receive a haplo-identical related kidney. The optimum number of blood transfusions to obtain an effect is still under discussion although some centers, including our own, have observed this effect already after only 1 or a few blood transfusions.

The composition of the transfusion appears to be important. Leukocytes in the transfusate seem to be a pre-requisite to induce a 'transfusion effect'. A reduced number of transfusions, especially of whole blood, has been recommended. In our opinion the best policy would be to give 1 single transfusion of leukocyte poor blood to the recipient. Of course, it would be ideal to transfuse HLA-A and -B matched leukocyte poor blood to the kidney patient. It might be that, especially, the never-transfused female patients with previous pregnancies would benefit the most by this approach. Very recently, pure platelets seem to be effective in prolonging kidney graft survival in the Rhesus monkey (41). What the clinical relevance of this will be, has to be investigated in well designed protocols. The optimal time-interval might be within 200 days before transplantation. Per-or peri-operative transfusions might be beneficial but this is still controversial. However, they seem to be not harmful on kidney graft outcome. Finally, the mechanism underlying the blood transfusion effect in renal transplantation is still unclear. Although much of the work done in humans suggests that non-specific suppressor cells are responsible for this effect, other possibilities like the production of enhancing antibodies, antigen-antibody complexes or anti-idiotype antibodies or the induction of specific anti-donor cytotoxic clones cannot be excluded.

## Acknowledgement

This work was in part supported by the Dutch Foundation for Medical Research (FUNGO) which is subsidized by the Dutch Organization for the Advancement of Pure Research (ZWO), the J.A.Cohen Institute for Radiopathology and Radiation Protection (IRS) and the Kuratorium fur Heimdialyse, Neu-Isenburg, Germany.

## References

1. Hooff JP van, Kalff MW, Poelgeest AE van, Persijn GG, Rood JJ van: Blood transfusions and kidney transplantation. Transplantation 22:306, 1976.
2. Hooff JP van, Schippers HMA, Steen GJ van der, Rood JJ van: Efficacy of HL-A matching in Eurotransplant Lancet 2:1385, 1972.
3. Opelz G, Mickey MR, Terasaki PI: Blood transfusions and unresponsiveness to HL-A. Transplantation 16:649, 1973.
4. Dossetor JB, MacKinnon KJ, Gault MH, Maclean LD: Cadaver Kidney transplants. Transplantation 5:844, 1967.
5. Michielsen P: EDTA. Proc 3:162, 1966.
6. Es AA van, Marquet RL, Rood JJ van, Kalff MW, Balner H: Blood transfusions induce prolonged kidney allograft survival in rhesus monkeys. Lancet 1:506, 1977.
7. Abouna GM, Barabas AZ, Pazerderba V, Kinninburg D, Kovithavongs T, Lao V, Schlout J,

Dossetor JB: The effect of Treatment with Multiple Blood Transfusion and with skin grafts on the survival of renal allografts in unmatched Mongrel Dogs. Transplant Proc. 9:265, 1977.

8. Obertop H, Bijnen AB, Niessen GJCM, Joling P: The influence of number and timing of pretransplant blood transfusion on the beneficial effect of renal allograft survival in immunosuppressed dogs. Eur Surg Res 13:21, 1981.

9. Morris PJ, Oliver D, Bischop M, Cullen P, Fellows G, French M, Ledingham JG, Smith JC, Ting A, Williams K: Results from a new renal transplantation unit. Lancet 2:1353, 1978.

10. Williams GM, Ting A, Cullen PR, Morris PJ: Transfusions: Their Influence on Human Graft Survival. Transplant Proc 11:175, 1979.

11. Borleffs JCC, Marquet RL, Balner H: Pretransplant blood transfusions have an additive positive effect on kidney graft prognosis in D/DR-matched rhesus monkeys. Transplantation 32:48, 1981.

12. Opelz G, Terasaki PI: Enhancement of Kidney Graft Survival by Blood Transfusions. Transplant Proc 9:121, 1977.

13. Opelz G, Terasaki PI, Graver B, Sasaki N, Langston M, Cohn M, Mickey MR: Correlation between number of Pretransplant Blood Transfusions and Kidney Graft Survival. Transplant Proc 9:145, 1979.

14. Opelz G, Terasaki PI: Blood Transfusions and Kidney Transplants: Remaining Controversies. Transplant Proc 13:136, 1981.

15. Opelz G, Graver B, Terasaki PI: Induction of high kidney graft survival rate by multiple transfusion. Lancet 1:1223, 1981.

16. Opelz G, Terasaki PI: Importance of preoperative (not peroperative) transfusions for cadaver kidney transplants. Transplantation 31:106, 1981.

17. Buy-Quang D, Soulillou JP, Fontenaille Ch, Guimbretiere J, Guenel J: Role benefique des transfusions sanguines et des grossesses dans la survie des allogreffes renales. La Nouv Presse med 6, 3503, 1977.

18. Persijn GG, Hooff JP van, Kalff MW, Lansbergen Q, Rood JJ van: Effect of Blood Transfusions and HLA Matching on Renal Transplantation in The Netherlands. Transplant Proc 9:503, 1977.

19. Buhlmann H, Largiader F, Uhlschmid G, Binswanger U, Binz H: Verlangertes Nierentransplantat-Uberleben dank Bluttransfusionen. Dtsch med Wschr 103, 293, 1978.

20. Hourmant M, Soulillou JP, Buy-Quang D: Beneficial effect of blood transfusion. Transplantation 28:40, 1979.

21. Oei LS, Thompson JS, Corry RJ: Effect of Blood transfusions on survival of cadaver and living related renal transplants. Transplantation 28:482, 1979.

22. Betuel H, Touraine JL, Malik MC, Traeger J: Pretransplant Protocols: Thoracic Duct Drainage, Transfusions Programmed and Random, Their Effect on Kidney Graft Survival. Transplant Proc 13:167, 1981.

23. Opelz G, Terasaki PI: Prolongation effect of blood transfusions on kidney graft survival. Transplantation 22:380, 1976.

24. Vincenti F, Duca RM, Amend W, Perkings HA, Cochrum KC, Feducka NJ, Salvatierra O: Immunologic a factors determining survival of cadaver-kidney transplants. N Engl J Med 299:793, 1978.

25. Alexandre GPJ, Van Cangh PJ: Influence of Blood Transfusion on Kidney Transplantation. Dial Transpl. 7:392, 1978.

26. Opelz G, Terasaki PI: International study of Histocompatibility in renal transplantation. Transplantation 33:87, 1982.

27. Diepenhorst P, Sprokholt R, Prins HK: Removal of leukocytes from whole blood and erythrocyte suspensions by filtration through cotton wool. I. Filtration technique. Vox Sang 23:308, 1972.

28. Briggs JD, Canavan JSF, Dick HM, Hamilton DNH, Kyle KF, Macpherson SG, Paton AM, Titterington DM: Influence of HLA matching and blood transfusion on renal allograft survival. Transplantation 25;80, 1978.

29. Sirchia G: Blood Transfusion and Kidney Transplantation. Dial Transpl 7:390, 1978.
30. Blamey RW, Knapp MS, Burden RP, Salisbury M: Blood transfusion and renal allograft survival. Br Med J 1, 138, 1978.
31. Fehrman I, Ringden O, Moller E, Lundgren G, Groth CG: Is Cell-Mediated Immunity in the Uremic Patient Affected by Blood Transfusion? Transplant Proc 13:164, 1981.
32. Opelz G, Terasaki PI: Poor Kidney-transplant survival in recipients with frozen-blood transfusions or no transfusions. Lancet 2:696, 1974.
33. Safwenberg J, Backman-Bave U, Hogmann CF: The effect of blood transfusions on cadaver kidney transplants - an analysis of patients transplanted in Uppsala. Scand J Urol Nephrol -Suppl 42:59, 1977.
34. Hunsicker LG, Oei LS, Freeman RM, Thompson JS, Corry RJ: Effect of Blood Transfusions on Cadaver Renal Allograft Survival. Transplant Proc 11:156, 1979.
35. Hamilton DNH, Watson MA, Briggs JD: Interrelation of Pretransplant Cell-Medicated Immunity, Blood Transfusion, and Kidney Transplant Survival. Transplant Proc 13:194, 1981.
36. Spees EK, Vaughn WK, Niblack G, Williams GM, Amos DB, Filo RS, McDonald JC, Mendes-Picon G: The Effects of Blood Transfusion on Cadaver Renal Transplantation: A Prospective Study of the South-eastern Organ Procurement Foundation 1977–1980. Transplant Proc 13:155, 1981.
37. Polesky HF, McCullough JJ, Yunis E, Helgeson MA, Andersen RC, Simmons RL, Najarian JS: The effects of transfusion of frozen-thawed deglycerolized red cells on renal graft survival. Transplantation 24:449, 1977.
38. Fuller TC, Delmonico FL, Cosimi AB, Huggins CE, King M, Russel PS: Effects of Various Types of RBC Transfusions on HLA Alloimmunization and Renal Allograft Survival. Transplant Proc 9:117, 1977.
39. Nube MJ, Persijn GG, Kalff MW, Rood JJ van: Kidney Transplantation - transplant survival after planned HLA-A and -B matched blood transfusions. Tissue Antigens 17:449, 1981.
40. Albert ED, Scholz S, Meixner U, Land W: HLA-A, B Matching of Pretransplant Blood Transfusion is Associated with Poor Graft Survival. Transplant Proc 13:175, 1981.
41. Borleffs JCC, Neuhaus P, Rood JJ van, Balner H: Platelet transfusions have a positive effect on kidney allograft survival in rhesus monkeys without inducing cytotoxic antibodies. Lancet 1:1117, 1982.
42. Editorial: Blood transfusions and Renal Transplantation. Lancet 2:193, 1978.
43. Werner-Favre C, Jeannet M, Harder F, Montadon A: Blood transfusions, cytotoxic antibodies, and kidney graft survival. Transplantation 28:343, 1979.
44. Fauchet R, Wattelet J, Genetet B, Campion JP, Launois B, Cartier F: Role of Blood Transfusions and Pregnancies in Kidney Transplantation. Vox Sang 37:222, 1979.
45. Persijn GG, Cohen B, Lansbergen Q, Rood JJ van: Retrospective and prospective studies on the effect of blood transfusions in renal transplantation in The Netherlands. Transplantation 28:396, 1979.
46. Uldall PR, Wilkinson R, Dewar PJ, Murray S, Morley AR, Baxby K, Hall RR, Taylor RMR: Factors affecting the outcome of cadaver renal transplantation in Newcastle upon Tyne. Lancet 2:316, 1977.
47. Stiller CR, Lockwood BL, Sinclair NR, Ulan RA, Sheppard RR, Sharpe JA, Hayman P: Beneficial effect of operation-day blood-transfusions on human renal-allograft survival. Lancet 1:169, 1978.
48. Persijn GG, Rood JJ van: Operation-day blood-transfusion and renal transplantation. Lancet 1:495, 1978.
49. Solheim BG: The Role of Pretransplant Blood Transfusions. Transplant Proc 11:138, 1979.
50. Brynger H, Frisk B, Sandberg L, Gelin LE: Renal graft rejection and blood transfusion before and during the transplant operation. Scand J Urol Nephrol 12:271, 1978.
51. Fassbinder W, Frei U, Persijn G, Bechstein PB, Schopow K, Dathe G, Jonas D, Weber W,

Kuehnl P, Schoeppe W: Graft Survival in Renal Allograft Recipients Transfused Perioperatively Only. Transplant Proc 14:164, 1982.

52. Glass NR, Felsheim G, Miller DT, Sollinger HW, Belzer FO: Influence of pre and peri-operative blood transfusions on renal allograft survival. Transplantation 33, 4:430, 1982.

53. Joysey VC, Roger JH, Evans DB, Herbertson BM: Differential kidney graft survival associated with interaction between recipient ABO group and pretransplant blood transfusion. Transplantation 24:371, 1977.

54. Bore PJ, Sells RA, Jamieson V, Burrows K: Transfusion-Induced Renal Allograft Protection. Transplant Proc 11:148, 1979.

55. Festenstein H, Pachoula-Papasteriadis C, Sachs JA, Jaraquemada D, Burke JM: Collaborative Scheme for Tissue Typing and Matching in Renal Transplantation. X.Effect of HLA-A, and B, D, and DR Matching and Pretransplant Blood Transfusion on 769 Cadaver Renal Grafts. Transplant Proc 11:752, 1979.

56. Fehrman I, Groth CG, Lundgren G, Magnusson G, Moller E: Pretransplant Dialysis and Blood Transfusion-Correlation with Cadaveric Kidney Graft Survival. Transplant Proc 11:152, 1979.

57. Guttmann RD: Interrelationship of Time of Dialysis-Dependent Uremia and Pretransplant Blood Transfusions. Nephron 22:196, 1978.

58. Andrus CH, Betts RF, May AG, Freeman RB: Cytomegalovirus infection blocks the beneficial effect of pretransplant blood transfusion on renal allograft survival. Transplantation 28:451, 1979.

59. Tiilikainen A, Kock B, Kuhlback B, Wallenius M: Transfusions and kidney graft survival in Finland. Scand J Urol Nephrol -Suppl 42:70, 1977.

60. Ferrara GB, Tosi RM, Azzolina G, Carminati G, Longo A: HL-A unresponsiveness induced by weekly transfusions of small aliquots of whole blood. Transplantation 17:194, 1974.

61. Zimmerman CE: Enhancing Potential of Whole Blood. Transplant Proc 9:1:1081, 1977.

62. Ettinger RB, Terasaki I, Opelz G, Malekzadeh M, Pennisi AJ, Uittenbogaart C, Fine R: Successful renal allografts across a positive cross-match for donor. Lancet 2:56, 1976.

63. Iwaki Y, Terasaki PI, Park MS, Billing R: Enhancement of human kidney allografts by cold B-lymphocyte cytotoxins. Lancet 1:1228, 1978.

64. Jeannet M, Vassali P, Hufschmid MF: Enhancement of human kidney allografts by cold B lympocyte cytotoxins. Transplantation 29:174, 1980.

65. Rood JJ van, Balner H: Blood transfusion and transplantation. Transplantation 26:275, 1978.

66. Es AA van, Marquet RL, Rood JJ van, Balner H: The influence of a single blood transfusion on kidney allograft survival in unrelated rhesus monkeys. Transplantation 26:325, 1978.

67. Fisher E, Lenhard V, Seifert P, Kluge A, Johannsen R: Blood transfusion induced suppression of cellular immunity in man. Hum Immunol 3:187, 1980.

68. Keown PA and Descamps B: Improved renal allograft survival after blood transfusion: a non-specific, erythrocyte mediated immunoregulatory process? Lancet 1:20, 1979.

69. Goulmy E, Persijn GG, Blokland EC, D'Amaro J Rood JJ van: Cell-mediated lympholysis studies in renal allograft recipients. Transplantation 31:210, 1981.

# 5. The development of immunosuppression

T.E. STARZL, B.W. SHAW and S. IWATSUKI

## Introduction

In this contribution I will deal with the development of immunosuppression as this occurred with renal transplantation and then was applied to the transplantation of other organs. This was an entirely natural sequence because with the other organs (liver, lung, heart, heart-lung, and pancreas grafts) the technical requirements and technical complications were so high that the evaluation of new immunosuppressive drugs was not really feasible.

With the simple kidney transplantation model, it was possible to define the patterns of rejection without the artifacts caused by the surgical complications and to assess how immunosuppression changed these patterns.

## Cell mediated versus humoral rejection

It became obvious in the early 1960's that cell mediated rejection was not the only kind of immunologic problem which we had. James Cerilli (see Chapter 00) has alluded to the fact that in hyperacute rejection the signal event is devascularization of the kidney cortex despite the main renal vessels being open. It was recognized that hyperacute rejection was precipitated by antibodies such as the isoagglutinins that attach to renal cells if transplantation is performed across red blood cell group barriers (1) or more importantly if the recipient has antigraft cytotoxic antibodies (2). The avoidance of hyperacute rejection is not dependent upon immunosuppression but rather on the avoidance of antibodies by tissue typing.

## Modified cell mediated rejection

In 1962 and 1963 it was recognized that azathioprine and prednisone could be used together to modify cell mediated renal rejection. In Figure 1 are shown the events following transplantation from a brother who probably was well matched at the

40

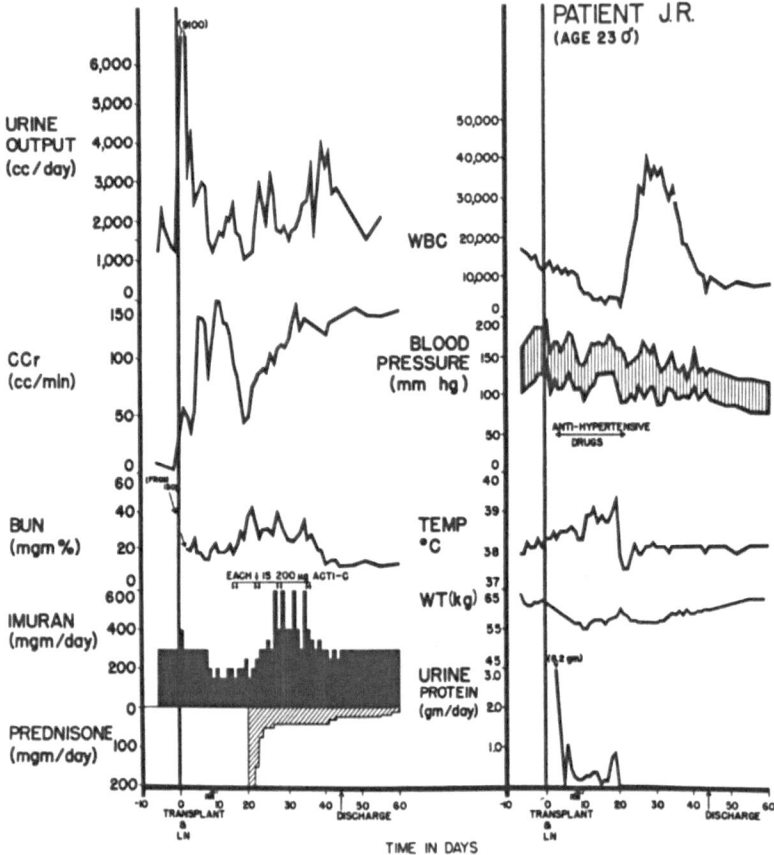

*Fig.1.* Classic rejection crisis in patient treated 20 years ago. The donor was a sibling. Deterioration of renal function began more than 2 weeks after transplantation. All stigmata of rejection were present except for acute hypertension and weight gain, which were successfully prevented by medical treatment. Acti-C-Actinomycin C; LN - Left nephrectomy at time of transplantation; RN - Right nephrectomy. Imuran is synonymous with azathioprine. (By permission of Surg Gynec Obstet 117:385, 1963).

A, B, and DR loci although we did not know this at the time. The creatinine clearance which was near zero before went to super normal levels after operation. The recipient had a massive diuresis which was typical in those days because of the generally poor condition of the recipients which in turn was explained by the fact that chronic hemodialysis was not generally available. The patient had a magnificent recovery and felt better for about 2 weeks than he had for several years.

The sense of well being was temporary. Secondary deterioration of graft function followed with a rise in BUN, and a decline in creatinine clearance. A finding that is not much seen any more because of the extensive use of steroid therapy today was fever (Fig.1). Also, the patient gained weight and developed proteinurea. In our earliest kidney recipients, azathioprine was used alone at first (Fig.1) and steroids were reserved to treat proven or presumed rejection (3).

With the institution or prednisone therapy (Fig.1), renal function improved and the other adverse findings including fever were ameliorated. As these patients were successfully treated it was realized that rejection was a reversible process (1, 3). An additional interesting observation in some of these early patients was that it became possible to greatly reduce or in a few instances to even stop the prednisone therapy within a surprisingly short time. This implied the induction of an altered host-graft relationship which we rashly called 'tolerance' (3). The kidney whose function is depicted in Figure 1 is still functioning more than 20 years later.


**Alternative immunosuppressive regimens**

Experiences in 1962 and 1963 such as those shown in Figure 1 constituted the beginning of the so-called double drug therapy with azathioprine and prednisone that has become the standard throughout the world. Before this time, 6 mercaptopurine and azathioprine had been used as single agents, but the success rate was miniscule (4).

Subsequently, a number of deviations from the original double drug programs have been described (Table 1), as summarized elswhere (5). Perhaps the most important was the use of antilymphocyte globulin (ALG) as adjunctive therapy during the first few postoperative days or weeks (6). The addition of ALG to base therapy with azathioprine and prednisone has been called 'triple drug therapy'. It was of considerable interest to note a few years later that cyclophosphamide, the widely used anticancer agent, could be substituted freely for azathioprine (7) (Table 1). Cyclophosphamide had been (and is still) thought to be a fairly specific drug against B lymphocytes for which reason some people thought it surprising that the drug was as effective as the azathioprine to which anti-T-lymphocyte activity had been attributed.

Prior to 1962, the literature about renal transplantation was uniformly pessimistic in all except twin cases. For this reason, it was remarkable how well our first wave of patients did under treatment with azathioprine and prednisone. After consanguineous transplantation (excluding twin cases) in 1962 and 1963, the one year graft and patient survival was almost 70% (1). More than half of the kidney grafts were still functioning at 10 years (8) and now with 20 years of followup the number is still almost half.

It was interesting that in our subsequent experience (1964–1966) using double drug immunosuppression for consanguineous transplantations was not quite as good in spite of the fact that an effort was made to prospectively tissue match all donors and recipients (8). These disappointing results were prophetic of those in later and much larger trials which also showed that tissue matching (at least at the

*Table 1.* Immunosuppressive drug regimens and adjuncts for kidney transplantation.

| Agent | Year (Ref.) | Place | Deficiencies |
|---|---|---|---|
| Azathioprine | 1962 (4) | Boston | Ineffective, dangerous |
| Azathioprine-steroids | 1963 (3, 22–24) | Denver, Richmond, Boston, Edinborough | Suboptimal |
| Thoracic duct drainage as adjunct | 1963 (17)[a] | Stockholm | Nuisance: requires 20 to 30 days pretreatment |
| Thymectomy as adjunct | 1963 (1) | Denver | Unproven value |
| Splenectomy as adjunct | 1963 (1) | Denver | No longer necessary |
| ALG as adjunct | 1966 (6) | Denver | Suboptimal |
| Cyclophosphamide substitute for azathioprine | 1970 (7) | Denver | No advantage except for patients with azathioprine toxicity |
| Total lymphoid irradiation | 1979 (14, 15) | Palo Alto, Minneapolis | Dangerous; extensive preparation; not quickly reversible |
| Cyclosporine alone | 1978–1979 (19) | Cambridge | Suboptimal |
| Cyclosporine-steroids | 1980 (5, 20, 21) | Denver | Under evaluation |

[a] It was not realized until much later that pretreatment for 3 to 4 weeks before transplantation was a necessary condition (16).

A and B loci) was a poor instrument of donor and recipient selection except for sibling combinations.

The use of the triple drug combinations provided better results after related transplantation and it became common year after year to have graft survival after related transplantation at or above 80% (8).

## The non-related donor

The defect in renal transplantation and one which of course was transferred to all extrarenal organs was that the results were so poor after cadaveric transplantation or transplantation from living non-related donors. In our 1962–63 series, two thirds of the recipients of non-related kidneys died during the first postoperative year of graft rejection or of complications of the immunosuppression used to control the rejection (1). Most of these donors were living unrelated volunteers, and thus the quality of the grafts was generally better than could be obtained under the condition of cadaveric donation which pertained in those early years. At that time, chronic dialysis was not generally available, and because of this, patient and renal graft survival were very nearly synomymous.

The one year survival after transplantation from nonrelated volunteers or cadaveric donors in our Series 2 (1964–1966) rose to 50%. In subsequent series from 1966 to 1972 in which the triple drug programs were used, including ALG, the one year patient survival rose to the more satisfactory levels of 80% or better (8). However, this increased survival was explained in part by the more and more common practice of returning patients to dialysis in the event of irreversible rejection; many of these patients underwent retransplantation (8).

During the decade beginning in 1970 it became a common practice to look at graft (not patient) survival in assessing the effectiveness of immunosuppression. In this same decade, there was a drying up of reports of cadaveric renal transplantation from individual centers. I suspect that the reason was that many surgeons who were using double drug therepy were having such poor graft survival that they labored under the impression that other people must be doing better. This perception of things was undoubtedly aided by a tendency from a few centers to issue what have been termed 'See what a big boy am I' reports which at times were based upon imcomplete data or upon data pools that were diluted by unspecified numbers of related transplantations in addition to the cadaveric cases.

The true state of affairs was revealed by reports from Dr.Paul Terasaki's center at the University of California, Los Angeles. Terasaki provided a mechanism for more than 100 centers to report their results under a cloak of anonymity. It was found that the one year cadaveric graft survival under conventional (for the most part double drug) therapy was 50% or less (9). As recently as 1981, another multicenter report from the Southeastern Organ Procurement Foundation has shown the same thing (10).

Finally, reports from centers known for the quality of patient care such as the Peter Bent Brigham Hospital, showed one year cadaveric kidney survival of considerably less than 50% in recipients who were surviving for one year at better than a 90% rate (11). Individual centers which had higher cadaveric graft survival almost invariably paid a price of an increased one year patient mortality (12). Thus differences in graft survival from center to center reflected in part differing philosophies about what kind of patient mortality to accept, and the extent to which immunosuppression was pushed to the limit.

**The watershed year of 1978**

The need for fundamental changes in immunosuppression or some other aspect of the strategy of cadaveric transplantation was widely acknowledged by the time the International Transplantation Society met in Rome in early September, 1978. The possible value of matching at the DR locus was at center stage for the first time, and in addition Terasaki's concept of recipient preparation with multiple blood transfusions (1, 3) had been increasingly accepted. However, both of the foregoing approaches would have tended to restrict the numbers of patients

treated with transplantation.

In particular, it was obvious that the practice of preoperative transfusions improved the statistics after cadaveric transplantation but at the cost of rendering many patients nontransplantable who developed widely reacting cytotoxic antibodies. What was happening was that part of the 'transfusion effect' was the weeding out of strong immunologic responders. The transfusion approach had the capability of making the transplant surgeons' statistics look better, but the aims of society partially were being subverted by consigning a significant number of patients to permanent dialysis.

In the field of immunosuppression, three major topics dominated the 1978 meeting. One was the use of total lymphoid irradiation for preoperative recipient preparation. The techniques had been worked out at Stanford University by Strober et al. (14) and the first clinical trials had been begun at the University of Minnesota (15). A second technique was also based on lymphoid depletion prior to transplantation and was a re-examination of thoracic duct drainage (TDD) (16) which was first used clinically by Franksson of Stockholm more than 15 years earlier (17).

The earlier trials of thoracic duct drainage had not been successful, partly because the pace of the immunologic changes caused by TDD in humans was not understood. In his original studies in rats, James Gowans of Oxford had shown profound immunodepression within 5 days after beginning TDD and it was assumed that the same applied in humans. It was not until the late 1970's that it became clear that 20 to 30 days of effective thoracic duct drainage was necessary in man before an advantage was created for a new transplant (16).

The necessity for such a prolonged preparation for cadaveric transplantation implied a high cost and excessive inconvenience. In spite of these disadvantages, thoracic duct drainage undoubtedly would have undergone a clinical renaissance were it not for the fact that the possibility of better drug therapy also came to the fore at the same time. The incidence of rejection with appropriate TDD pretreatment was reduced to less than 5% in the first three months after primary cadaveric transplantation (16).

The most important subject at the 1978 Rome meeting was the potential value of the new immunosuppressive drug cyclosporine which had been discovered by scientists at the Sandoz Corporation, Basel, Switzerland. The immunosuppressive qualities of cyclosporine had been described by Borel et al. (18). The drug was capable of inhibiting a number of experimental auto-immune diseases and was spectacularly effective in preventing skin graft rejection in rodents. The drug was described as having weak myelotoxicity, and subsequent observations have suggested that there may be no bone marrow toxicity at all. Calne and his associates of Cambridge, England reported the first clinical trials with cyclosporine, and a little more than a year later they published a classical series of observations in recipients of cadaveric kidneys, livers and pancreases (19). For clinical use, Calne et al. (19) recommended that cyclosporine be used as the sole immunosuppressive

agent. In late 1979, our own trials with cyclosporine were begun, with the conclusion that the optimal use of cyclosporine depended upon its combination with steroid therapy (20).

Our usual practice has been to begin prednisone on the day of operation in a dose for adults of 200 mg on the first postoperative day and with daily decrements of 40 mg/day until 20 mg/day is reached as a maintenance dose in the noncomplicated case after 5 postoperative days. If rejection supervenes in spite of this therapy a second burst of steroid therapy is given. The dose of cyclosporine which we have used has been about 17.5 mg/kg/day.

Less than half of the patients treated in this way have a completely untroubled convalescence. In the rest, adequate renal function either is not obtained at the outset or else graft deterioration occurs after initially satisfactory function (21). When a secondary decline in renal function occurs, it is necessary to devise changes in therapy that can accommodate either the possibilities of rejection or of cyclosporine nephrotoxicity. The most serious and consistent side effect of the agent has been renal injury, but fortunately this has almost always been responsive to reductions in dose. Our own hypothesis has been that nephrotoxicity and rejection can occur simultaneously (21).

Our initial trials with cyclosporine were in 1979 and 1980. The results were compared with historical controls. In spite of the fact that we were engaged in a learning process, the one year actual graft survival after primary cadaveric transplantation was nearly 80% (Table 2).

At the University of Pittsburgh in 1981 a randomized trial was carried out in which the results under cyclosporine-steroid therapy were compared to those with conventional double drug treatment using azathioprine and prednisone. The divergence in results was so great that the trial had to be discontinued within less than a year. The one year primary graft survival was 90% under the experimental protocol compared to than less than 50% using conventional therapy (Table 3). The mortality during 1981 in all groups of patients was 1%.

An important feature of the improved immunosuppression with cyclosporine and steroids has been the ease with which cadaveric retransplantation has been

Table 2. Cadaveric graft and patient survival in first cyclosporine trial, from December 1979 to September 1980.

|  | At 6 months | At 12 months | At 18 months | At 24/25 months | At 36 months |
|---|---|---|---|---|---|
| First grafts (57 in 57 patients) | 48 (84.2%) | 45 (79%) | 44 (77.2%) | 43 (75.4%) | 39 (68.4%) |
| Retransplants (10 in 9 patients) | 6 (60%) | 6 (60%) | 6 (60%) | 6 (60%) | 6 (60%) |
| Survival of the 66 patients | 58 (87.9%) | 57 (86.4%) | 57 (86.4%) | 56 (84.8%) | 52 (78.8%) |

*Table 3.* Cadaveric graft and patient survival in second cyclosporine (and control) trial (1981).

|  | At 3 months | At 6 months | At 9 months | At 11 months | At 11 to 21 months |
|---|---|---|---|---|---|
| Primary grafts with cyclosporine-steroids (N = 38) | 36 (94.7%) | 35 (92.1%) | 35 (92.1%) | 35 (92.1%) | 35 (92.1%) |
| Primary grafts with azathioprine-steroids (N = 32) | 22 (68.6%) | 17 (53.1%) | 16 (50%) | 15 (46.9%) | 14 (43.8%) |
| Retransplants with cyclosporine-steroids (N = 29 patients) | 24 (80%) | 23 (76.6%) | 23 (76.6%) | 23 (76.6%) | 20 (66.7%)[b] |
| Survival in all 99 patients[a] | 98 98 | 98 | 97 | 96 (97%) | |

[a] Two deaths after 2 weeks and 18 months were with functioning grafts (one each in the cyclosporine and retransplantation series) and were caused by myocardial infarction and ruptured abdominal aneurysm. The third patient (azathioprine series) was anephric and died of gastrointestinal hemorrhage 9 1/2 months after transplantation.
[b] Two of the 3 late graft losses were from chronic rejection after 12 and 13 months; the third was from death (ruptured aneurysm) after 18 months.

possible. After retransplantation, our results in the pilot trials at the University of Colorado and subsequently at the University of Pittsburgh have resulted in about a 75% one year cadaveric graft survival (Table 2 and 3), almost double that usually reported and in comparison with the outcome in our own institution for several preceding years. The fact that retransplantation can be so readily carried out with this improved immunosuppression has virtually eliminated any incentive to carry out persistant or excessive attempts at salvaging kidneys undergoing protracted or unusually severe rejection.

## Future policies in transplantation

The conclusions which have been reached from observations in the last several years have opened up some areas for lively discussions. Thus what I will speculate upon might be considered to be controversial. My own feeling is that the use of living related donors will become obsolete as a result of the great improvements in immunosuppression and particularly those made possible with cyclosporine-steroid therapy. The role of tissue matching will be diminished in transplantation practices, since it has been so easy to override the immunologic problems caused by mismatches. At the same time it will be increasingly important to have accurate crossmatching techniques since there is no reason to believe that pre-formed antibody states can be successfully dealt with with cyclosporine-steroid therapy. The importance of sensitization will be an important objective in future times and because of that the preparation of patients by transfusion which I discussed earlier will become a less and less desirable practice. Diabetics will be easier to treat and the same applies to other patients currently considered to have an increased risk. Thus the criteria for candidacy will be liberalized. It seems certain that the drain of patients from the dialysis centers will become more rapid, but we have been told recently that the numbers entering dialysis will also increase and thus the dialysis pools will not dry up. In any case the interface between dialysis and transplantation will undoubtedly change.

It has been often remarked that the ambience between the transplant surgeons and the nephrologists has sometimes been a hostile one. This will have to change. The nephrologists are going to have to face the fact that transplantation is a reliable service and probably safer than dialysis. Physicians who have withheld patients from cadaveric transplantation because of their dissatisfaction with the results to the present time will be in a position to change their minds. The question which is so paramount in importance here is the extent to which the organ supply will be a critical limitation in renal transplantation. I think it is vitally important for all nations who wish to serve their own citizens to create a legal structure which will permit and even openly encourage the donation of organs from cadavers and under the appropriate circumstances (including brain death) which will permit a high expectation of success.

### Acknowledgement

Supported by Research Grants from the Veterans Administration; by project grant AM–29961 from the National Institutes of Health and by grant RR–00084 from the General Clinical Research Centers Program of the Division of Research Resourches, National Institutes of Health.

### References

1. Starzl TE: Experience in Renal Transplantation Philadelphia, WB Saunders, 1964.
2. Terasaki PI, Marchioro TL, Starzl TE: Sero-typing of human lymphocyte antigens: Preliminary trials on long-term kidney homograft survivors. In: Histocompatibility Testing, Washington, DC, National Acad Sci - National Res Council, 1965, pp 83–96.
3. Starzl TE, Marchioro TL, Waddell WR: The reversal of rejection in human renal homografts with subsequent development of homograft tolerance. Surg Gynec Obstet 117: 385–395, 1963.
4. Murray JE, Merrill JP, Dealy JB Jr, Alexandre GW, Harrison JH: Kidney transplantation in modified recipients. Ann Surg 156: 337–355, 1962.
5. Starzl TE, Rosenthal JT, Hakala TR, Iwatsuki S, Shaw BW Jr, Klintmalm GBG: Steps in immunosuppression for renal transplantation. Kidney Int 23:S60–S65, 1983.
6. Starzl TE, Marchioro TL, Porter KA, Iwasaki I, Cerilli GH: The use of heterologous anti-lymphoid agents in canine renal and liver homotransplantation and in human renal homo-

transplantation. Surg Gynec Obstet 124: 310–318, 1967.

7. Starzl TE, Putnam CW, Halgrimson CG, Schroter GP, Martineau G, Launois B, Corman JL, Penn L, Booth AS Jr., Porter KA, Groth CGS: Cyclophosphamide and whole organ transplantation in humans. Surg Gynecol Obstet 133: 981–991, 1971.

8. Starzl TE, Weil R, Putnam CW: Modern trends in kidney transplantation. Transplant Proc 9: 1–8, 1977.

9. Opelz G, Mickey MR, Terasaki PI: HLA matching and cadaver transplant survival in North America. Transplantation 23: 490–497, 1977.

10. McDonald JC, Vaughn W, Filo RS, Picon GM, Niblack G, Spees EK, Williams GM: Cadaver donor renal transplantation by centers of the Southeastern Organ Procurement Foundation. Ann Surg 193:1–8, 1981.

11. Tilney NL, Strom TB, Vineyard GC, Merrill JP: Factors contributing to the declining mortality rate in renal transplantation. N Eng J Med 299:1321–1325, 1978.

12. Najarian JS, Sutherland DER, Simmons RL, Howard RJ, Kuellstrand CM, Ramsay RC, Goetz FC, Fryd DS, Sommer BG: Ten year experience with renal transplantation in juvenile onset diabetics. Ann Surg 190:487–500, 1979.

13. Opelz G, Sengar DPS, Mickey MR, Terasaki PI: Effect of blood transfusions on subsequent kidney transplants. Transplant Proc 5:253–259, 1973.

14. Strober S, Slavin S, Fuks Z, Kaplan HS, Gottlieb M, Bieber C, Hoppe RT, Grument FC: Transplantation tolerance after total lymhpoid irradiation. Transplant Proc 11:1032–1038, 1979.

15. Najarian JS, Ferguson RM, Sutherland DER, Slavin S, Kim T, Kersey J, Simmons RL: Fractional total lymphoid irradiation (TLI) as preparative immunosuppression in high risk renal transplantation. Ann Surg 196:442–452, 1982.

16. Starzl TE, Weil R III, Koep LJ, Iwaki Y, Terasaki PI, Schroter GPJ: Thoracic duct drainage before and after cadaveric kidney transplantation. Surg Gynecol Obstet 149:815–821, 1979.

17. Franksson C: Survival of homografts of skin in rats depleted of lymphocytes by chronic drainage from the thoracic duct (Letter). Lancet 1:1331–1332, 1964.

18. Borel JF, Feurer C, Gubler HU, Stahelin H: Biological effect of cyclosporin A: A new anti-lymphocytic agent. Agents Actions 6:468–475, 1976.

19. Calne RY, Rolles K, White DJG, Thiru S, Evans DB, McMaster P, Dunn DC, Craddock GN, Henderson RG, Aziz S, Lewis P: Cyclosporin A initially as the only immunosuppressant in 34 patients of cadaveric organs: 32 kidney, 2 pancreases, and 2 livers. Lancet 2:1033–1036, 1979.

20. Starzl TE, Weil R III, Iwatsuki S, Klintmalm G, Schroter GPJ, Koep LJ, Iwaki Y, Terasaki PI, Porter KA: The use of cyclosporin A and prednisone in cadaver kidney transplantation. Surg Gynecol Obstet 151:17–26, 1980.

21. Starzl TE, Hakala TR, Rosenthal JT, Iwatsuki S, Shaw BW: Variable convalescence and therapy after cadaveric renal transplantations under cyclosporin A and steroids. Surg Gynecol Obstet 154:819–825, 1982.

22. Hume DM, Magee JH, Kauffman HM, Rittenbury MS, Prout GR Jr: Renal transplantation in man in modified recipients. Ann Surg 158:608–644, 1963.

23. Murray JE, Merrill JP, Harrison JH, Wilson RE, Dammin GJ: Prolonged survival of human kidney homografts with immunosuprressive drug therapy. N Engl J Med 268:1315–1323, 1963.

24. Woodruff MFA, Robson JS, Nolan B, Lambie AT, Wilson TI, Clark JG: Homotransplantation of kidney in patients treated by preoperative local radiation and postoperative administration of an antimetabolite (Imuran). Lancet 2:675–682, 1963.

# 6. Antilymphocyte Globulin (ALG) infusion in the treatment of acute renal allograft rejection: a prospective study

M.S.A. KUMAR, A.G. WHITE, P. JOHN and G.M. ABOUNA

## Introduction

Acute allograft rejection is the most common problem in clinical transplantation. Administration of increased oral doses of steroids or large intravenous doses of methyl Prednisolone have been widely used as the standard antirejection treatment. However, steroid therapy is limited by its serious side effects and its success rate remains unsatisfactory. Antilymphocyte Globulin (ALG) or Antithymocyte Globulin (ATG) was first used in clinical renal transplantation, prophylactically, by Starzl et al. (1) in 1967 and since that time it has been used by several investigators both prophylactically and in the treatment of established acute renal allograft rejection (2–6). In the Kuwait transplantation programme steroid therapy was initially used in the treatment of acute renal allograft rejection and ALG was tried in a few patients and found to be successful. Subsequently a prospective study was undertaken to evaluate the effect of ALG in the treatment of established acute renal allograft rejection in humans and compared with standard high dose steroid therapy.

## Patients and methods

A consecutive series of 66 patients were entered into the study. Thirty-six patients received ALG infusion for the treatment of 61 episodes of established acute rejection while in another 30 patients high pulse-doses of steroid therapy were used for 58 episodes. All patients received a kidney transplant in Kuwait using standard prophylactic immunosuppressive therapy, with azathioprine and Prednisolone. The same prophylactic immunosuppression was continued during the antirejection therapy.

Patients in the two groups were comparable in age, sex, HLA matching and graft source (Table 1).

Acute allograft rejection was diagnosed by clinical and biochemical criteria. Fever, graft tenderness, hypertension, reduced urinary output and increase in body weight associated with a sustained increase in the serum creatinine levels of

*Table 1.* Description of patients in the study.

|  | ALG Group | Steroid group |
|---|---|---|
| No. of patients | 36 | 30 |
| Age | 12–40 years | 15–45 years |
|  | (mean 33.6) | (mean 35.5) |
| *Sex* |  |  |
| Male | 22 | 15 |
| Female | 14 | 15 |
| *Graft source* |  |  |
| L.R.D. | 28 | 28 |
| C.F. | 8 | 2 |
| *HLA matching* |  |  |
| HLA identical | 3 | 3 |
| No HLA mismatch | 4 | 5 |
| 1 Mismatch | 11 | 11 |
| 2 or more mismatches | 18 | 11 |

25% or more and/or a sustained fall in 24 h creatinine clearance of 25% or more was taken as diagnostic of acute rejection, after exclusion of other causes. In doubtful cases transplant biopsy was performed to confirm the diagnosis.

The ALG used in the study was obtained from two sources. Lymphoglobulin from Institute Merieux, France, and Pressimmune from the Behring Institute, Germany. Both contained 50 mg/ml of globulin and were equine in origin. The cells used for immunisation were thoracic duct lymphocytes in case of lympho-globulin and cultered lymphoblasts for the production of Pressimmune. The rosette inhibition titre of lymphoglobulin was 1:2400 and that of Pressimmune was 1:2000. They contained no antired cell or anti-human protein antibodies. Both prolonged skin allograft survival in monkeys to more than 13 days. Anti-thymocyte globulin used in the study was raised in rabbits by immunising with human thymocytes (ATG) This was obtained from Fresenius of Germany. Lym-phoglobulin was used in 41 rejection episodes. Pressimmune in 12, and ATG Fresenius in 8. Our policy was to give lymphoglobulin at first if the patient showed sensitivity reactions then Pressimmune or Rabbit ATG were used.

ALG/ATG was administered according to the following protocol: On the day of diagnosis of acute rejection, patients received one gm. of methyl Prednisolone as an intravenous infusion, over one hour. Following this ALG/ATG was infused intravenously through a central vein catheter or via the arteriovenous fistula slowly over a period of 8 h. The dose of equine ALG used was 18–26 mg/kg body weight/day and that of rabbit ATG was 2.5 to 3 mg/kg body weight/day. (The maximum dose was achieved by 3 days). On the second and subsequent days, only ALG/ATG was infused in similar doses after an initial intramuscular injection of 5 mg chlorpheniamine maleate, an antihistamine, to minimise the hypersentitivity reactions. The treatment was continued for 10 to 12 days. Patients in the steroid group were given one gm. of methyl Prednisolone as an intravenous infusion on days 1, 2 and 3 and in some cases, additional doses of 1 gm were given on 5th and 7th day.

During the antirejection therapy, all patients were monitored as follows: daily body weight, urinary output, vital signs. Clinical examination for any hypersensitivity reaction to ALG/ATG, daily complete haemogram which included haemoglobin, white cell count, platelet count. Daily estimation of serum creatinine and 24 h creatinine clearance in patients receiving ALG/ATG and the 'T' lymphocyte count was performed twice weekly.

## Results

### Reversal of rejection

The 66 patients who entered the study have been followed up for 12 to 36 months. Of the 61 acute rejections treated by ALG infusion 36 were first, 18 were second and 7 were third episodes. ALG reversed or controlled 32(89%) first rejection episodes, 18(100%) 2nd rejection episodes and 6(86%) third rejection episodes. The overall number of rejections controlled or reversed was 56 or 92%. Four patients in whom the first rejection episode did not respond to ALG infusion continue to have grafts functioning but with serum creatinine level ranging from 2.5 mg to 3 mg%. One patient in whom 3rd rejection episode could not be controlled, lost the graft and is back on haemodialysis. There was no patient death in the ALG group. The type of ALG/ATG used did not influence the outcome of therapy.

In the steroid group, 58 rejection episodes were treated of which 30 were first, 16 were 2nd and 12 were third rejection episodes. Steroid therapy controlled or reversed 24(80%) first rejection episodes, 14 (85%) 2nd rejection episodes and 8 (66%) third rejection episodes. Overall number of rejections reversed or controlled was 46 or 80%. In 5 patients steroid therapy failed to control the first rejection episode, and these patients subsequently developed 2nd and 3rd rejection episodes. In two of these patients, the 2nd rejection episode was controlled but the remaining 3 patients subsequently lost their grafts due to rejection. One patient, in whom the 1st rejection episode could not be controlled, developed chronic rejection and lost the graft. There was 1 patient death due to reactivation of pulmonary tuberculosis (Table 2). The rate of reversal of rejection between the ALG and steroid group by the student test show no significant difference (p> 0.1).

*Table 2.* Results of anti-rejection therapy.

| | ALG group | | | Steroid group | | |
|---|---|---|---|---|---|---|
| No. of patients | 36 | | | 30 | | |
| Total no. of acute rejections treated | 61 | | | 58 | | |
| Total no. of acute rejections controlled or reversed | 56(92%) | | | 46(80%) | | |
| No. of 1st, 2nd & 3rd rejections | 36 | 18 | 7 | 30 | 16 | 12 |
| No. of 1st, 2nd & 3rd rejections controlled or reversed | 32 (89%) | 18 (100%) | 6 (86%) | 24 (88%) | 14 (85%) | 8 (66%) |
| Mean time of reversal of rejection in days | 7.6 days | | | 9 days | | |
| No. of patients lost | 0 | | | 1(3%) | | |
| Patient survival at 6 months | 36(100%) | | | 29(97%) | | |
| Patient survival at 1, 2, 3 years | 36(100%) | | | 29(97%) | | |
| No. of grafts lost | 1(3%) | | | 5(16%) | | |
| Graft survival at 6 months | 35(96%) | | | 26(87%) | | |
| Graft survival at 1, 2, 3 years | 35(96%) | | | 25(80%) | | |

## Graft survival

Overall graft survival in the ALG group was 96% at 6 months and remained at this level upto 3 years. In the steroid group, it was 87% at 6 months and 80% at 1, 2 and 3 years (Fig. 1). The difference in graft survival between the two groups was not statistically significant at any time interval ($p > 0.1$).

## 'T' lymphocytes

In patients receiving ALG infusion there was a marked decrease in 'T' lymphocyte count in the peripheral blood. From a mean count of 753 cells/cmm before ALG therapy the 'T' lymphocyte count fell to 125 cells/cmm after therapy. This fall in 'T' lymphocyte count was seen in all rejection episodes after every ALG infusion. The T-cell lymphopenia was not predictive of the outcome of therapy. There was no drop in haemoglobin, total white cell, count or platelets.

## Complications

Non-infective complications in the ALG group were mainly in the form of mild hypersensitivity reactions. There was fever in 11, local thrombophlebitis in 6 and a skin rash in one patient. All these reactions responded to additional doses of antihistamine or small doses of intravenous hydro cortisone. In none of the patients,

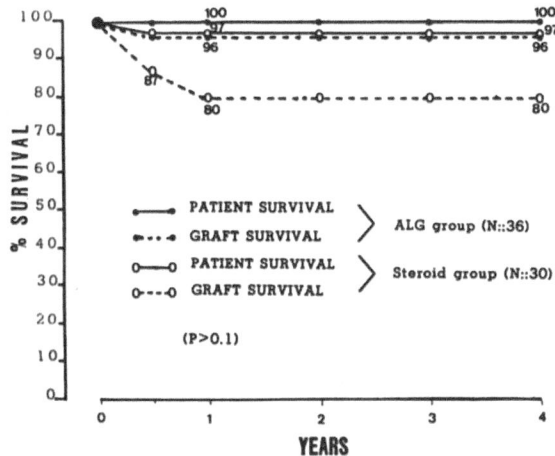

*Fig.1* . Patient and graft survival after treatment with ALG or steroid.

were the reactions severe enough to discontinue ALG therapy.

In the steroid group non infective complications included development of diabetes mellitus in 6, cushingoid facies in 12 and lower limb skeletel pain in 2. Of the 6 patients who developed diabetes mellitus, 3 had temporary diabetes lasting for 6 months. The remaining three continue to be insulin dependent diabetics. Some of the 12 patients with Cushingoid facies showed some improvement in time. None of the complications were fatal.

Infective complications in the two groups include bacterial, viral and fungal infections. Viral infections were more common in the ALG group, while bacterial infections were predominant in the steroid group (Table 3).

In the ALG group 19 (53%) of patients developed infections during therapy or within a month after completion of therapy. Bacterial infections were caused. Urinary tract infection in 3 and septicemia in 3 and all responded rapidly to appropriate antibiotic therapy. Viral infections included *Herpes simplex, Herpes zoster, Cytomegalovirus (CMV) & Varicella zoster. Herpes simplex* cleared spontaneously. *Herpes zoster* and CMV were a reactivation of previous infections and diagnosed by serological tests. However, both were self limiting and regressed spontaneously. Fungal infection due to *Candida albicans* was seen in 5 patients mainly in the oral cavity and pharynx, which rapidly responded to oral mycostatin suspension. All infections in the ALG group were controlled.

In the steroid group 17(56%) patients developed bacterial, viral and fungal infections. Bacterial infections were most common. They usually manifested as urinary tract infection and were controlled by antibiotic therapy. Reactivation of pulmonary tuberculosis in one patient resulted in patient death. Viral infections were minimal and were seen in 8 patients who developed *Herpex simplex*. Three patients had oral candidiasis and were controlled by mycostatin.

*Table 3.* Infective complications of anti-rejection therapy.

|  | ALG Group | Steroid group |
| --- | --- | --- |
| Total no. of patients | 36 | 30 |
| No. of patients with infection | 19 (53%) | 17 (56%) |
| *Bacterial* |  |  |
| Pseudomonas pyocyaneus | 4 | 12 |
| Pseudomonas aerogenosa | 0 | 6 |
| Eschericia coli | 2 | 7 |
| Reactivation of tuberculosis | 0 | 1 |
| Enterococci | 0 | 3 |
| *Viral* |  |  |
| Herpes simplex | 12 | 8 |
| Herpes zoster | 3 | 0 |
| C.M.V. | 3 | 0 |
| Varicella zoster | 1 | 0 |
| *Fungal* |  |  |
| Candida albicans | 5 | 3 |

## Cumulative steroid dose

For patients receiving only baseline immunosuppression without antirejection treatment, the mean cumulative steroid dose was 24 mg/kg body weight at 30 days and 39 mg/kg body weight at 60 days. For patients in ALG group, the mean cumulative steroid dose was 41 mg/kg body weight at 30 days and 75 mg at 60 days and for those in the steroid group it was 75 mg/kg body weight at 30 days and 125 mg/kg at 60 days.

## Discussion

Acute allograft rejection is a common problem in clinical renal transplantation and is the most frequent cause of graft loss. Administration of high pulse doses of methyl prednisolone or increase of the oral steroids dose have been the main stay in the treatment of acute renal allograft rejection. This increased steroid therapy is not always successful in reversing acute rejection and is frequently associated with significant side effects (7) and long term complications. High steroid therapy is usually effective in about 70% of acute rejection episodes. The combination of serious side effects and limited success of steroids has prompted a search for a better therapy for the treatment of acute allograft rejection.

Many workers have used ALG or ATG as an adjunct to steroids (3, 8, 10, 11) and some of these have reported a more rapid reversal of rejection (3, 8, 11) and better long term graft survival (3, 8). Others (2, 5, 6) have used ALG or high dose steroids and have demonstrated improved graft survival in their ALG treated patients. In our study we used ALG as the sole therapy from the second day of treatment.

Our result clearly indicates that with the ALG alone the rate of reversal of rejection was considerably higher than with high dose steroids. This was noted in the first, second and third rejection episodes. However, the difference between ALG and steroid was not statistically significant (Table 2). Likewise graft survival was higher with ALG than with steroid treatment at all intervals (Fig.1).

Again the differences were not statistically significant at 1–3 years. However, the majority of our patients received living related donor grafts in whom the overall graft survival at 4 years exceed 87% and a much larger number of patients will be required to show a statistical difference. Filo (8, 9) using ATG as an adjunctive therapy found a significant difference with ATG plus steroids than with steroids alone (67% vs 34%) at 3 years. Nowygrod (6) also reported a significantly better graft survival using similar ATG adjunctive protocol 73% vs 47% at one year.

On the other hand, Howard (5), Hong (10) and Birkeland (11) reported no significant difference in graft survival in their controlled randomized trials. Various investigators used different sources of ALG and ATG.

In our study we employed the Horse ALG from Merieux and from Behring, as well as the rabbit ATG from Fresenius but found no apparent difference in efficacy amongst the three but the numbers are of course small. However, it was observed that the sensitivity reactions were less and the quantities required smaller when rabbit ATG was used.

In our study infective complications were similar in the 2 groups (Table 3) although there was a tendency for more viral infections in the ALG group and more bacterial infections in the steroid group. Cosimi (2) noted a detrimental effect regarding CMV infections in ATG treated patients whereas Howard *et al.*(5) and Launois *et al.* (12) found no increased incidence of infections in ALG treated patients. The incidence of non-infective complications in our study was dramatically different in the ALG and in high dose steroid treated groups. Our ALG treated patients suffered mainly mild hypersensitivity reactions but not severe enough to discontinue therapy. In the steroid group, 6 patients developed diabetes and 12 became Cushingoid. In fact the major advantage of ALG treatment appears to be its steroid sparing effect.

The mean cumulative steroid dose at 60 days in our ALG treated patients (75 mg/kg) was just over half that of the steroid treated patients (125 mg/kg). Shiels *et al.* (4) have commented that the major advantage of using ATG to reverse rejection is the marked decrease in the cumulative steroid dose. At 60 days their ATG group had a cumulative dose of 52 mg/kg compared with 121 mg/kg in the steroid group. They also noted no serious side effects in the ATG treated patients and further emphasized the problems associated with high dose steroids including a patient who died of diverticulitis in their steroid group.

In conclusion, the use of ALG alone is as effective as high dose steroid therapy for the treatment of acute allograft rejection. It is safe and it reduces dramatically the non-infective complications seen with steroid therapy and should seriously be considered as a substitute for high dose steroid therapy, as well as an adjunct to steroids in resistant rejections.

## References

1. Starzl TE, Marchioro TL, Hutchinson DE et al: The clinical use of antilymphocyte globulin in renal homotransplantation. Transplantation 28:365, 1979.
2. Cosimi AB: The clinical value of antilymphocyte antibodies. Transplant Proc XIII:462, 1981.
3. Light JA, Alijani MR, Biggers JA: Antilymphocyte globulin reverses 'Irreversible' allograft rejection. Transplant Proc XIII: 475, 1981.
4. Sheild CF III, Cosimi AB, Tolkoff - Rubin N et al: Use of antilymphocyte globulin for reversal of acute allograft rejection. Transplantation 28:461, 1979.
5. Howard RJ, Condie RM, Sutherland DER et al: The use of antilymphoblast in the treatment of renal allograft rejection. Transplant Proc XIII:473, 1981.
6. Nowygrod R, Appel G, Hardy MA: Use of ATG for reversal of acute allograft rejection. Transplant Proc XIII:469, 1981.
7. McDougal BA, Whitter FC, Cross DE: Sudden death after bolus steroid therapy for acute rejection. Transplant Proc VIII:493, 1976.
8. Filo RS, Smith EJ, Leabman SB: Reversal of acute renal allograft rejection with adjunctive ATG therapy. Transplant Proc XIII: 482, 1981.
9. Filo RS, Leapman SB, Smith EJ: Efficacy of ATG treatment of acute renal allograft rejection - a second look. 9th Annual Scientific Meeting of American Society of Transplant Surgeons. June 1983 (Abstract).
10. Hong JH, Desai P, Hanson RN, Rossal A, Manis T, Butt KMH: Adjunctive ATG treatment for reversal of acute allograft rejection: Long term assessment by a prospective randomized single center trial. 9th Annual Scientific Meeting of American Society of Transplant Surgeons. June 1983 (Abstract).
11. Birkeland SA: A controlled clinical trial of treatment with ALG in established rejection of renal allografts. Acta Med Scand 198:289, 1975.
12. Launois B, Campion JP, Fauchet R et al: Prospective randomized clinical trial in patients with cadaver kidney transplants. Transplant Proc IX: 1023, 1977.

# 7. Cyclosporin in renal transplantation: results of the Minnesota randomised trial

D.E.R. SUTHERLAND, J.S. NAJARIAN, M. STRAND, D.S. FRYD,
R.M. FERGUSON, R.L. SIMMONS and N.L. ASCHER

## Introduction

In 1980, at the University of Minnesota, we introduced Cyclosporin (CsA) as an immunosuppressant for renal transplantation. We had an advantage in being able to call on the experience of Professor Calne in Cambridge, England, who had been using CsA as a sole immunosuppressant and also the experience of Dr.Starzl in Denver who had commenced using CsA together with low dose steroids for immunosuppression. The relatively high doses of CsA used by Calne had revealed a nephrotoxic effect especially with a non-diuresing kidney. Prior to embarking on a trial of CsA, analysis of our renal transplant results over a 13 year period showed an overall graft survival rate at 4 years of about 70%. Obviously this was achieved using heavy immunosuppression, including steroids and the penalty we paid was a high incidence of osteonecrosis. In the period upto 1980, 88 patients required treatment, the incidence being highest in the cadaver group (7.1%) compared to 3.8% in the related recipient group. This side effect together with the other side effects of steroids is an indication for some form of alternative immunosuppression or at least a reduction in steroid dose.

In order to investigate the best immunosuppressive regime for our patients we decided to embark on a randomised trial of CsA in comparison with our established immunosuppressive treatment in September 1980(1).

## Patients

All patients in the trial were adults who had been splenectomised and had received five or more transfusions from unrelated donors at least one month before transplantation. Kidneys were obtained from either cadavers or from non-HLA identical related donors. The two immunosuppressive regimes used were (a) CsA and a relatively low dose of prednisone and (b) Azathioprine (AZA) and a relatively high dose of prednisone plus anti-lymphocyte globulin (ALG) in the immediate post transplant period. The patient breakdown in each group was as follows. Of 92 patients in the CsA group, 53 had cadaver kidneys and 39 received kidneys from living related donors. Fifty-two of the patients were diabetic and 8 of the patients were retransplants. There were 90 patients in the AZA group, 57 of which had a cadaver kidney and 33, related grafts. Forty-nine patients were diabetic and there were 7 retransplants. The period of study covered in this report was from September 1980 to April 1983.

Treatment with CsA consisted of an oral dose of 14 mg/kg daily for the first post transplant week. The dose was then adjusted to approximately 12 mg/kg/day according to CsA blood levels and also the serum creatinine values. An attempt was made to maintain the CsA blood levels between 100–200 ng/ml and the serum creatinine at less than 2 mg/100ml but this was not always achieved. At 1 year after transplantation the mean dose of CsA in those with functioning grafts was 6.3 ± 3.6 mg/kg/day and the prednisone dose was 0.2 mg/kg/day. Rejection episodes were treated with intravenous methyl prednisolone for 3 days or with a prednisone increase to 2 mg/kg.

In the conventional immunosuppression group, AZA was given at 5 mg/kg before operation and tapered to 2.5 mg/kg/day at one week. Initial prednisone dose was 2 mg/kg/day and this was tapered to 0.3 mg/kg/day at one year. Intravenous ALG at 30 mg/kg/day was given for a total of 14 doses in the immediate post transplant period.

Actuarial analysis was used to calculate the patient and graft survival rates, graft loss being defined as either return to dialysis or patient death. Seventeen patients in the CsA group were changed to AZA treatment because of nephrotoxicity, severe rejection, prolonged acute tubular necrosis (ATN) or severe thrombocytosis. These patients were still considered as belonging to the CsA group for analysis. In those patients treated with AZA, 1 patient was changed to cyclophosphamide and 2 patients were changed to CsA. Again these patients were considered as belonging to the AZA group for analysis.

**Results**

Table 1, summarises the actuarial patient and graft survival rates in the two treatment groups. Patient survival in the CsA and AZA groups was 92% and 95% respectively at one year and the graft survival 87% and 80%. There were no significant differences between the treatment groups ($p > 0.1$) or when the patients were divided into subgroups on the basis of diabetes or donor source.

In the recipients of cadaver grafts, 25% of those in the CsA group and 22% in the AZA group required dialysis in the immediate post transplant period. The number of dialysis required in the CsA group was significantly greater ($p < .05$) than in the AZA group. In the recipients of living related grafts only 5.1% in the CsA group and 3.2% in the AZA group required dialysis immediately post transplant.

In the follow up period of 1–32 months, 31% of the CsA patients and 58% of the AZA patients were treated for rejection and the onset of rejection after trans-

*Table 1.* Actuarial analysis of results of renal transplantation in subgroups randomized to Cyclosporine (CsA) or Azathioprine (AZA) at the University of Minnesota between September 1, 1980 and April 1, 1983.

| Donor | Diabetic (N) | | Non-diabetic (N) | | All recipients (N) | |
|---|---|---|---|---|---|---|
| Source | CsA | AZA | CsA | AZA | CsA | AZA |
| One year *graft* survival rates (%) | | | | | | |
| CAD | 84%(30) | 67%(30) | 81%(23) | 85%(27) | 83%(53) | 76%(57) |
| REL | 88%(22) | 94%(19) | 100%(17) | 77%(14) | 94%(39) | 87%(33) |
| All sources | 86%(52) | 77%(49) | 89%(40) | 82%(41) | 87%(92) | 80%(90) |
| One year *patient* survival rates (%) | | | | | | |
| CAD | 84%(30) | 91%(30) | 95%(23) | 96%(27) | 89%(53) | 94%(57) |
| REL | 92%(22) | 94%(19) | 100%(17) | 100%(14) | 96%(39) | 97%(33) |
| All sources | 87%(52) | 92%(49) | 97%(40) | 97%(41) | 92%(92) | 95%(90) |

plantation was slower in the CsA group (94 days compared with 62 days). Irreversible or chronic rejection occurred in 10% of the CsA patients and in 12% of the AZA group. The mean serum creatinine measured at 3, 6, 12 and 24 months in both patient groups, was higher in the CsA group. Overall the CsA group had a serum creatinine of approximately 2.0 mg/100 ml and the AZA group of 1.5 mg/100 ml.

There were significantly more viral infections in the AZA group ($p < .05$) and in particular the incidence of Cytomegalovirus was increased. The incidence of other viruses, of mainly the Herpes group, was 13% in the CsA patients and 29% in the AZA group. There were no significant differences in the incidence of bacterial infections in the 2 groups - 16% in the CsA and 24% in the AZA group respectively.

Evidence of CsA nephrotoxicity was present in 74% of the CsA patients. These patients had serum creatinine levels above 2 mg/100 ml or had elevations of serum creatinine that decreased when the CsA dose was lowered. Biopsy revealed histological features of CsA nephrotoxicity in 26 out of 28 specimens. There was no statistically significant differences in the hospitalisation times at the time of transplantation or on readmission of in the numbers of readmissions between the two groups.

## Discussion

The renal allograft survival rates were slightly better (7%) in the CsA group compared to those patients treated with AZA. This difference was not significant. It is therefore necessary to consider the advantages and disadvantages of the

CsA treatment. CsA patients had a similar incidence of ATN to the AZA patients but it is of longer duration in the CsA patients. Renal function as evidenced by serum creatinine values was reduced in the CsA group and there was more difficulty in managing the hypertension and hyperkalemia in these patients. However, there were fewer bacterial and viral infections, shorter hospitalisation and a few rejection episodes in the CsA group although some of these differences did not approach statistical significance. It has been commented that the use of CsA reduces the advantages of using related donors for transplantation (2). Our results do not support this. Graft survival in the CsA group who received related donor kidneys had a better survival rate than cadavers (94% v. 83% at one year), this relative difference also being found in the AZA group (87% v. 76%).

Our results with AZA-prednisone and ALG are similar to those achieved with CsA in the European randomised trial of CsA compared with conventional immunosuppression (3). The European trial gave one year graft survival rates of 53% for AZA and 73% for CsA. The European trial was able to show a significant difference between the two groups but it should be emphasized that the results are not strictly comparable to those in Minnesota. In Minnesota we used prednisone prophylactically in our CsA patient group whereas in the European trial prednisone was only added when rejection occurred. Furthermore the AZA patients in the European trial had neither splenectomy or received ALG. The significant difference obtained in the European trial could possibly be explained because their conventional immunosuppressive regimen did not contain features that can maximise graft survival rates such as splenectomy and the administration of ALG.

## Conclusion

Immunosuppression with CsA-prednisone or AZA-prednisone-ALG can give good patient and graft survival rates. Each regimen has advantages and disadvantages and only longer term analysis will reveal whether one or the other is more cost effective and which is optimal for long term renal allograft function.

## References

1. Ferguson RM, Rynasiewicz JJ, Sutherland DER et al.: Cyclosporin A in renal Transplantation. A prospective randomised trial. Surgery 92: 175–182, 1982.
2. Starzl TE, Hakala TR, Iwatsuki S et al.: Variable Convalescence and therapy after cadaveric renal transplantation under Cyclosporin A and Steroids. Sur Gyn Obst 154:819, 1982.
3. European Multicenter Trial. Cyclosporin A as sole immunosuppressive agent in recipients of kidney allografts from cadaver donors. Lancet 2: 57–60, 1982.

# 8. Antilymphocyte globulin and thoracic duct drainage in renal transplantation

J. TRAEGER, J.L. TOURAINE, J.M. DUBERNARD and M.C. MALIK

## Introduction

Despite absence of major modifications in the treatment of patients with a renal transplant, significant improvement, in terms of both patient and transplant survival, has been recorded over the last decade. Hopes that methods leading to the specific acceptance of the transplant by the host would be very shortly applicable in the clinic have not yet been fulfilled. More experience in the handling of previously available immunosuppressive drugs or procedures has, however, been associated with a decrease in the complication rate and a increase in transplant successes to a larger extent than usually anticipated (1, 2).

The lymphocyte depletion induced by thoracic duct drainage (TDD) and the treatment with antilymphocyte serum injections have potent immunosuppressive effects, as demonstrated in the rat skin graft model (3). In man, as opposed to rodents, the quantitative aspects of lymphocyte recirculation are somewhat different (4) and proportional doses of administered antilymphocyte globulins (ALG) are lower. The applicability of Sir Michael Woodruff's findings to human renal transplantation had thus to be ascertained. Several transplantation centers, including ours have studied the efficacy of ALG in human renal allotransplantation. We have previously shown that relatively 'large' doses of intravenous ALG, in clinical use, led to better transplantation results than low doses administered by the intramuscular route (5). In addition, we have used TDD prior to transplantation in some patients, since 1966, both to obtain lymphocytes for ALG preparation and as an adjunct to other immunosuppressants (6). In this paper we review the methods for thoracic duct fistula and for ALG treatment, then we present the efficacy of these methods, based on the results observed in our different groups of patients.

## 1. Methods of thoracic duct drainage

*Surgical procedure for TDD*

The thoracic duct cannulation was performed in uremic patients waiting for renal transplantation, one or two days after an hemodialysis. The terminal portion of the thoracic duct was exposed by an incision in the subclavicular region (7). A teflon and silastic catheter was carefully introduced into the duct and a sub-cutaneous tunnel was performed. Mainly for anatomical reasons (e.g. very small duct or presence of many divisions), lymph drainage was satisfactory in only one half of the 250 thoracic duct fistulae attempted.

*Post operative course*

To obtain a good lymph drainage and to avoid complications, several precautions were taken. Patients were hemodialysed the day before surgery and, in case of hypovolemia, it was carefully corrected. Soon after the operation the patients were fed with a lipid-rich meal, by a gastric tube if needed. To avoid clotting, heparin was initially used in some cases, but it is no longer felt necessary. Lymph, collected by simple siphoning, was centrifuged, then lymphocytes were discarded (or injected into horses for ALG preparation) and the supernatant was infused back to the patient while its sterility was verified. Additional infusions included plasma, salt, calcium, lipids and glucose.

Very few complications were observed. The prevention of infection was assured by measures comparable to those used immediately after transplantation. Patients were isolated and bacteriologic monitoring was undertaken. When a contamination of lymph was found after it had been infused back, the patient was treated according to the antibiotic sensitivity of the organism.

After two weeks, the thoracic duct drainage was stopped by progressive clamping of the catheter and the induction of thrombosis. No prolonged fistulae were noted but hypertension in the thoracic duct was sometimes ill-tolerated. This hypertension was responsible for local and abdominal pains and, when no other lymph-vein anastomosis was present, for lipid malabsorption. It may have contributed, with other factors, to 3 acute pancreatitis syndromes, one of which led to the patient's death. Currently, when such complications occur, we unclamp the catheter and sometimes reimplant the thoracic duct into a vein. We have performed such a reimplantation eleven times into the internal jugular vein and once into the external jugular vein.

If adequate prevention of complications is performed, the thoracic duct drainage is thus a relatively safe technique. With the exception of the one death due to pancreatitis, we have not observed severe complications after 250 such operations and infections have been few and moderate. The drainage has never been prolonged more than three weeks. It should, however, be stressed that a 'good' drainage was accomplished in only half of the patients in which it was attempted.

Lymph output generally averaged 1 to 3 l/24 h (up to 7l/25 h). Lymphocyte output reached a peak (5 to 16 × $10^9$ lymphocytes/14 h) on the first or second day, then decreased during the first week before plateauing at 1 to 5 × $10^9$ lymphocytes/24 h (4). The average amount of lymphocytes collected by this technique was 50 × $10^9$/patient.

## Preparation of ALG

*Antigen choice.* The properties of ALG depend to a large extent on its method of preparation. ALG can be prepared against a wide variety of antigens: thoracic duct or blood lymphocytes, cultured lymphoblasts, tonsillar cells, subcellular fractions of lymphocytes, human or monkey thymocytes, lymph node or spleen cells. ALG batches prepared from either thoracic duct lymphocytes or from thymocytes appeared to be generally more effective and less toxic than the other preparations (8, 9).

*Human thymocytes.* They usually came from pieces of thymuses from young children undergoing cardiac surgery.

Thymuses were immersed in Parker's or RPMI–1640 medium and cooled to + 4°C (10), then aseptic extraction of cells was performed. Thymocytes were then enumerated and their viability checked by the trypan blue exclusion test (85 to 95% viable cells on the average). Contamination by red blood cells is low (≤5%).

*Animal immunization and serum collection.* Rabbits, sheep and horses can be immunized with human lymphocytes. However, the more frequently used ALG batches have been prepared in horses in view of the large amounts of serum obtainable in this species.

Horses were immunized according to Monaco's method (11) with human thymocytes and thoracic duct lymphocytes. Animals were injected with $10^9$ cells mixed with complete Freund's adjuvant, by the intradermal route the first day. Three weeks later, 3 booster injections of $10^9$ cells were done intravenously, renewed every week there after.

Plasmaphereses were performed from the 4th week till the 6th month of immunization. Plasma was decomplemented, then stored at −20°C until fractionation.

*ALG purification, absorptions and controls.* Fractionation was performed in three stages:

Precipitation with rivanol-alcohol. The precipitate was dissolved in a solution of pH 5 acetic acid then dialyzed against distilled water.

Absorptions with human placental tissue (12). The absorbed serum was concentrated by precipitation with 28.5% ethanol, dissolved in a solution of pH 5.5 acetic acid and dialyzed again.

Chromatography using QAE Sephadex A 50 (Pharmacia) in 0.015 M phosphate buffer, pH 6.8 (Na2HP04 : 2, 72/1000 : K2HP04 : 1/1000). The free fraction was precipitated with 28.5% ethanol at low temperature, solubilized in acetic solution, dialyzed and filtered. The obtained material is an équine IgG2 with antilymphocyte activities.

## 3. Tests of activity and safety

*In vitro safety tests.* The absence of any significant anti-erythrocyte activity contained in ALG preparations was checked by detection and titration of hemolysins ($< 1/16$) and hemagglutinins ($< 1/16$) active on human erythrocytes of A and O groups. Incomplete anti-erythrocyte antibody titration has also been performed by indirect Coomb's test using an anti-equine globulin serum.

Anti-thrombocytic activity was evaluated by assaying complement fixing anti-thrombocyte antibodies (titre <1:80 is acceptable) and thromboagglutinins ($\leqslant +/++++$).

The absence of precipitating anti-human serum protein antibodies was checked through immunoelectrophoresis and agar immuno-diffusion. Protein content, pH, and sterility were also verified.

*In vitro activity tests.* The lymphocytotoxicity test gave an indication, though imperfect, of this activity. We used a micromethod in two stages derived from the technique of Amos (13). The dilution of ALG giving a significantly increased cytotoxic index was determined, using rabbit complement and trypan blue. The ALGs employed for administration to patients exhibited a lymphocytotoxic titre $\geqslant 1/1024$.

The rosette inhibition test was performed by introducing various dilutions of ALG into an E. rosette assay (14). The active ALGs had inhibition titres $> 1/128$.

The mixed lymphocyte reaction inhibition test (15) also enabled evaluation of the immunosuppressive potency of ALG. Active preparations suppressed the proliferative response to allogeneic stimulation by more than 50%, even when diluted 1/1000.

Direct lymphoagglutination did not enable one to predict the immunosuppressive activity of an ALG batch. On the other hand, the results of an indirect lymphoagglutination test with titres (16, 17) 1 : 2048 and in addition, immunofluorescent titration, also determining the binding ability of antibodies on lymphocytes, gave results in good correlation with the degree of *in vivo* immunosuppression (18).

Lymphocyte opsonization (19, 20) or lymphocyte-mediated cytotoxicity inhibition (21) also gave interesting results.

*In vivo safety tests.* To ascertain the lack of toxic effects of ALG, tests were performed in several animal species:

Pyrogenicity was tested in rabbits. Animals received 1 ml of ALG per kg intravenously. No temperature rise exceeding 0.6°C should be noted.

ALG was also injected subcutaneously (0.5 ml) into 20 g mice. Platelets were counted after 48h and animals were sacrificed after 8 days. The anatomical examination of viscera should not reveal any lesion and especially any hemorrhagic suffusion of the peritoneus and mesentery.

The search for anti-glomerular basement membrane (GBM) antibodies was performed by injecting intravenously 120 mg of ALG per kg into rats. Animals were sacrificed 6 h after the injection: their kidneys were subjected to an immunofluorescent examination (fluorescein-labeled anti-equine globulin serum). Anti-GBM antibodies would be revealed by a linear fluorescence.

Monkeys such as *Macacus rhesus* and *Macacus speciosa* were treated according to a therapeutic protocol described by Balner (8, 9, 22) and by Bonneau (23) : ALG was given intramuscularly at a dose of 80 mg protein per kg daily for a pretreatment period of 5 days; two skin allografts were done and intramuscular injections were continued three times a week. For the detection of possible renal toxicity, the treatment described (the total duration of which is three weeks) was completed by an intravenous injection performed 6 h before the kidney removal and the immunofluorescent examination. Linear deposits along glomerular basement membranes were taken as evidence of anti-GBM antibodies in one batch of anti-lymphoblast serum which was never used in humans. The presence of a granular fluorescence along the basement membrane or in the mesangium revealed deposits of antigen-antibody complexes resulting from an immunization of the monkey against equine protein. This situation was much more frequent, being found in more than half the animals given no other associated immunosuppressive therapy.

*In vivo activity tests.* The survival time of skin allografts in monkeys was determined by daily examination. The changes in the gross appearance and consistency of the grafts established the date of rejection. A skin graft survival longer than 13 days was regarded as significantly prolonged. Blood cell and platelet counts were performed throughout the treatment period. In some cases the animals were subjected to complete autopsy.

Although the test of skin graft prolongation in the monkey is at present the most reliable of the tests performed before the use in man, the existence of an absolute relationship between the results obtained and the survival of skin allografts in man has not been fully demonstrated, nor has it been established whether the survival of skin grafts in man is faithful and consistently reliable reflection of the fate of a renal transplant.

After the various tests, an evaluation of the activity in man was performed as often as possible. The degree of lymphopenia provided a gross and imperfect but important indication of *in vivo* activity. The effects on delayed hypersensitivity skin reaction (DHSR) to several recall antigens (5) and on skin allograft survival, when they could be studied, were taken as significant reflections of the immunosuppressive activity of ALG, although the decrease in DHSR may be partially dependent on an anti-inflammatory mechanism (24).

When these various *in vitro* and *in vivo* tests in animals and humans had been performed, it became possible to select the most effective and least toxic batches of ALG to administer to the recipients of renal transplants.

## 4. Clinical tolerance of ALG - immunization against ALG

The treatment with heterologous ALG entails a number of drawbacks, but the complications caused by this biological agent, associated with other immunosuppressive drugs, are less serious and frequent than some experimental work and most predictions would have indicated. Clinical intolerance and manifestations of toxicity vary according to batches, patients, routes of administration, treatment duration, and associated medications. The improvement in preparation, absorption and purification techniques has resulted in less frequent adverse reactions.

*Clinical tolerance.* In two-thirds of cases, pain and inflammatory phenomena with erythema and induration develop at intramuscular injection sites. These phenomena often, but not always, tend to decrease in intensity with continued therapy. Their precise mechanism is unknown; however, it is to be noted that the injection of non-immune heterologous sera does not cause these local reactions. In some patients treated for several weeks and having developed an immune response to equine globulin, important local reactions of a some-what different type may occur; they are comparable to an Arthus phenomenon. The lesions of aseptic muscular necrosis that appear in these cases may be mistaken for an 'abscess'. Although we have not observed it ourselves, some authors have described the development of a malignant tumor at the injection site (25).

When ALG was injected into a high-flow vein, no local reaction occurred but, if a small peripheral vein was used, venous and perivenous inflammatory signs were sometimes noted.

Of the systemic manifestations noted, fever was the most frequent, appearing 4 to 6 h after nearly half the intramuscular injections and 2 to 4 h after nearly a quarter of the intravenous infusions when infusions were rapid. In a few cases, fever was accompanied by chills and tachycardia. The frequency and intensity of these reactions were decreased by the administration of small doses of prednisone and anti-histamines or by applying Besredka's technique when performing injections.

More severe, but fortunately much much rarer, have been anaphylactoid manifestations with hypotension, asthmatiform dyspnea, arthralgias, lumbar pain, vomiting and pruritic skin rashes. These signs, isolated or associated, often required an intravenous injection of corticosteroids. The chronology of these incidents has been variable and we were unable to establish a consistent and absolute relationship between their occurrence and the degree of immunization of the patient against equine globulin (26).

*Hematological tolerance.* After the first ALG injections, a lymphopenia developed much more marked and rapid in the case of intravenous infusions. Despite continued therapy, the lymphocyte count then tended to return more or less rapidly to normal. Within hours of injection, a marked but transient increase in the granulocyte count was also noted.

A significant thrombocytopenia (peripheral and rapidly corrected within two days) could be noted only in a few cases. This thrombocytopenia, rare with anti-thoracic duct lymphocyte or anti-thymocyte globulin, was more frequent with anti-blood lymphocyte globulin. We never observed hemorrhages related to this thrombocytopenia, but we routinely performed platelet counts and adjusted the daily dose of ALG based on the results of these counts. As opposed to other authors, we never found hyperthrombocytosis (27).

In some cases, Coombs'tests with various antiglobulins showed the presence on red blood cells of complement, sometimes associated with equine globulin.

Repeated lymph node biopsies performed in patients with intramuscular ALG treatment showed no consistent lymphocyte depletion, notably in the deep cortex perifollicular and paracortical areas. Besides, these nodes displayed histological changes testifying to the patient's immune and inflammatory reaction against the administration of heterologous protein: significant increase in germinal centres and proliferation of plasma cells. Bone marrow examination showed no evidence of toxicity; at most a distinct eosinophilia was often noted, and occasionally an increase in all of the granular series and plasma cells.

*Immunization against horse globulin.* The host immunization against heterologous protein should result in a loss of effectiveness of ALG and occasionally, in some complications, serum sickness, anaphylactic shock, possible glomerulonephritis due to deposits of antigen-antibody complexes.

As serological tests, we mainly used the titration of anti-horse protein precipitins and heterologous anti-sheep red blood cell hemagglutinins; less often, we assayed agglutinins of group 0 human erythrocytes coated with horse gamma-globulin (28).

The study of the intravascular life-time of equine IgG labelled with $I^{131}$ and injected into the patients gave us more sensitive and apparently more reliable results. The immune elimination of heterologous globulin showed itself as a break in the linear decline of the plasma radioactivity when the test was performed at the time of appearance of this immunization or as an immediate elimination when the test was performed later (26). Frequency of anti-horse globulin immunization has been differently appreciated by various authors (26, 29, 30).

Attempts at inducing a state of immunological tolerance to horse globulin in man have given sometimes encouraging (29, 31), and other times disappointing results (32, 33). A more easily applied method consists of substituting ALG prepared in another animal species for horse globulin in immunized patients. The rabbit seems to be the animal of choice; it can easily be immunized with a moderate number of lymphocytes (34), its serum is relatively well tolerated clinically (35), and above all its globulins do not show any cross-antigenicity with those from the horse (36).

*Renal tolerance.* ALG may be toxic to the kidney by either of two mechanisms: fixation of anti-glomerular basement membrane antibodies leading to development of an heteroimmune glomerulonephritis of the Masugi type that evolves in two stages (heterologous then autologous), or deposits of antigen-antibody complexes when the recipient has developed immunity to heterologous protein (serum glomerulonephritis).

## 5. Effectiveness of ALG in human renal transplantation

The remarkable immunosuppressive effect of ALG in animals is generally accepted (37, 38). It has especially been well-established that ALG prolongs and improves the survival of renal allografts in dogs (39, 40, 41) and rats (42).

Arguments in favor of the effectiveness of ALG in human renal transplantation are as follows:

*ALG and transplant survival.* Ideally patient survival and transplant survival should be the best criteria for evaluating the efficacy of any treatment in transplant recipients. According to this criteria ALG has been usually shown to be beneficial. However, in many reports, as well as in our initial experience, sequential series of patients were compared. (43)

More recently randomized studies have been performed (44, 45). In a current analysis of four treatment protocols in LYON, a suggestive but not significant improvement of results appears to depend of ALG therapy (Table 1).

*ALG and the frequency of rejection crises.* The decrease in the frequency of rejection crises attributable to ALG administration has been noted by many authors (45, 46, 11, 47) since the initial reports (48, 41).

Furthermore, in the opinions of most authors (49, 50) the development of rejection was somewhat modified: clinical signs became more insidious, changes

*Table 1.* Randomized analysis of ALG and placental eluates after renal transplantation.

|  | A (0) | B (ALG) | C (PE) | D (ALG + PE) |
|---|---|---|---|---|
| Death | 0 | 1 | 0 | 0 |
| Failures | 1 | 1 | 6 | 3 |
| No rejection crises (1st. month) | 13 | 10 | 18 | 9 |
| Average date 1st. reject. | 8 d | 23 d | 13 d | 14 d |
| Mean dose steroids (mg/kg/day, 1st. month) | 1.7 | 1.2 | 2.1 | 1.2 |
| No. E-RFC/mm³ blood | 520 | 30 | 404 | 123 |

Four groups of 20 patients' each received azathioprine and steroids for a renal transplant. Group A had no additional treatment, groups B, C and D had ALG (10 mg/kg/day for 1 month), placental eluates (PE, containing anti-HLA DR antibodies and inhibiting MLC, 25 mg/kg/day for 1 month) or both.

in renal function occurred more slowly, initial oliguria was less frequent.

*ALG and the treatment of rejection crises.* The most obvious aspect has been the effectiveness of ALG in the treatment of severe acute or subacute rejection crises (51). A decrease in serum creatinine was usually observed. This effect, less remarkable than that achieved with high doses of corticosteroids, was often apparent by the second of third day of treatment, associated with a stabilization of renal function which then improved gradually during the next 2 to 4 weeks.

However, in some cases serum creatinine increased again after the decrease in ALG dose.

The effectiveness of ALG in the treatment of rejection crises has also been observed by other authors (52, 53). The mechanism of action underlying this effect remains open to discussion, for it is not certain whether a genuine immunosuppression or an anti-inflammatory effect is mainly responsible for such an improvement of the transplant function. When ALG was associated with steroids for the treatment of rejection crises the rate of therapy effectiveness appeared to be higher than with steroids alone but the difference was not statistically significant (54).

*ALG and dosage of other immunosuppressive drugs.* The doses of corticosteroids and Azathioprine required were lower in patients treated with ALG (55 and Table 1).

## 6. Effectiveness of thoracic duct drainage (TDD)

A few years ago we analysed two comparable groups of patients with or without TDD prior to transplantation (6).

*Patient groups (TDD + and TDD −).* The two groups of patients were transplanted in similar conditions and during the same period of time between 1966–1976.

Arbitrarily and *a priori* we have included in the first group (TDD +) only those patients who had a lymphocyte depletion of more than $20 \times 10^9$ cells via thoracic duct fistula, during the three months prior to renal transplantation. In this group of thirty-seven patients, the mean duration of TDD was 12 days and the mean number of lymphocytes removed by TDD was $57 \times 10^9$ cells. In most patients, the lymphocyte output was high (above $5 \times 10^9$ cells/day) during the first four to six days only. The second group (TDD-) included all patients transplanted during the same period, without prior TDD or with a low lymphocyte depletion or else with a remote TDD. The two groups were identical in respect to periods considered for analysis, surgical procedure, sex ratio mean number of blood transfusions and pregnancies, and average doses of immunosuppressive drugs. The mean number of HLA specificities shared by the kidney donor and the recipient was lower in group TDD + as poorer HLA compatibilities were accepted for cadaver donor transplant in this group to avoid long delays between TDD and renal transplantation. The incidence of positive HBs antigenemia was lower in group TDD + because, for some time, patients with serum HBs antigen were not subjected to TDD. Two other bias to analysis were discovered and they concern age and clinical condition. If the mean age is comparable in both groups, the few small children and older patients that we transplanted were not subjected to TDD. Similarly, the average clinical condition of the patients was approximately comparable in both groups, but a few patients in poor condition were not subjected to TDD. Two other bias to analysis were discovered and they concern age and clinical condition. If the mean age is comparable in both groups, the few small tained. Ideally these studies should only compare TDD + patients to those patients in whom TDD was attempted and failed for surgical reasons, but the latter group is still too limited in size for statistical analysis. Even better will be a completely randomized and prospective study but the results will only be known in several years.

*Mortality and morbidity.* Comparing TDD + and TDD − groups, no significant difference was found in the death rate, the incidence of malignancies, or the incidence of infectious complications, including septicemias and all infections with facultative intracellular parasitic organisms. Specifically, the frequency of infections with fungi, *cytomegalovirus, herpes simplex, herpes zoster,* and *papilloma* virus were the same in both groups of patients. In each group, mortality and morbidity were comparatively lower in recipients of related living donor kidneys than in recipients of cadaver kidneys.

*Transplant survival.* Among recipients of kidneys from HLA-A, -B, and -D identical sibling donors, two had been subjected to TDD : one failure and one

*Table 2.* Survival of kidney allotransplants from haploidentical, related, living donors, 3 months to 5 years after transplantation, in patients subjected (TDD +) or not subjected (TDD −) to prior thoracic duct drainage.

| Pretreatment[a] | 3 months | 6 months | 1 year | 2 years | 3 years | 5 years |
|---|---|---|---|---|---|---|
| TDD + | $^{14}/_{16}$=87% | $^{13}/_{16}$=81% | $^{13}/_{16}$=81% | $^{10}/_{14}$=71% | $^{9}/_{14}$=64% | $^{8}/_{13}$=62% |
| TDD − | $^{30}/_{41}$=73% | $^{30}/_{41}$=73% | $^{28}/_{40}$=70% | $^{24}/_{38}$=63% | $^{22}/_{38}$=58% | $^{20}/_{38}$=53% |

[a] All patients received antilymphocyte globulins (ALG), azathioprine, and prednisone.

*Table 3.* Survival of kidney allo-transplants from unrelated cadaver donors, 3 months to 5 years after transplantation in patients subjected (TDD +) or not subjected (TDD −), to prior thoracic duct drainage.

| Pretreatment[a] | 3 months | 6 months | 1 year | 2 years | 3 years | 5 years |
|---|---|---|---|---|---|---|
| TDD+ | $^{15}/_{19}$=79% | $^{13}/_{19}$=68% | $^{10}/_{15}$=67% | $^{7}/_{10}$=70% | $^{6}/_{10}$=60% | $^{5}/_{10}$=50% |
| TDD − | $^{61}/_{99}$=62% | $^{52}/_{99}$=53% | $^{43}/_{91}$=48% | $^{38}/_{86}$=44% | $^{30}/_{70}$=43% | $^{27}/_{70}$=39% |

[a] All patients received antilymphocyte globulins (ALG) azathioprine and prednisone.

eight -year success have been recorded. Twenty TDD-patients have had 2 failures and 18 successes (9 months to 9 years). The first group was obviously too small for any comparison.

HLA haploidentical living donors included patients' parents and patients' haploidentical siblings. In this category of transplants, the kidney graft survival appeared slightly better in the TDD + group than in the TDD − group (Table 2). The difference, however, was very minimal.

In recipients of kidneys from cadaver donors, a larger difference was noted (Table 3). Those patients with a prior TDD had a higher incidence of transplant survival. The difference was already apparent 3 months after transplantation, was maximal at 2 years, and was slightly less prominent at 5 years. Results obtained in TDD + recipients of cadaver kidneys were very close to results obtained in recipients of kidneys from haploidentical living donors.

To avoid subjective interpretation, all failures, whatever the cause, were included in these studies. However, as shown below, the incidence of rejection crises was lower in TDD + and, when analyzing the main causes of failure, intractable rejection was indeed responsible for the observed difference in overall results.

Comparable results have been reported by the other transplant centers which used TDD (56,59). A significantly improved transplant survival has especially been noticed in TDD + patients receiving cadaver kidneys. A beneficial effect of TDD on results of living donor kidney transplants was observed several years ago, at a time when results obtained with 'classical' immunosuppression were poorer than they are now. A question raised in some studies (56) is whether the improved cadaver transplant survival is a long-term effect or whether TDD merely delays and modifies rejection of poorly compatible kidney grafts. No definitive answer will be available until significant numbers of TDD + recipients of cadaver transplants are analyzed with a 10-year follow up. However, for the first three years, the difference between TDD + and TDD − is apparent in all series.

*Incidence of rejection.* Because the diagnosis of rejection is somewhat more subjective than that of transplant survival, a 'blind study' was performed, rejection episodes being retrospectively defined in case-reports by physicians unaware of prior TDD.

The percentage of patients from each group with at least one rejection crises during the first 6 months is shown in Table 4. For this analysis, the total number of rejection crises per patient was used, as separating close episodes may be somewhat difficult, artificial, and inadequate. Criteria defining rejection crises are those derived from Williams's classification (60). Only those rejection episodes with an increase of plasma creatinine concentration above 2 mg/dl were considered as significant and included in this study.

A relatively low percentage of patients developed acute rejection crises, even in the TDD − groups, perhaps because of routine ALG therapy in all patients. This incidence was still lower in the TDD + groups, the difference being more significant in those receiving cadaver donor transplants (Table 4). Again, the figures obtained in TDD + recipients of cadaver kidneys were comparable to that of TDD − recipients of haploidentical living donors.

*Mechanisms of action of TDD and ALG.* From our results, it can be concluded that TDD performed prior to renal transplantation leads to an increased graft survival and to a decreased incidence of early acute rejection crises, especially in recipients of cadaver kidneys. These data confirm and extend our previous

*Table 4.* Incidence of rejection episodes of kidney allo-transplants from haploidentical living donors or from cadaver donors, in -patients subjected to (TDD+) or not subjected to (TDD-), prior thoracic duct drainage.[a]

| Pretreatment[b] | HLA haploidentical living donor[c] | Cadaver donors[c] |
|---|---|---|
| TDD+ | $5/_{14}=36\%$ | * $6/_{15}=40\%$ |
| TDD- | * * * $15/_{13}=45\%$ | * * $47/_{68}=69\%$ |

[a] Patients who presented transplant failure unrelated to rejection during the first six months were excluded from this analysis of rejection incidence in the various groups of patients.

[b] All patients received antilymphocyte globulins (ALG), azathioprine, and prednisone.

[c] Statistical comparisons: Comparison between values denoted by a single or double asterisk showed $p<0.05$: between values denoted by two and three asterisks showed $p<0.05$: comparisons between all other values were not significant.

suggestive evidence a beneficial effect of TDD on the outcome of kidney allotransplants (5). They are in complete agreement with results obtained in other
centers (56, 59). All our patients from TDD + and TDD − groups also received
ALG at the time of transplantation and for several weeks or months thereafter.
The better results observed in the TDD + group may thus be considered as
consequent either to the TDD itself or to the synergistic efficiency of ALG and
prior TDD.

In our patients, thoracic duct lymphocyte depletion by TDD induced a moderate decrease in peripheral blood lymphocytes, T lymphocytes being generally
more decreased than B lymphocytes. However, the diminution of T lymphocytes
bearing surface differentiation antigens and capable of E-rosette formation was
not very significant. The decrease of *in vitro* proliferative responses of peripheral
blood lymphocytes to mitogens, antigens, and allogeneic stimuli was more pronounced. The finding in peripheral blood of a population of T lymphocytes with
characteristics of early differentiation stages (61, 62) without properties of more
mature T lymphocytes suggests that the long-lived, recirculating, immunocompetent T lymphocytes removed by TDD are replaced by comparatively immature T
lymphocytes. Alternatively, they may have been replaced by a subpopulation of
T lymphocytes with a suppressive effect on the other subsets of T lymphocytes.
These two hypotheses are not mutually exclusive, as some thymic or immediately
postthymic lymphocytes do behave as suppressor cells in various experimental
models.

In addition to these consequences, TDD also resulted in diminished delayed
hypersensitivity skin reactions to antigens and decreased cell concentration in the
thymus-dependent areas of spleen and lymph nodes, but did not induce significant alterations in systemic antibody production (although a subset of B lymphocytes is depleted by TDD).

A recent modification of lymphocyte-labelling with 99m Tc has enabled us to
improve fixation and yield (63). After injection of labelled lymphocytes into
patients with TDD, measurements of radioactivity could be performed on lymphocytes separated from sequential blood or lymph specimens. In addition, using
a gammacamera, it was possible to follow the body distribution of labelled
lymphocytes over the 24-h period following injection. In brief, results showed
patterns of recirculation comparable to that of rodents (64, 65) and confirmed
results obtained in man by the use of H³ uridine lymphocytes (4). A wide organ
distribution was found and the rate of lymphocyte passage from blood to lymph
appeared to be lower than it was in rats. Simple extrapolation of these results to
the physiologic pattern of normal lymphocyte recirculation needs a word of
caution, as the verification of cell viability alone (above 93%) after labelling
cannot be considered as sufficient. The continuous circulation of lymphocytes
between blood and lymph has indeed been shown to be altered by many things,
including *in vivo* treatment with antigens, *B.pertussis,* dextrans, cortisone, X-ir-
radiation, and *in vitro* treatment of lymphocytes with substances altering their

surface, i.e., enzymes, lectins, ALG, LPS, etc.

In our patients, the immunosuppressive effect of TDD was reinforced by subsequent ALG treatment. ALG acts primarily in the blood circulation and potently depresses circulating lymphocytes and T lymphocytes in particular. Some of the cells are rapidly eliminated by cytotoxicity and opsonization followed by trapping in the reticuloendothelial system. Other cells remain in the circulation, but their functions are altered by antilymphocyte antibodies. Furthermore, after ALG treatment, the T cell subsets appear to be modified with the development of a large population of suppressor T lymphocytes. In view of this experimental data, an additional, and perhaps synergistic, effect of TDD and ALG in man can be envisioned. Furthermore, in renal transplant recipients, several other major factors of immunosuppression should be taken into account: azathioprine and steroid treatments, cell-mediated immunodeficiency secondary to renal failure, etc..

In conclusion, TDD and ALG in man are significantly immunosuppressive, as they are in rats, although lymphocyte recirculation is quantitatively different in both species. T lymphocyte subpopulations are modified which results in an improved transplant survival and a decreased incidence of rejection in transplant recipients. Such a beneficial effect favors the use of TDD prior to transplantation, in association with ALG and other immunosuppressants (66). Although methods for specific tolerance must be defined in the future, this therapeutic regimen induces a profound immunosuppression allowing increased survival of cadaveric kidney grafts, with a relatively moderate risk. We presently use this method in those patients requiring rapid transplantation when a well-matched donor cannot be found. In this group of patients subjected to the combination of immunosuppressive measures, the mortality has been reduced below 5% and the one year transplant survival exceeds 78% (2), despite a poor HLA compatibility with the donors. Its will be of interest to analyse long term results.

## References

1. Tilney NL, Murray JE: The thoracic duct fistula as an adjunct to immunosuppression in human renal transplantation. Transplantation 5: 1204, 1967.
2. Betuel H, Touraine JL, Bonnet MC, Carrie J, Traeger J: Biological and practical implications of programmed blood transfusions before kidney transplantation. In: Transplantation and Clinical Immunology. Amsterdam, Excerpta Medica, 1979.
3. Woodruff MFA, Anderson NF: Effect of lymphocyte depletion by thoracic duct fistula and administration of lymphocytic serum on the survival of skin homografts in rats. Nature (Lond) 200: 702, 1963.
4. Revillard JP, Brochier J, Durix A, Bernhardt JP, Bryon PA, Archimbaud JP, Fries D, Traeger J: Drainage du canal thoracique avant transplantation chez des malades atteints d'insuffisance rénale chronique. Nouvell Revue Française d'Hématologie 8: 585, 1968.
5. Touraine JL, Traeger J: In: Human Renal allotransplantation and antilymphocyte globuline. Simep ed. Villeurbanne, France, 1974.

6. Touraine JL, Archimbaud JP, Malik MC, Dubernard JM, Guey A, Neyra P, Mongin D, Bauraud B, Traeger J: Improved results of human renal transplantation after thoracic duct drainage and antilymphocyte globulin treatment. In: Transplantation and Clinical Immunology. Amsterdam, Excerpta Medica, 1977.

7. Archimbaud JP, Bansillon V et G, Bernhardt JP, Revillard JP, Perrin J, Traeger J, Carraz M, Fries D, Saubier EC, Bonnet P, Brochier J, Zech P: Technique, surveillance et intérêt du drainage du canal thoracique effectué en vue d'une transplantation rénale. J Chir Pari 98: 211, 1969.

8. Balner H: Recommendations for the production of anti-human lymphocyte sera based on in vitro testing in sub-human primates. In: Propriétés immuno-dépressives et mécanisme d'action du sérum antilymphocytaire, pp 125. CNRS Ed, 1 vol, 1971.

9. Balner H, Dersjant H, Betel I, Van Kekkum DW: Current state of evaluating anti-human lymphocyte sera by 'in vivo' testing. In: Symp Series immunobiol. 16, 179. Standard., Karger Ed, Basel/München/New-York, 1970.

10. Pollini J: Globulines anti-thymocytes. Préparation et essais cliniques (A propos de l'étude de 15 observations).Thèse, Marseille, 1971.

11. Monaco AP, Lewis EJ, Latzina A, Hardy M, Quint J, Schlesinger R, Mc Donough E, Latham W, Madoff M, Edsall G: Clinical use of equine anti-human lymph node lymphocyte serum: preliminary results in twenty-one mismatched cadaveric renal transplant. In: Symp Series immunobiol 16, 355. Standard, Karger Ed, Basel/München/New-York, 1970.

12. Bonneau M, Touraine JL, Traeger J: Préparation et propriétés d'IgG2 antilymphocytaires absorbés. In: Transplantation and Clinical Immunology, 132. Simep ed Publ, Villeurbanne, France, 1977.

13. Amos DB, Peacoke N: Leukoagglutination technique. In: Histocompatibility Testing. Nat Acad Sci, Dubl, 1965.

14. Pang GTM, Baguley DM, Wilson JD: Spontaneous rosettes as T lymphocyte marker. A modified method giving consistent results. J Immunol methods 4: 41, 1974.

15. Revillard JP, Brochier J, Traeger J, Balner H: In vitro asay of suppressive properties of antilymphocyte sera (ALS) on lymphocyte stimulation. Transplantation 9: 592, 1970.

16. Touraine JL: Un nouveau test d'activité in vitro des globulines antilymphocytaires. Lyon Medical 225: 1253, 1971.

17. Touraine JL, Touraine F: Antiglobulin test for titration of antilymphocyte globulin. ZI Forsch Bd 149: 28, 1975.

18. Rolland JM, Naurn RC, Davies DJ: Assay of antilymphocyte serum by membrane immunofluorescence. Journal of Immunological Methods 1: 83, 1971.

19. Greaves MF, Tursi A, Playfair JHL, Torrigiani G, Zamir R, Roitt IM: Immunosuppressive potency and in vitro activity of antilymphocyte globulin. Lancet i:68, 1969.

20. Roitt IM, Greaves MF, Tursi A, Torrigiani F, Playfair JHL, Berbi W: Correlation between immunosuppressive potency of antilymphocyte globulin and its activity in an opsonic adherence test in vitro. In: Pharmacological treatment in organ and tissue transplantation, p 284 Bertelli A, Monaco AP eds). Excerpta Medica, Amsterdam, 1970.

21. Moller G, Lundgren G, Balner H: An in vitro test of the immunosuppressive activity of antilymphocyte serum. Transplantation 9: 166, 1970.

22. Balner H, Dersjant H, Van Bekkum DW: Testing of anti-human lymphocyte sera in chimpanzees and lower primates. Transplantation 8: 281, 1969.

23. Bonneau M, Latour M, Plan R, Beranger G, Triau R: Survie des allogreffes de peau chez le Macaque Rhésus traité par le sérum antilymphocytaire humain: étude statistique et quantitative. In: Symp Series immunobiol 16, 215. Standard, Karger Ed, Basel/München/New-York, 1970.

24. Perper RJ, Glenn EM, Yu TZ, Monovich RE, Brunden MN: Analysis of the biological activities in antilymphocyte serum. In: Pharmacological treatment in organ and tissue transplantation, p 298 (Bertelli A, Monaco AP eds). Excerpta Medica, Amsterdam, 1970.

76

25. Deodhar SD, Kuklinca AG, Vidt DG, Robertson AL, Hazard JB: Development of reticulum-cell sarcoma at the site of antilymphocyte globulin injection in a patient with renal transplant. New England J Med 180: 1104, 1969.
26. Berthoux F: Etude de la distribution et de l'élimination des globulines antilymphocytaires ches l'homme par la méthode des traceurs nucléaires: critères, fréquence et conséquences de l'immunisation en transplantation rénale. Thèse, Lyon, 1971.
27. Josso F, Hors J, Bach JG, Kamoun P, Dormont J: Activité antiplaquettaire des sérums anti-lymphocytes. In: Symp Series immunobiol 16, 333. Standard, Karger Ed, Basel/München/New-York, 1970.
28. Vincent C, Revillard JP: Antibody response to horse gamma globulin in recipients of renal allografts. Transplantation 2: 141, 1977.
29. Butler WT, Rossen RD, Reisberg MA, Mazov JB, Trentin JJ, Judo KP: Antibody formation to equine antilymphocytic globulins (ALG) in man: effect on absorption, distribution and effectiveness of the ALG. J Immunol 106: 1, 1971.
30. Weksler ME, Rull G, Schwartz GH, Stenzel KH, Rubin AL: Immunologic responses of graft recipients to antilymphocyte globulin: effect of prior treatment with agregate free gamma-globulins. J Clin Invest 49: 1589, 1970.
31. Brendel W, Lob G, Seifert J: Indications et résultats des SAL en dehors des transplantations rénales. In: Cours International de Transplantation Lyon, p 301. Simep Ed, Lyon, 1972.
32. Gewurz H, Moberg AW, Johnson D, Simmons RL, Najarian JS: Induction of tolerance to horse gammaglobulin (HoGG) and antilymphocyte globulin (HoALG) in humans and experimental animals. Transplant Proc 3: 737, 1971.
33. Najarian JS, Simmons RL, Moberg AW, Gewurz H, Soll R, Tallent MB: Immunosuppressive assay of antilymphoblast globulin in man: effect of dose histocompatibility and serologic response to horse gammaglobulin. In: Symp Series Immunobiol 16, 199 Standard, Karger Ed, Basel/München/New-York, 1970.
34. Gozzo JJ, Wood ML, Monaco AP: Use of minimal doses of lymphoid cells for production of heterologous antilymphocyte serum. Transplant Proc 3: 779, 1971.
35. Davis RC, Glasgow AH, Williams LF Jr, Nabseth DC, Olsson CA, Schmitt GW, Idelson BA, Cooperband SR, Harrington JT, Mannick JA: Trial of rabbit anthuman ALG in cadaver kidney transplantation. Transplant Proc 3: 766, 1971.
36. Amemiya M, Kashiwagi N, Putnam CW, Starzl TE: Cross-reactivity studies of horse goat and rabbit antilymphocyte globulin. Clin exp Immunol 6: 279, 1970.
37. Bach JF: Les sérums antilymphocytes. Rev Europ études clin et biol 15: 28 et 258, 1970.
38. James K: The preparation and properties of antilymphocytic sera. Progr Surg 7: 140. Karger Ed, Basel/New-York, 1969.
39. Abaza HM, Nolan B, Watt JG, Woodruff MFA: Effect of antilymphocytic serum on the survival of homotransplants in dogs. Transplantation 4: 618, 1966.
40. Pichlmayr R, Brendel W, Zenker R: Production and effect of heterologous anti-canine lympho-cyte serum. Surgery 61: 774, 1967.
41. Starzl TE, Marchioro TL, Porter KA, Iwasaki Y, Cerilli GJ: The use of heterologous anti-lymphoïd agents in canine renal and liver homotransplantation and in human renal homo-transplantation. Surg Gynec Obstet 124: 301, 1967.
42. Guttmann RD, Lindquist RR, Ockner SA, Merrill JP: Mechanism of long-term survival of renal allografts after treatment with antilymphocyte antibody. Transplant Proc 1: 463, 1969.
43. Launois B, Campion JP, Fouchet R, Kerbaol M, Cartier F: Prospective Randomized clinical trial in Patients with cadaver kidney transplants. Transplant Proc 9: 1027, 1977.
44. Galle P, Hinglais N, Crosnier J: Reccurence of an original glomerular lesion in three renal allografts. Transplant Proc 3: 368, 1971.
45. Birtch AG, Carpenter CB, Tilney NL, Hampers CL, Hager FB, Levine L, Wilson RE, Murray JE: Controlled clinical trial of antilymphocyte globulin in human renal allografts. Transplant Proc 3: 762, 1971.

46. Doak PB, Dalton NT, Meredith J, Montgomeri JL, North JDK: Use of antilymphocyte globulin after cadaveric renal transplantation. Brit Med J 4: 522, 1969.

47. Sheil AGR, Stewart JH, Johnson JR, May J, Charles-Worth J, Kalowski S, Sharp AM, Bashir H: Evaluation of cadaver-donor renal transplantation. Transplant Proc 3: 347, 1971.

48. Traeger J, Perrin J, Fries D, Saubier E, Carrez M, Bonnet P, Archimbaud JP, Bernhardt JP, Brochier J, Betuel H, Veysseyre C, Bryon PA, Prevot J, Jouvenceaux A, Bansillon V, Zech P, Rollet A: Utilisation chez l'homme d'une globuline antilymphocytaire: résultats cliniques en transplantation rénale. Lyon Médical 219: 307, 1968.

49. Hamburger J, Corsnier J, Dormont J, Bach JF: La transplantation rénale. 1 vol. Ed Flammarion, Paris, 1971.

50. Toussaint C, Kinnaert P, Vereerstraeten P, Buchin R, Tagnon A, Geertruyden J: Semiologie de la crise de rejet du premier trimestre de la greffe rénale. Influence de l'administration de globuline antilymphocytaire. In: Cours International de Transplantation, Lyon Simep Ed, Lyon, p 221, 1972.

51. Traeger J, Touraine JL, Fries D, Berthoux F: Evaluation of intravenous route for administration of antilymphocyte globulins in humans. Transpl Proc 3: 749, 1971.

52. Brendel W, Land W, Pichlmayr R: Intravenous treatment with horse antihuman lymphocyte globulin (ALG) in organ transplantation and autoimmune diseases. p 208 Pharmacological treatment in organ and tissue transplantation.(Bertelli AP. Monaco, Excerpta Medica, Ed, Amsterdam), 1971.

53. Toussaint C, Ban Geertruyden J, Govaerts A, Plan R, Latour M, Kinnaert P, Vereerstraeten P, Depelchin A, Bonneau M, Buchin R, Wybran J: Administration intraveineuse d'une globuline antilymphocytaire chez cinq patients porteurs d'une greffe rénale. In: Symp series immunobiol 16, 371, 1970. Standard. Karger Ed Basel/München/New-York.

54. Touraine JL, Traeger J: Mode of administration of steroïds in treatment of renal allograft rejection. Lancet 1, 607, 1978.

55. Starzl TE, Brettschneider L, Penn I, Schmidt RW, Bell P, Kashiwagin N, Townsend CM, Putnam CW: A trial with hererologous antilymphocyte globulin in man. Transplant Proc 1: 448, 1969.

56. Franksson C, Lundgren G, Magnusson G, Ringden O: Thoracic duct drainage in renal transplantation in man. In: Transplantation and Clinical Immunology, Lyon, Vol 9, 1977. Amsterdam, Excerpta Medica.

57. Tilney NC: Lymphocyte depletion by thoracic duct drainage in clinical transplantation. In: Transplantation and Clinical Immunology, Lyon vol. 9, 1977. Amsterdam, Excerpta Medica.

58. Fish JC, Sarles HE, Remmers AR, Tyson KRJ, Conales CO, Beathard GA, Fukushima M, Ritzmann SE, Lewin WE: Circulation lymphocyte depletion in preparation for renal allotransplantation. Surg Gynecol Obstet 128: 777, 1969.

59. Niblac GD, Johnson HK, Richie RE, Tallent MB: Immunologic parameters of patients subjected to chronic thoracic duct drainage. Fed Proc 36: 1211, 1977.

60. Williams GM, White HJO, Hume DM, Factors influencing the long term functional success rate of human renal allografts. Transplantation 5: 837, 1967.

61. Touraine JL: Induction of human T-lymphocyte differentiation antigens. In: Leukocyte Membrane Determinants Regulating Immune Reactivity 711, 1976. (Eijsvoogel VP, Roos D, Zeijlemaker WR, eds). New-York, Academic Press.

62. Touraine JL, Hadden JW, Good RA: Sequential stages of human T lymphocyte differentiation. Proc Natl Acad Sci USA 74: 3414, 1977.

63. Touraine JL, Guey A, Traeger J: Marquage des lymphocytes humains par le Technetium 99m: application au diagnostic précoce des rejets d'allogreffes? Bull de l'Acomen 3: 1, 1979.

64. Gowans JL, Knight JE: The route of recirculation of lymphocyte in rat. Proc R Soc Lond (Biol) 159: 257, 1974.

65. Rannie GH, Ford WL: Physiology of lymphocyte recirculation in animal models. In: Transplantation and Clinical Immunology, Lyon, vol 9, 1977. Amsterdam, Excerpta Medica.
66. Starzl TE, Koep JL, Weil R, Halgrimson CG, Kranks JJ: Thoracic duct drainage in organ transplantation: will it Permit Better immunosuppression? Transplant Proc 1: 276, 1979.

# 9. Monitoring of organ allograft rejection by fine needle aspiration cytology

P. HÄYRY, J. AHONEN and E. VON WILLEBRAND

## 1.Introduction

Most diagnostic problems in clinical transplantation focus in the graft. An obvious need for a closer monitoring of the organ allograft has therefore, emerged. Although several attempts have been made to monitor the intra-graft events in the blood, no reliable method has been developed so far and needle biopsy (NB) has remained as the only method to assess the graft and the intra-graft parameters in clinical practice.

Excluding hyperacute rejection, which may be avoided by a negative crossmatch, histological analysis of the allograft has demonstrated two major forms of early organ allograft failure: 'cellular rejection' and 'vascular rejection'. The characteristic feature in *cellular rejection* is accumulation of inflammatory cells, lymphocytes, blast cells and mononuclear phagocytes, around the blood vessels and later, throughout remaining structures of the graft. Most rejections with this pattern of inflammation occur during the first months after transplantation and most of them are reversible (1, 2). The characteristic features of *vascular rejection* are fibrointimal thickening of the graft arteriolar endothelium leading eventually to 'onion skinning' and final obliteration of the graft arteries and destruction of the glomeruli (2, 3). In contrast to cellular rejection, most vascular rejections are irreversible. It has also been demonstrated that immunoglobulin deposits, fibrinogen and complement are nearly always found in these grafts; therefore, this type of rejection has been suggested as being due to humoral immunity (4). Needless to say, it is important to realize that both major arms of the immune response function usually concomitantly and that most rejections of, e.g., a human renal allograft, are mixtures of these two major pathways.

The risks related to the NB and to open biopsy, have necessitated the development of another, alternative method to assess the intra-graft events. This cytological method is based on a sizeable amount of experimental research primarily in the rat (5, 6) and applies a fine needle aspiration biopsy (FNAB). Instead of NB, which is always a risky procedure, the FNAB can be performed daily or even hourly to, e.g., human renal allografts without risk to the graft or to the graft recipient (7, 8, 9). From these cytological specimens, it is possible to evaluate many intra-graft events, in particular the cellular integrity of the graft, the presence, size and type of inflammation and, what is very important, the impact of anti-inflammatory and immunosuppressive drugs on these two major parameters.

It is well-documented by now that both liver and kidney allografts are easily accessable by the FNAB. Heart allografts, due to their hard consistency are probably not accessable. However, endomyocardial biopsy may be safely performed to heart allografts and essentially similar information is obtained (10). An alternative cytological approach, the broncho-alveolar lavation (BAL) has been developed for lung allografts. This method employs basically the same cytological method as the FNAB and supplies essentially the same information from the lung parenchyma as the FNAB gives from the kidney and the liver (11).

## 2. Technical aspects

The technical details of performing of the FNAB, processing of the material, reading of the results and superimposition of monoclonal antibody techniques of the transplant aspiration cytology (TAC), have been described in earlier communications (12, 13). It should, however, be emphasized that the reading of the FNAB specimen is based on cytological criteria rather than on histological evaluation and that the frequently-needed immunological methods place this approach in an interdisciplinary area between classical cytology and immunology.

It should also be emphasized that the FNAB aspirates are always contaminated by variable amounts of blood. Therefore, the evaluation of inflammation requires adjustment to blood background. This has been difficult to achieve, and the currently-used method may still be far from excellence. At present this is done by performing white cell differential counts separately from the graft and from the blood. It has been documented that after deduction of the blood differential from the graft differential, the remaining 'increment' rather faithfully describes the inflammatory events in situ (13). However, further adjustments in the quantitation of the inflammatory infiltrate are necessary and require that also the representativity of the sample, i.e., the number of parenchymal cells obtained in each specimen, must be taken into account.

## 3. Cytological evaluation of the transplant

As stated, aspiration cytology gives substantially less information on the graft than does the NB. However, certain parameters of the graft can be assessed in detail also from the cytological specimens. These include the overall integrity of the graft, acute tubular necrosis in the kidney and cyclosporin-induced nephrotoxicity in the kidney and the liver. Moreover, the presence of cholestasis in a liver allograft and viral infections in the lung and (possibly) in a kidney allograft may also be evaluated.

### 3.1 Acute tubular necrosis

After, e.g., arterial thrombosis and/or venous occlusion the transplant parenchymal cells die and appear necrotic in the cytological specimens. Under these circumstances no inflammation may be recorded because due to a massive accumulation of granulocytes in the necrotic graft, the specimen closely resembles blood background with granulocyte predominance.

In acute tubular necrosis, a frequent complication of renal transplantation, the tubular cells appear swollen and vacuolized (12). These changes disappear when the graft resumes its function.

### 3.2 Cyclosporin nephrotoxicity

In cyclosporin-induced nephrotoxicity similar but more pronounced changes are seen in the allograft tubular and endothelial cells (14): the tubular cells appear strongly swollen, vacuolized and contain frequently amorphous inclusions and even erythrophagocytosis is not uncommon. The most distinct morphological changes in the graft vascular endothelial cells are swelling and vacuolization. Concomitantly with these morphological changes, deposits of CyA (and/or its metabolites) are demonstrated in the renal tubular cells by indirect immunofluorescence (14). Similar changes have been observed in the kidney of bone marrow transplant recipients in cases of clinical CyA toxicity (unpublished). As yet we have not been able to demonstrate any inflammation accompanying the early CyA deposits. If inflammation is present and especially if there is a distinct blast cell component in the inflammatory lesion, this indicates ongoing rejection. These different patterns make it possible to perform an accurate differential diagnosis between the three most commonly encountered post transplantation disorders of a renal allograft: acute tubular necrosis, drug toxicity and rejection (Table 1). After reduction of the dose, the cyclosporin deposits usually rapidly disappear from the graft and the transplant resumes normal function (14). Normalization of renal tubular cell morphology requires, however, a longer period of time.

### 3.3 Parenchymal components of the liver

The major parenchymal cell component in the liver, the hepatocytes, are easily

*Table 1.* Differential diagnosis between cyclosporin nephrotoxicity and other reasons of renal transplant failure by FNAB.

| S-Creat | FNAB | | | Explanation |
|---------|------|-----------|-----------|-------------|
| | Inflammation | Tubular cell changes | CyA deposits in graft | |
| Normal | − | + | ± | Well-to-do-graft |
| Elevated | − | + + | − | ATN |
| Elevated | −[a] | + + + | + + + | CyA toxicity |
| Elevated | + + + | + | − | Rejection |
| Elevated | + + + | + + + | + + + | Rejection and CyA toxicity |

[a] The possibility that CyA deposits induce occasionally some inflammation, is not entirely excluded. (From v. Willebrand and Häyry, Transplant Proc, 1983 in press).

damaged during the aspiration procedure. This makes their morphological evaluation more difficult than, e.g., that of the renal tubular cells. However, very prominent changes, such as e.g., vacuolization associated with fatty liver, are recognized. Aspirates of a liver allograft contain sometimes liver sinusoidal endothelial cells. Changes like cholestasis may also be evaluated as bile deposits in the hepatocytes. Accumulation of cyclosporin (and/or its metabolites) in the liver can be demonstrated, as in the kidney, by indirect immunofluorescence although the liver transplant appears usually less sensitive to cyclosporin than the recipient's own kidney (Lautenschlager *et al.*, unpublished results).

## 3.4 Aspiration cytology in bone marrow transplantation

One important application of aspiration cytology is bone marrow transplantation in man. Currently, methods are being worked out for the differential diagnosis of virus infection vs graft-versus-host (GVH) reaction and/or irradiation damage in the recipient lung. Using broncho- alveolar lavation, viral antigens can be demonstrated by indirect immunofluorescence in the alveolar epithelial cells and viral infection is frequently associated with a clear lymphocytosis *in situ*. Most of these lymphocytes are of the T suppressor/killer type, representing possibly a cellular response towards the virus-infected cells (Ekblom *et al.*, unpublished results). The cytological criteria for GVH and irradiation damage in the lung, are still under investigation.

## 4. Evaluation of the inflammatory lesion

The size, type and duration of the inflammatory episodes of rejection, may be evaluated more precisely from the aspiration cytology specimens than from an ordinary NB. Quantitation of inflammation must, however, as stated above, be performed against blood background. The current method of doing this, is to perform separate white cell differential counts from the aspirate and from the blood, and subtract the blood differential count from the aspiration differential. In ordinary acute renal allograft rejection the granulocytes, being frequent in the blood but few in the graft, appear as negative figures while the remaining mononuclear cell types appear positive. The arithmetic sum of the positive 'increment' values, the 'total increment' represents the degree of inflammation (13).

### 4.1 Cellular components of rejection

In May-Grünwald-Giemsa (MGG) stained specimens, the following inflammatory cell types may be identified in these preparations: lymphoblasts, representing primarily T blast cells, plasmablasts representing primarily B blast cells, plasma cells, 'activated lymphocytes', large granular lymphocytes (LGL) representing the allograftinfiltrating natural killer (NK) cells, small lymphocytes, monoblasts, monocytes and tissue macrophages at varying degrees of maturation (12). It has recently been observed that blood eosinophilia is frequently associated with rejection (von Willebrand, unpublished observation) as well as in other non-immunological inflammatory episodes within the graft (15); however, the eosinophilia is usually stronger in the blood and none of the remaining types of granulocytes have so far been demonstrated in the increment.

Further dissection of the inflammatory lesion may be performed by using monoclonal antibody techniques applied either by the *Staphylococcus aureus* rosette assay (12) or by the indirect immunoperodixase method on the cytological specimen (16). Application of proper marker antibodies to white cell subsets has made it possible to evaluate the type(s) of blast cells and lymphocytes present in the specimens and to define more exactly the degree of mononuclear phagocyte maturation. Use of anti-MHC antibodies, directed either to the backbone molecule or to the allelic specificity of the AB subregion, makes it possible to evaluate whether the graft vascular endothelial cells display the major histocompatibility complex antigens on the cell surface (17). Finally, the origin of blast cells *in situ* may be identified by alloantibodies directed to the donor vs the recipient allelic specificities or the AB locus (unpublished).

## 4.2 Profiles of inflammation

Studies on renal transplantation in man, have demonstrated that the underlying immunosuppressive drug therapy may influence the frequency and especially the patterns of the inflammatory episodes of rejection. In well-to-do allografts very little inflammation is recovered. Under azathioprine and low postoperative steroid regimens, the first inflammatory episodes of rejection occur earlier and are higher in magnitude than in regimens employing high postoperative steroid administration (18). The 'low' steroid inflammatory pattern follows most closely the pattern observed in drug-unmodified renal allograft rejection in the rat (6). The first cells to invade the allograft are lymphocytes and monocytes (Fig. 1) Before clinical signs of rejection appear, a distinct (T cell) lymphoblastogenesis and (B cell) plasmablastogenesis are observed *in situ*. Along with advancing rejection more lymphocytes and monocytes appear in the graft. The blast cell-dominated episodes usually subside within days or a week concomitantly with the application of intensified glucocorticosteroid therapy. Alternatively, more lymphocytes and monocytes appear in the graft, and a rapid transformation of monocytes into tissue macrophages is usually a hallmark of irreversible rejection (9).

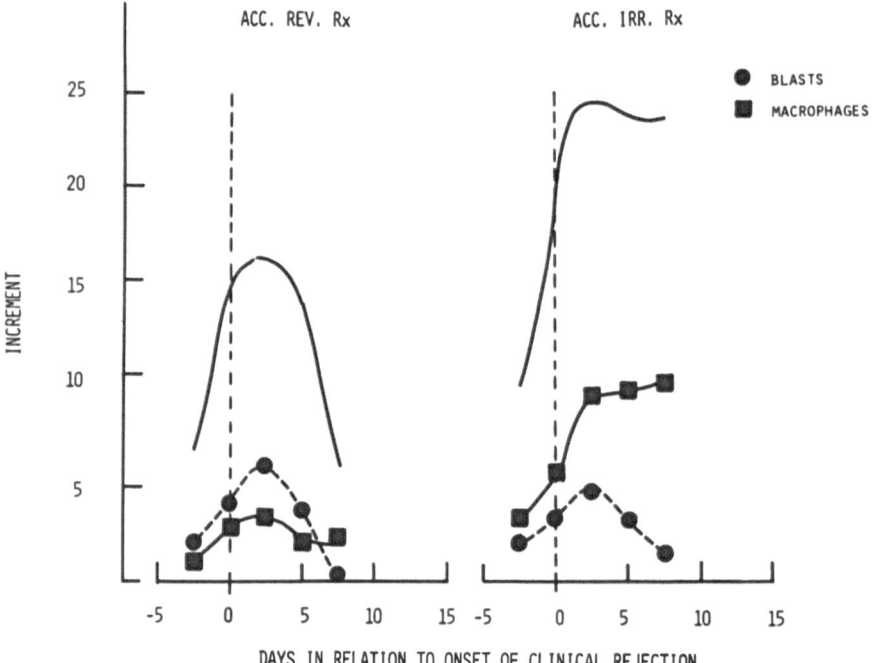

*Fig. 1.* Profiles of inflammation in acute reversible rejection (left) and in acute irreversible rejection (right) under azathioprine and 'low initial' steroid regimen. Total inflammation given as solid line, number of blast cells as closed circles and dashed line, and number of macrophages as closed quadrangles and solid line. (Based on Häyry and von Willebrand, Scand J Immunol 13:87, 1981).

Needless to say, the profiles of inflammation vary considerably from one case to another. On some occasions, the inflammation mounts up slowly and the inflammatory cells are seen *in situ* prior to any clinical signs of rejection becoming apparent. In other cases, the graft may be cytologically tranquil in the morning but may be undergoing a fulminant inflammation in the evening of the same day. On most occasions the inflammatory episode subsides shortly, within days and the graft assumes normal function. In other cases, inflammation may persist for weeks together with exacerbations and remissions (Fig. 2). These changes are usually, though not always, accompanied by changes in the clinical patterns of the recipient.

These different profiles of inflammation are not inconceivable, if one takes into account the sizeable cellular traffic between the graft and the host taking place during episodes of rejection (19). The cohort of white cells, migrating into and out from the graft is comparable, if not equal, to the size of the whole allograft-responding inflammatory cell pool in the recipient (19). Thus even relatively small changes in the influx/outflux ratio may result in a rapid accumulation of inflammatory cells in the graft and explain why the inflammatory episodes of rejection may be mounted on some occasions within hours. However, it should be also understood that a renal transplant may tolerate a certain amount of inflammation without clinical signs (13) and that the inflammation is accompanied by clinical signs only if it exceeds the critical level. We believe that many of the weak inflammatory episodes of rejection, at least in renal transplantation in man, have thus been overlooked in the past.

### 4.3 Further patterns of inflammation

Further dissection of the inflammatory lesion may be done by employing monoclonal antibody markers to the inflammatory cell subsets (20). This analysis has demonstrated that on most occasions the T suppressor/killer lymphocytes dominate over the T helper lymphocytes in the graft. Occasionally, however, the T helper lymphocyte subset may dominate, and preliminary evidence suggests that many of the grafts with this type of inflammation are lost because of rejection (20).

It is also likely that many of the inflammatory episodes of 'rejection' are not rejections but may represent acute graft vs host episodes *in situ*. We have used the *Staphylococcus aureus* rosette assay and alloantibodies directed to the donor or to the recipient and found (unpublished) that in at least some of the episodes of inflammation most, or a good portion of blast cells in the graft derive not from the graft recipient but from the graft donor. Alternatively, the response may be 'split' resembling a bi-directional mixed lymphocyte culture reaction *in vitro*. In the absence of systematic analysis we do not know how frequent these type of inflammatory episodes are or whether they should be treated by drugs.

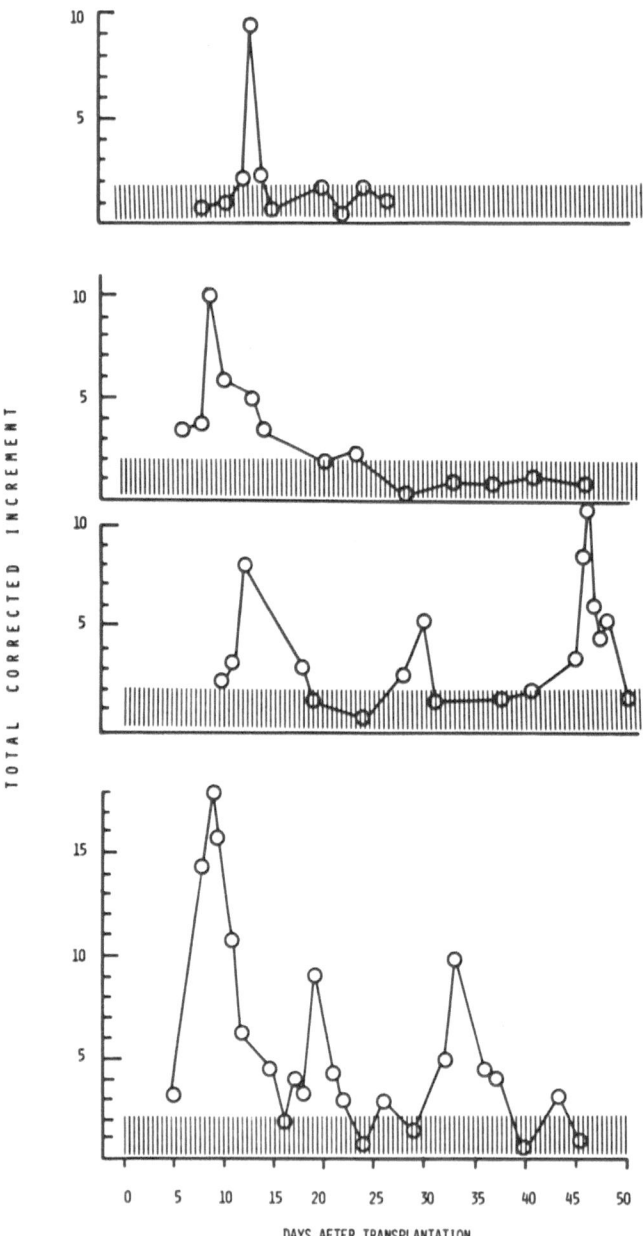

*Fig. 2.* Different profiles of inflammation. Shaded area represents background inflammation in well-to-do grafts ±SD. For details, see the text. (From Häyry and von Willebrand, Proc of the 15th International Course on Transplantation and Clinical Immunology, in press 1983 (27)).

As stated, the underlying immunosuppressive therapy greatly modifies the onset, type and frequency of the early inflammatory episodes of rejection. These changes are clearly demonstrable by transplant aspiration cytology in randomized clinical trials. For example, high initial administration of glucocorticosteroids immediately after transplantation (see later) both significantly postpones the first episode of inflammation and reduces the size of the episode. The inflammatory components which are significantly depleted from the inflammatory lesion under high (compared to low initial) steroid regimen are (B) plasmablasts and macrophages.

Administration of cyclosporin, without steroids, is nearly invariably accompanied with a prominent inflammatory response in the graft during the first few days after transplantation (15). This type of inflammatory lesion consists nearly exclusively of lymphocytes and mononuclear phagocytes with a prominent absence of T and B blast cells. It subsides spontaneously within days and concomitantly, the graft resumes a normal function (15). It is unlikely that the inflammatory response is due to cyclosporin as such, as similar inflammatory episodes are not seen when cyclosporin is administered together with glucocorticosteroids (unpublished). However, such inflammations are invariably seen in rat renal autografts unmodified by immunosuppressive treatment (6). We therefore interpret that this type of inflammation represents a normal physiological response to the surgical manipulation but it is not seen in ordinary circumstances because of the masking effect of routinely-administered anti-inflammatory glucocorticosteroids.

Administration of cyclosporin A both alone and combined with a small dose of glucocorticosteroids, may also be accompanied by a persistent inflammation in a kidney allograft consisting of lymphocytes, monocytes and occasional monoblasts but not lymphoid blast cells. This is often seen even months after transplantation and is (usually) accompanied by somewhat improper graft function. We do not know yet whether this type of inflammation, which may accompany cyclosporin deposits in the kidney, represents: (a) an inflammatory lesion towards cyclosporin and/or drug-modified parenchymal cells or, alternatively; (b) is an uncommon cytological manifestation of 'rejection'. A systematic study must, therefore, be performed whereby grafts are aspiration biopsied at very frequent intervals and the dose of the drug reduced, until the kidney resumes its normal function or ends up in clear clinical rejection.

### 4.4 Drug sensitivity of different inflammatory patterns

It is also quite apparent that some inflammatory episodes of rejection, seemingly resistant to high dose treatment with glucocorticosteroids (GS), may rapidly respond to cyclosporin A (21) or, to (monoclonal) anti-lymphocyte antibody (Goldstein, personal communication). We have now systematically treated rejection episodes occurring under azathioprine plus steroids, which do not respond to high dose GS, with cyclosporin (Table 2). Of 18 episodes treated so far, 16 responded to cyclosporin administration within days and the inflammatory cells disappeared from the graft with normalization of its function. All cases which responded to cyclosporin, represented typical blast cell-dominated inflammatory episodes. Of the two unresponding cases one was a blast-cell dominated episode which subsided 'spontaneously' two days after discontinuation of cyclosporin treatment and the other a case of chronic rejection devoid of any blastogenic component. Needless to say, these observations are still anecdotal (21), but they possibly warrant a clinical trial to be performed.

## 5. Monitoring of individual patients

In renal transplantation in man, rejection is usually easy to diagnose provided that the graft functions well. However, certain other clinical conditions, such as drug nephrotoxicity and viral infections (22) may mimick rejection. Thus on most occasions aspiration cytology is not necessary to establish the diagnosis of rejection but rather to exclude this possibility. However, other transplants, complicated by prolonged acute tubular necrosis are more difficult to treat as the signs of rejection are more difficult to visualize. Also in CyA-trial patients (in combination with steroids), clinical signs of rejection may often be weak or absent. On these occasions, frequent FNA biopsies and analysis of the intra-graft events have proven invaluable in the treatment of renal transplant recipients (Fig. 3).

Aspiration cytology is even more important in the monitoring of rejection episodes in the transplantation of the liver. In liver transplantation the episodes of rejection are more difficult to monitor than in the transplantation of kidneys, primarily because of the absence of reliable laboratory methods reflecting early

Table 2. Current experience in Transplantation Center Helsinki on the use of cyclosporine in the treatment of acute episodes of rejection.

Material
53 renal consequtive transplantations
39 patients had a rejection episode
18 rejection episodes treated with CyA
21 rejection episodes treated with MP
2/18 grafts lost in the CyA-treated group
6/22 grafts lost in the MP-treated group

Indications to CyA-treatment
9 cases - no response to MP
5 cases - 'blast' dominated FNAB finding
4 cases - rejection episodes appeared while azathioprine was stopped
          because of leukopenia

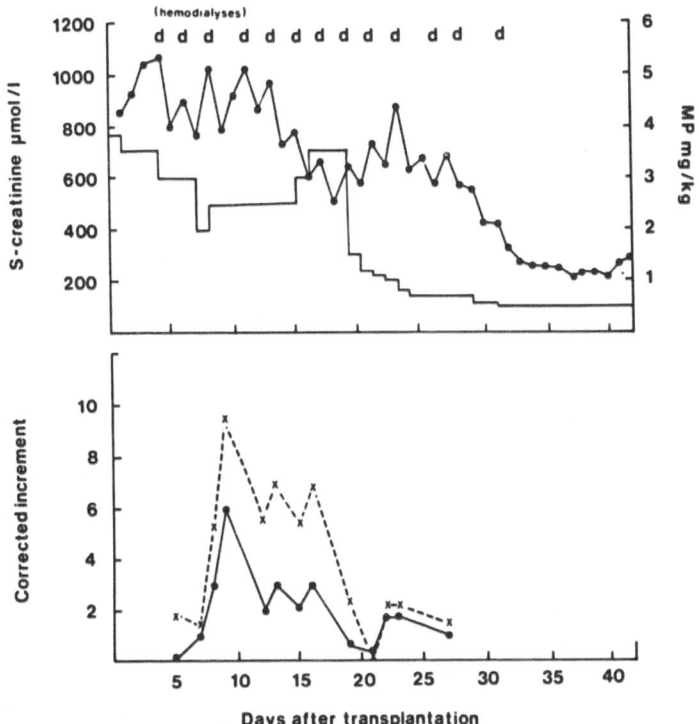

*Fig. 3.* The pattern of inflammation during a strong inflammatory episode duri g acute tubular necrosis while the patient was still on hemodialysis (d). The main features of the c inical course are given in the upper section: Serum creatinine is indicated with closed circles and solid ine and the dose of methyl-prednisolone (MP) with columns. The inflammation in the transplant aspi ation cytology is given in the lower section. Crosses and dashed line indicate total inflammation (i.e., he total number of all types of inflammatory cell elements in the corrected increment) and closed cir les and solid line the proportion of blast cells in the corrected increment. Note that the inflammation has been treated on the basis of the TAC finding only. (From Häyry et al: Ann Clin Res 13:264–287, 1981).

changes in hepatocyte function. Although certain labile coagulation factors rapidly indicate changes in the hepatocyte function, large fluctuations are common and, needless to say, these methods cannot differentiate between different causes of hepatocyte failure. Enzymatic signs of liver failure appear later and, e.g., S-ALAT and S-ASAT levels are unreliable, as they are high throughout the postoperative course due to the operation itself. Monitoring of the liver transplant at 1–2 day intervals by the FNAB has, at least in our hands, been superior to any other test system alone or combined in the transplant follow-up both in experimental transplantation in the pig (Lautenschlager, unpublished results) and clinical transplantation in man (Lautenschlager, unpublished results and Fig. 4).

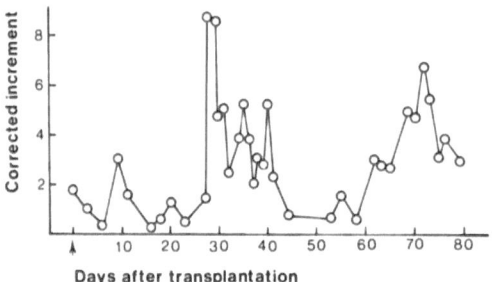

*Fig. 4* Three inflammatory episodes in a human liver allograft occurring in a patient immunosuppressed with cyclosporin. The first episode consisted of lymphocytes and mononuclear phagocytes without any clear blastogenic component, and was associated with some cytological evidence of cholestasis. This inflammatory episode was probably non-immunological in nature and represented most likely a 'background' response to surgical handling of the graft. The following two episodes were typical blast cell-dominated episodes of inflammation, which were followed by laboratory evidence of hepatocyte failure and which subsided concomitantly with elevated administration of glucocorticosteroids. (Lautenschlager et al., unpublished results).

## 6. Applications of aspiration cytology in clinical trials

In all clinical trials the endpoint of titration is naturally graft and patient survival. With the present level of success in renal transplantation in man, ranging approximately from 50 to 80% of one year graft survival in different centers, small improvements to the pre-existing protocol are difficult to visualize even in randomized trials. Therefore, large numbers of patients must be transplanted before these differences become statistically significant.

Application of aspiration cytology, which quantitates simultaneously several parameters of the anti-graft response, may reveal these differences earlier and against a higher level of significance. Moreover, if a comparison is made between two protocols differing in one single parameter as should usually be the case, differences in the structure of the inflammatory infiltrate may reveal or hint the site(s) of action of drug or regimen employed. This may be exemplified in the light of the following two examples.

### 6.1 Impact of 'high dose' steroids

After the Belfast team went to very low administration of steroids and McGeown (23) reported the apparent beneficial effects of her regimen, most transplant centers in the world abandoned the high-dose post operative steroid administration and confined to very low prophylactic steroid regimens (24). However, they still employed the high-dose bolus therapy in the treatment of acute episodes of rejection. In the light of these observations, we designed an opposite experiment;

we performed a randomized trial where- without increasing the total amount of postoperative administration of GS - the steroids were distributed in a different manner: instead of giving large doses of GS during rejection, we administered most of the GS immediately after transplantation and treated the established episodes of rejection by a moderate oral dose of GS, only (18).

Cadaveric renal transplant recipients immunosuppressed with 2.1 mg/kg/d of azathioprine (AZA), were randomized for two steroid protocols. The basic leg employed a low (0.5 mg/kg/d) dose of methyl-prednisolone (MP) for prophylactic immunosuppression and 14 mg/kg/d alternate day boluses during rejection. In the experimental leg the patient received 3.6 mg/kg/d of MP on days 1...3 tapered to 0.5 mg/kg/d by day 15, and the episodes of rejection were treated by 3.6 mg/kg/d of oral MP divided in four doses. The results of this trial are summarized in Table 3. High initial administration of steroids significantly postponed the first inflammatory episode, and reduced the size of the episode. Significantly fewer episodes of rejection were recorded in those patients who were treated with 'high dose' postoperative steroid regimen. However, we had to randomize 200 more patients (unpublished) before the differences in graft survival, 72% vs 41%, respectively (p=0.003), became significant.

## 6.2 Impact of cyclosporin A

In another randomized experiment we compared azathioprine and 'high initial' steroid administration to cyclosporin (CyA) as the only immunosuppressive drug (15). In the basic leg azathioprine and steroids were administered as above while the control group received only cyclosporin as suggested by Calne et al. (25). The dose of CyA was 17 mg/kg/d intramuscularly for the first 1...3 days followed by 17

Table 3. Effect of 'high initial' (compared to 'low initial') steroid administration on the inflammatory cell components of first rejection.[a]

| Component | Effect | p |
|---|---|---|
| Onset of inflammation | delayed | 0.000 |
| Size of inflammation | reduced | 0.001 |
| (T) lymphoblasts | not affected | 1.000 |
| Monocytes | not affected | 0.200 |
| (B) lymphoblasts | depressed | 0.040 |
| Lymphocytes | depressed | 0.040 |
| Macrophages | depressed delayed | 0.070 |
| Duration of inflammation | reduced | 0.020 |

[a] From Häyry et al: Scand J Immunol 16:39, 1982.

mg/kg/d peroral dose from the 3rd day onwards. Acute episodes of rejection were treated in both groups with 3.5 mg/kg/d of MP in four peroral doses per day. The first episodes of inflammation were observed earlier in the CyA group compared to the azathioprine plus steroid group, and significantly more episodes of inflammation were recorded in the former. When the serum levels of CyA were quantitated retrospectively, we found that cyclosporin was released only slowly from the intramuscular depot resulting in very low plasma levels during the first few days postoperatively.

Because the patients in the CyA group were thus virtually unimmunosuppressed during the first days post transplantation, we found it necessary to repeat this trial. In the second cyclosporin trial (to be published) we randomized 96 patients in three treatment groups, azathioprine plus 'high initial' steroids, cyclosporin only and cyclosporin plus steroids. Cyclosporin was given initially at a dose of 10 mg/kg/d as intravenous infusion and tapered to the plasma level of 200 ng/ml after transfer to peroral administration on day three. In the CyA+MP group, the patients received also 3.6 mg/kg/d of MP tapered to 0 mg/kg/d on day 9. The impact of the different drug regimens on the first episode(s) of inflammation are summarized in Table 4. The first episode of inflammation occurred significantly earlier in the CyA group compared to the patients receiving AZA+MP or CyA+MP. The frequency of inflammatory episodes, quantitated as the number of days with inflammation in the graft, was significantly higher in the CyA group compared to the control or to the patients receiving CyA plus MP. Needless to say, these differences were also visible in graft survival, the 10-month graft survival being approximately 80% in the control group and in the patients receiving CyA+MP, and only 62% in the group receiving CyA only.

## 7. Future

We believe that the advantages of intragraft diagnostic methods are so obvious that *in situ* diagnostic approaches will probably replace most of the indirect diagnostic methods in organ transplantation in the future. It is, however, possible that the cytological approach suggested in this review, need not be the final one in the assessment of the intragraft events. Furthermore, such organs which cannot be reached by aspiration cytology, must be analyzed by other invasive but nontraumatic procedures, such as transvenous endomyocardial biopsy in cardiac transplantation (10, 26) and the broncho-alveolar lavation in the transplantation of the lung (11).

Further dissection of the inflammatory events, by applying subclassspecific markers for leukocyte subsets, will undoubtedly reveal still further patterns of inflammation in the future. If these different inflammatory patterns are responsive to different modes of therapy, as may now be expected, this will further add to the impact of aspiration cytology and other methods of this type.

*Table 4.* Onset and duration of the (first) episodes of inflammation in patients treated with azathioprine plus methylprednisolone, cyclosporin or cyclosporin plus methyl prednisolone[a].

| | Treatment group | | | | |
|---|---|---|---|---|---|
| | AZA + MP (n = 32) | | CyA (n = 32) | | CyA + MP (n = 32) |
| **A.** Onset of the first episode of inflammation (day of onset ± SD) | | | | | |
| – initially non-functioning grafts excluded[b] | 11.8 ± 8.7 | | 7.4 ± 5.4 | | 12.3 ± 7.4 |
| – significance in Student's t-test | | p = 0.021 | | p = 0.005 | |
| – initially non-functioning grafts and grafts displaying no evidence of inflammation excluded | 9.1 ± 8.3 | | 6.7 ± 3.4 | | 12.3 ± 7.4 |
| – significance in Student's t-test | | p = 0.172 | | p = 0.001 | |
| **B.** Duration of the episodes of inflammation during the immediate postoperative period of 30 days | | | | | |
| – number of functioning grafts at 30 d | 30 | | 28 | | 29 |
| – number of patient days | 900 | | 840 | | 870 |
| – number of days with significant[c] inflammation in the graft | 179 | | 271 | | 190 |
| – significance (p in $\chi^2$-test) | | p = 0.000 | | p = 0.000 | |
| – total period of inflammation per patient (± SD) | 6.0 ± 5.2 | | 10.0 ± 6.1 | | 6.2 ± 5.2 |
| – significance (p in Student's t-test) | | p = 0.010 | | p = 0.018 | |

[a] These results should be considered preliminary, as they are based on manual analysis and will be re-analyzed by computer.
[b] No evidence of inflammation: day of onset taken as day 30.
[c] Increment >2.0.

94

Finally we should also emphasize some of the difficulties in the aspiration cytology. Needless to say, the method falls in an interdisciplinary area between cytology, histology and immunology. Although performing of the biopsy is easy, reading of the result and evaluation of the intragraft events is more difficult to do than in the histological approach and needs a considerable amount of training. Most of the centers applying this method in routine clinical practice, have been trained either by Dr Eeva von Willebrand in Helsinki or by Dr Claus Hammer in Munich. For obvious reasons this assay is also relatively expensive: our Department is performing approximately 140 renal transplantations per year, and a full time cytologist is needed for the evaluation of these specimens and two technicians to prepare and screen them. On the other hand, substantial savings may be achieved not only by optimizing the patient care but also by a sizeable reduction of the costs of the other more expensive and indirect diagnostic methods, in particular the use of nuclear scintigrams, urographies and transplant angiograms.

## Acknowledgements

We wish to thank the staff of the Transplantation Laboratory, and the Division of Transplantation Surgery, Department IV of Surgery and Division of Hematology, Helsinki University Central Hospital, in particular Drs Bjo"rn Eklund, Krister Ho"ckerstedt, Irmeli Lautenschlager, Tapani Ruutu and Marja Ekblom for cooperation. This study was supported by grants 26882–02 and –03, and 31730–01 from the National Institutes of Health, Bethesda, Maryland, and by grants from the Sigrid Juselius Foundation, The Finnish Medical Research Council, the Association of Finnish Life Insurance Companies, Helsinki, Finland. Lyon, France, June 1983.

## References

1. Dunnill MS: A review of the pathology and pathogenesis of acute renal failure due to acute tubular necrosis. J Clin Pathol 27:2–13, 1974.
2. Porter KA: Rejection in treated renal allografts. J Clin Pathol 20:518–534, 1967.
3. Andres GA, Accinni L, Hsu KC, Penn I, Porter KA, Randall JM, Seegal BC, Starzl TE: Human renal transplants. III. Immunopathologic studies. Laboratory Investigation 22:588–604, 1970.
4. Porter KA, Andres GA, Colder MW, Dossitor JB, Hsu KC, Randall JM, Seegal BC, Starzl TE: Human renal transplants: II. Immunofluorescent and immunoferritin studies. Laboratory Investigation 18:159–171, 1968.
5. von Willebrand E, Soots A, Häyry P: In situ effector mechanisms in rat kidney allograft rejection. I. Characterization of the host cellular infiltrate in rejecting allograft parenchyma. Cell Immunol 46:309–326, 1979.
6. Häyry P, von Willebrand E, Soots A: In situ effector mechanisms in rat kidney allograft rejection. III Kinetics of the inflammatory response and generation of donor-directed killer cells. Scand J Immunol 10:95–108, 1979.

7. Pasternack A, Virolainen M, Häyry P: Fine needle aspiration biopsy in the diagnosis of human renal allograft rejection. J Urol 109:167–172, 1973.

8. von Willebrand E: Fine-needle aspiration cytology of human renal transplants. Clin Immunol Immunopathol 17:309–322, 1980.

9. Häyry P, von Willebrand E: Monitoring of human renal allograft rejection with fine needle aspiration cytology. Scand J Immunol 13:87-97, 1981.

10. Caves PK, Billingham ME, Stinson EB, Shumway NE: Serial transvenous biopsy of the transplanted human heart. Improved management of acute rejection episodes. Lancet 1:821–826, 1974.

11. Norin AL, Emeson EE, Kamholz SL, Pinsker KL, Montefusco CM, Matas AJ, Veith FJ: Cyclosporin A as the initial immunosuppressive agent for canine lung transplantation. Short- and long-term assessment of rejection phenomena. Transplantation 34:372–375, 1982.

12. Häyry P, von Willebrand E: Practical guidelines for fine needle aspiration biopsy of human renal allografts. Ann Clin Res 13:288–306, 1981.

13. Häyry P, von Willebrand E, Ahonen J, Eklund B, Lautenschlager I: Monitoring of organ allograft rejection by transplant aspiration cytology. Ann Clin Res 13:264–287, 1981.

14. von Willebrand E, Häyry P: Cyclosporin A deposits in renal allografts. Lancet 1983 (In press).

15. Häyry P, Ahonen J, von Willebrand E, Eklund B, Ho"ckerstedt K, Kauste A, Taskinen E, Lautenschlager I, Lalla M, Sarelin H: Effect of cyclosporin A on the in situ inflammatory response of human renal allograft rejection. A preliminary report. Scand J Immunol 16:135–149, 1982.

16. Wood RFM, Bolton EM, Thompson JF, Morris PJ: Monoclonal antibodies and fine needle aspiration cytology in detecting renal allograft rejection. Lancet II:278, 1982.

17. Häyry P, von Willebrand E, Ahonen J, Eklund B: Do well-to-do and repeatedly rejecting renal allografts express the transplantation antigens similarly on their surface? Scand J Urol Nephrol Suppl 64: 52–55, 1981.

18. Häyry P, von Willebrand E, Ahonen J, Eklund B: Glucocorticosteroids in renal transplantation. I. Impact of high vs low dose postoperative methyl-prednisolone administration on the first episode(s) of rejection. Scand J Immunol 16:39–49, 1982.

19. Nemlander A, Soots A, von Willebrand E, Husberg B, Häyry P: Redistribution of renal allograft responding leukocytes during rejection. 2. Kinetics and specificity. J Exp Med 156:1087–1100, 1982.

20. von Willebrand; OKT4/8 ratio in the blood and in the graft during episodes of human allograft rejection. Cell Immunol 77:196–201, 1983.

21. Häyry P, von Willebrand E, Taskinen E, Ahonen J, Eklund B, Ho"ckerstedt K, Pettersson E, Sarelin H: Cyclosporin A in the treatment of steroid-resistant episodes of rejection. Arch Surg 1983 (In press).

22. Matas AJ, Simmons RL, Kjellstrand CM, Najarian JS: Pseudorejection: factors mimicking rejection in renal allograft recipients. Ann Surg 198:51–59, 1977.

23. Mcgeown MG: Corticosteroid therapy for renal transplantation. Proc EDTA 17:385–391, 1981.

24. Salaman JR: Steroids in organ transplantation. Heart Transplantation II:118–121, 1983.

25. Calne RY, Rolles K, Thiru S, McMAster P, Craddock GN, Aziz S, White DJ, Evans DB, Dunn DC, Henderson RG, Lewis P: Cyclosporin A initially as the only immunosuppressant in 34 recipients of cadaveric organs: 32 kidneys, 2 pancreases, and 2 livers. Lancet II:1033–1036, 1979.

26. Billingham ME: Diagnosis of cardiac rejection by endomyocardial biopsy. Heart Transplantation I:25–39.

27. Häry P, von Willebrand E: Transplant aspiration cytology in the evaluation of a renal allograft. Proc. 15th International Course on Transplantation and Clinical Immunology. Excerpta Medica, Amsterdam, p1983 (In press).

# 10. Organ procurement and transportation

F.K. MERKEL and K.M. SIGARDSON

## Introduction

As transplantation of various organs has become successful for the treatment of a variety of clinical organ failures, the need for cadaver organs has increased dramatically. In the past, the attention of the surgeons was focused most often on the kidneys and little regard was given to the other vital organs. Because of this limited scope, kidneys were removed individually, often in haste, and with no regard towards use of other organs. This straightforward, but unsophisticated approach sometimes resulted in loss of one or both kidneys because of injuries inflicted on multiple renal arteries, trauma to the kidneys themselves and ureteral injury. Attempts to improve the technique of renal retrieval led to the development of the 'en bloc' (no touch) method of kidney removal (1). This technical advance which protected the kidneys from external trauma and injury to the renal artery was combined with *in situ* cooling (2), first using Ringers lactate, and then later with a modified Collins solution (3). This method provided cadaver kidneys that were uniformly of good quality, a fact which was essential to the establishment of the confidence between transplant centers so necessary for widespread national and international kidney sharing. The success of cadaver kidney transplantation has further increased the demand for kidneys and thus attention has been given to matters such as defining brain death (4), donor maintenance, organ preservation, use of procurement coordinators, investigation of cultural, social, ethnic, psychologic and religious factors effecting donation and development of better methods of organ distribution. More recently, the improved clinical success of cardiac and liver transplantation, and the increased interest in experimental clinical pancreas transplantation has refocused attention to techniques enabling removal of extra-renal organs without damaging the kidneys. Multi-organ donation has required solving additional logistical, socio-ethical, and procedural problems. This paper describes those factors we believe to be critical to a successful cadaveric organ procurement and distribution program.

## Establishment of the need

Because cadaveric organ transplants require the donation of the organs either by the patient prior to death or post-mortem by the family, it is necessary to establish the need for cadaver organs with the general public, religious leaders, and the physicians and nurses who care for potential donors. Increasing the public awareness involves the use of radio, television as well as meetings with civic and religious groups and schools and adult education classes. In general, it is difficult to measure the success of this aspect of the program because change in public awareness and acceptability takes years. Nevertheless, without such an approach, social progress will not occur.

In order to accomplish professional education, we have utilized contacts between the transplant personnel (surgeons, nurses and coordinators) and the physicians and nurses staffing the emergency rooms and intensive care units of regional trauma centers. We have found that it takes regular, repetitive professional visits with these donor hospital personnel in order to convince and remind them of the need for cadaver organs. The professional staff of the emergency room and intensive care units need to see facts and figures relating to the number of recipients awaiting transplantation, the number of transplants accomplished as well as the current success rates.

In order to facilitate staff compliance, we attempt to have organ donation become official hospital policy. Initially we negotiate with key administrative personnel at the donor hospital such as the chief executive officer, the president of the medical staff, the nurses, neurosurgeons and neurologists, the physician and nursing leaders of the emergency room and the intensive care units, and the hospital religious leaders. We then ask the hospital's administration to send letters to the physician and nursing staff to communicate the institution's favorable attitude towards transplantation and organ procurement. These actions legitimize our program in the eye of the professional staff.

A manual of instructions is provided to show how to identify a potential donor, determine when brain death has occurred, whom to call for organ retrieval, and how to support the donor until organ retrieval can be accomplished. Periodic in-services familiarize professional personnel with the need for organ donation and the necessary steps involved in a successful donation. Of paramount importance is for the emergency room and intensive care staffs to be able to identify potential organ donors (see section on donor selection). They must also know whom to call in order to initiate the process. Follow-up questionnaires allow us to assess the quality of our teaching and are helpful in developing changes in our procedures (5). Additional teaching is carried out for lay groups in the neighborhood of the hospital to acquaint the community with the program (6).

**Decreasing the workload of donor personnel**

A busy nursing and physician staff may look unfavorably upon organ donation because it requires an expenditure of additional time and effort. It is possible to minimize the workload of the donor hospital by providing trained coordinators. These transplant coordinators can be nurses, physician's assistants, medical technologist or public health specialists. Because there are many constraints on the time of transplant surgeons, because of the cost involved in having a physician do these duties, and because the coordinators often have a special ability to develop a colleagual relationship with donor hospital personnel, it has seemed reasonable to us to develop this approach. The functions of these transplant coordinators are many. They not only carry out important activities in the development of the organ procurement program but they also are initially involved with many activities leading up to the actual organ donation and follow-up work afterwards. During the developmental stages of the relationship between our transplant program and the donor hospital, the transplant coordinator meets with the personnel of the donor hospital described previously in the section titled 'Establishment of the Need'. In addition, the coordinator meets with local public officials such as the coroner or medical examiner; enlisting their support for the program, working out the specific details concerning organ donation in that area and developing a locally supported program for community relations. The transplant coordinator then obtains a protocol book for the donor hospital. By getting this support and working out the details of organ donation ahead of time, the process is simplified and made more acceptable to the donor hospital.

During the actual organ procurement process, the transplant coordinator can be of greatest assistance to the donor hospital personnel. Because the donor hospital personnel have been instructed to call the transplant coordinator by telephone whenever they suspect that they are caring for a potential donor, the transplant coordinator can provide immediate support by determining whether their patient really is a candidate and by giving helpful hints in donor management as described in the next two sections. The transplant coordinator then goes directly to the donor hospital, assists in donor resuscitation and participates in counselling the family of the prospective donor and obtaining permission for the organ donation. For the latter function, it is important that the coordinator be compassionate and understanding and yet be able to articulate the needs and values of donation to the family. Once permission has been obtained, the transplant coordinator can prepare the operating room staff so that the donor procedure will go smoothly. If necessary, operating privileges are obtained for the donor team and arrangements are made for the preservation of the organs. The transplant coordinator may also arrange for transportation of the donor team to the hospital, for obtaining and transporting lymphoid tissue for tissue matching and later, for the distribution of the kidneys and extra renal organs to appropriate recipient centers.

**Donor selection**

The criteria for donor selection are in some ways different for each organ.

*Kidney donors.* Nevertheless, suitable organ donors are previously healthy persons who have sustained an irreversible brain injury from acute trauma, subarachnoid hemorrhage, stroke, primary brain tumor, drug overdose, smoke inhalation, and hepatic coma. They must be free of malignancy (except for brain tumors) and systemic infection. In our experience, brain death is best established by a careful neurological examination that reveals absence of spontaneous breathing and movements, lack of response to painful stimuli, and absence of cranial reflexes including fixed and dilated pupils. Brain radio-nuclide blood flow studies and electroencephalographs are used primarily as confirmatory tests. Cadaver kidney donors generally must be under 65 years of age and be free from long standing diabetes and hypertension. Further, at the time of removal, the kidneys must produce urine and excrete creatinine. Our studies and others have shown that as long as donor homeostasis is achieved, the above criteria are the only necessary ones for obtaining uniformly useful cadaver kidneys. Some kidney transplant surgeons, however, hold more rigorous views of acceptability, i.e. no more than 2 arteries on each kidney, absence of injury to the kidneys, or their vessels, serum creatinines less than 2.5 mg%, and a variety of age requirements relating to preservation parameters. Our experience has not shown these considerations to be of great consequence. We have used kidneys from donors as young as 8 months (7) and as old as 69, with as many as five arteries, with complete decapsulation, and from donors with serum creatinine greater than 5.0 mg% all with excellent results (8).

The use of the new immunosuppressive agent, Cyclosporin A has heightened worldwide clinical interest in non-renal transplants, especially for liver, heart, heart/lung and pancreas transplants. Many new and active programs have been established, vastly increasing the demand for these organs. Because these programs depend for the most part on the established renal procurement systems, it is important that the methods used are safe for the kidneys (9, 10).

*Liver donors.* Special considerations important for liver transplantation effect the availability of useful organs. For example, size plays a greater role for liver transplantation than for kidney transplantation, in which case it is possible to place an adult kidney in a child and vice versa. In the case of liver transplantation, it is necessary that the donor liver be smaller than the recipient's own liver, in order to facilitate the multiple vascular anastomoses and to fit the new liver into the abdominal cavity of the recipient. Because many of the recipients are children, there is a high demand for pediatric donors. Unfortunately, children with Reyes Syndrome are acceptable as renal donors but their livers cannot be used. Naturally, there must be no evidence of liver disease or serious liver injury.

*Heart and heart/lung donors.* Today's requirements for cardiac donors include age under 30 years except for female donors, lack of evidence of arteriosclerosis, lack of acute injury to the heart, absence of arrythmias, and no severe hypertension. In some cases, size may play a role. For example, pediatric hearts are used for children because of the size of the vascular connection that must be made and similarly adult hearts are used in adults. Nevertheless, there may be some latitude regarding size. However, it is generally preferred to use a heart slightly larger than the recipient's original heart. In general, the same criteria used for heart donors apply for heart/lung donors, however, there must be no evidence of pulmonary disease or infection in both lungs. Because many victims of brain death have sustained severe trauma and have been on a respirator for one or more days, one or more lungs may not be in the excellent shape necessary for this procedure. For this reason, transplantation of a single lung may become a useful alternative to heart/lung transplant.

*Pancreas donors.* In the case of pancreas transplantation, donors must be younger than 35 years of age and be free of diabetes both by history and at the time of donation. Some would exclude donors with a strong family history of diabetes. Size does not play an important role here, however, since the organ itself is relatively small and is transplanted to an iliac fossa in a manner similar to that of a kidney transplant. Because of the interconnected blood supply of the liver and pancreas, it is rare that both organs are used from the same donor.

Finally, it is important to coordinate the various activities in preparation for organ donation as well as the actual proceedings. This coordination can be especially difficult when several different organs are being removed from one donor to be used at different recipient centers. Because the safe preservation times for heart, lung, pancreas and liver are much shorter than for kidneys, recipients for these organs must be readied during the removal. At the same time, care must be taken that the kidneys are not damaged while the other organs are being taken.

## Donor maintenance

Donor maintenance has, in our experience, been a key factor in consistently obtaining kidneys that are satisfactory for transplantation. It undoubtedly is at least as important in recovering useful extrarenal organs.

The standard care plan for the prospective cadaver donor has been designed so that it in no way adversely affects the patient. Our main objective is to ensure homeostasis, preferably by treating the donor in such a way that hypotension and electrolyte disturbances do not occur. Our work has demonstrated that early administration of concentrated colloid (preferably 25% albumin) will reduce cerebral edema and maintain vascular volume, thus preventing shock which could not only injure the transplantable organs, but might also cause a secondary brain injury. It is helpful to obtain central venous pressure measurements and to keep the CVP at a level of 12–14 cm $H_2O$. Careful periodic monitoring of the electrolytes should be done in all brain injured patients since prompt correction of electrolyte abnormalities will protect all the organs including the brain from injury. Naturally, other fluid losses such as blood from hemorrhage, nasogastric drainage, etc. are replaced with appropriate fluids. Urine output is replaced with equal volume of 5% D $^1/_2$NS if a normal electrolyte balance is present. Otherwise, the concentration of salts are altered to correct the specific problems that might exist such as hypo or hypernatremia, acidosis, hypokalemia, etc. Hypothermia and hyperthermia are corrected by the use of the temperature controlled blanket. Antibiotics are given as necessary. If the urine output is not adequate, mannitol and lasix are given, providing that the patient is well hydrated and volume expanded. In the case of adults, we expect them to produce at least 100 cc urine per hour. Although most donors can be resuscitated by fluid management alone, occasionally pressors are required, in which case dopamine is preferred. For dopamine to be effective acidosis must be corrected prior to its use.

Although many of our prospective donors are hypotensive when we are first called, in almost every case, it is possible to restore homeostasis by our method. Nevertheless, the longer a patient remains hypotensive and hypovolemic, the more difficult it becomes to restore cardiovascular normalcy.

We have discovered as noted previously, that provided donor homeostasis as described above is achieved prior to renal excision, a variety of conditions including donor serum creatinine, use of pressors, number of renal arteries, or method of preservation exert no effect on the outcome of the renal transplant. Similar information regarding other organs will be forthcoming as our experience with them increases. Thus donor resuscitation is the first step towards obtaining consistently effective cadaver kidneys.

**The donor operation**

Once donor homeostasis is achieved and permission for donation has been obtained, it is important to carry out organ retrieval with judicious dispatch. This is necessary because eventually, all brain dead individuals will become unstable. Since there is no way of being certain how much time is available prior to donor cardiovascular decompensation, the arrangements for operation are made by the coordinator as soon as is feasible. Two hours prior to the operation, Solumedrol, 30 mg/kg is administered slowly by the intravenous route as part of our pre-treatment protocol.

During the operation, crystalloid is given at a rapid rate in order to ensure diuresis. Dibenzylene is given at a rate of 2 mg/min providing protection against renal artery spasm, and mannitol, 25 g, followed by lasix, 100 mg are given 15 min prior to clamping the aorta. The operation is designed to minimize traima by an essentially 'no touch' technique which is satisfactory for removal of the kidneys alone or along with other extra renal organs such as the liver, pancreas, heart and lungs.

## Technique

A midline incision, xiphoid to pubis, is made using electrocoagulation in order to carry out a standard 'en bloc' nephrectomy. If extrarenal organs are also to be removed, the incision includes a complete sternal split. Occasionally, during donor hepatectomy, additional, lateral cruciate incisions are added.

The dissection commences with incising the right lateral peritoneum along the line of Toldt so that the right colon and cecum can be separated from the duodenum and the adjacent head of the pancreas. This manoeuvre exposes the vena cava which is separated from its adventitial attachments to the porta hepatis by sharp dissection. The peritoneal incision is then curved superiorly along the base of the small bowel mesentery dividing the ligament of Treitz, permitting the entire small intestine and right colon to be lifted out of the abdomen. The entire abdominal aorta below the superior mesenteric artery is now exposed, skeletonized, and the right and left iliac arteries are divided between large hemoclips. The ureters are next divided near the bladder and dissected superiorly, taking care to preserve the ureteral blood supply. In order to approach the left ureter, the sigmoid colon is freed from the lateral abdominal wall. If the liver is to be taken, its attachments to the abominal wall are next divided and a careful dissection is made of the porta hepatis. The common duct is divided as close to the duodenum as possible and an incision is made in the gallbladder in order to rinse out the bile. The dissection next exposes the celiac and superior mesenteric arteries by dividing the arcuate ligament and the adjacent diaphragm. The hepatic artery is dissected from the liver to the celiac artery, first making sure that there is a single blood supply to the liver and then suture ligating the gastroduodenal, left gastric and splenic arteries. Anomolous right lobe arteries arising from the superior mesenteric or gastroduodenal arteries are carefully preserved.

The portal vein and its branches are dissected so that the splenic vein can be used for flush cooling of the liver and so that the superior mesenteric vein is available, if needed, for the anastomosis with the recipient supra system.

The bare area of the liver is incised, skeletonizing the portal hepatic vena cava. Care is taken to suture ligate all side branches. Finally, the entire retrohepatic vena cava is dissected free from surrounding tissues.

If the pancreas is to be taken, the spleen is carefully preserved and used as a handle so that the pancreas is not traumatized. In this case, the portal, superior mesentery, and splenic veins are dissected at their junctions and the celiac artery with its splenic branches is carefully preserved for the transplant (11).

If the heart is to be removed, the superior and inferior vena cava are dissected as well as the pulmonary artery and the thoracic aorta, including all its branches.

When the kidneys alone are to be removed, the procedure is simplified by dividing the porta hepatis between clamps. The esophagus is then doubly ligated and divided, using umbilical tapes, the spleen is feed from its attachments, the left lateral peritoneum is incised, and the celiac, superior mesenteric, and inferior mesenteric arteries are clipped and divided. In one motion, the entire anterior viscera are removed from the abdomen, placed on the sterile drapes over the donors legs, and covered with a sterile, impermeable drape. This maneuver leaves the kidneys untouched and now easily accessible to removal.

After complete systemic heparinization (20,000 units I.V.), one of the iliac arteries is cannulated for retrograde perfusion with iced, modified Collins Solution (currently we use Euro-Collins). When the liver is to be preserved, several liters of iced Ringer's solution are first infused via the splenic vein in order to bring the temperature of the liver down to 30° C. When all is ready, the abdominal aorta is clamped at the diaphragm, divided, and retrograde perfusion of the kidneys, liver (if used) and pancreas (if used) is begun using the iced Collins solution. If the liver is to be used, additional iced Collins solution is perfused via the splenic vein cannula. The vena cava is opened above the renal veins and the kidneys can be excised rapidly, protected from external trauma by leaving them within Gerota's fascia. The kidneys, within Gerota's fascia, are separated from their lateral, abdominal wall attachments, and the dissection proceeds from above down using the aortic clamp for traction and staying right on the vertebrae. The adrenals are taken with the kidneys. As soon as the block of tissue is removed it is immersed in an iced saline basin where lumbar vessels are clipped and the renal vessels are dissected while gently distended with a slow infusion of iced Euro-Collins solution. The adrenals, and adventitious matter are then removed. If there are polar vessels with separate blood supply, they can be attached in the basin using micro surgical techniques (12). Preservation of the kidneys is then accomplished 'en bloc' by pulsatile preservation or individually by a cold infusion of iced Collins solution and cold storage.

The heart, liver and pancreas are preserved only by cold, infusion storage, placed on ice in plastic containers surrounded with Collins solution, and must be taken immediately to the recipients who have been synchronously prepared for transplant. Here, again the coordinators play an important role in organizing the complex arrangements.

The advantages of this technique are many. It permits routinization of the complex task of safely removing two kidneys and perhaps the heart, the liver and/or pancreas for transplant. In situ retrograde cooling via the iliac arteries avoids damage to the renal arteries, even when they are multiple, and provides excellent perfusion of the liver and pancreas. If pulsatile perfusion of the kidneys is used, this method avoids intimal damage to the renal vessels. This technique is thus the second important step in consistently obtaining useful organs for transplant.

**Distribution or transportation**

The logistics of organ distribution have become increasingly important as effective organ procurement programs are established and as organ sharing become widespread. As described in the previous sections, transportation of the heart, liver, and pancreas is carried out by the most rapid means possible to the center where, synchronously, the recipient has been prepared to receive the organ. Currently, the safe preservation time for hearts has been $4\frac{1}{2}$ h, 12–14 h for the liver, and 4–5 h for the pancreas. Because of these time constraints, helicopters and rented aircraft are used along with air to ground contact in order to carry out the process with precision.

Kidneys, of course, can be preserved for at least 50 h by the cold storage method with Collins solution and for at least 72 h when a preservation machine is used (13). Because of the enormous need for cadaver kidneys, we use them locally if an appropriate recipient can be found. If not, a national search for recipients is coordinated using a terminal hooked into U.N.O.S. (The United Network for Organ Sharing) and by calling Terasaki's recipient registry. If there are several centers that would like the kidney, donor lymphoid tissue is sent to their tissue typing lab for crossmatching. Then, depending on the time the kidneys have already been preserved as well as the method of preservation, the kidneys are sent, accompanied by a technologist, by either a scheduled airline or by rental aircraft.

Only when no suitable recipient can be found in America, are the kidneys shipped abroad. It has been possible to transport cadaver kidneys from Chicago to Europe, Greece, Turkey and Kuwait (14). In our view, it is laudatory and important to assist other countries by providing kidneys for their patients, but it does the United States transplant programs and their patients a gross disservice if kidneys are shipped abroad without a thorough search for candidates in America. Problems that remain to be solved are methods for rapid communication and making the international plane connections rapidly enough so that the kidneys and the accompanying lymphoid tissue are useful when they arrive.

Finally, for international cooperation to flourish, it is necessary for the nations receiving the kidneys to pay the expenses of not only transport, but also retrieval and preservation. It is not fair to expect the American organ procurement programs to support this endeavor.

**Conclusions**

1. Organ procurement is central to effective clinical transplant programs.
2. Coordinators provide valuable and essential services for these programs.
3. Donor resuscitation provides for uniformly acceptable organs for transplant.
4. Atraumatic organ harvest methods are essential.

5. Distribution requires experienced coordinators and national and international cooperation.

## References

1. Merkel FK, Jonasson O, Bergan JJ: Procurement of cadaver donor organs: evisceration technique. Transpl Proc 4: 585, 1972.
2. Schweitzer R, Sulphin BA, Bartus SA: Insitu cadaver kidney perfusion. Transpl 32: 482, 1981.
3. Collins GN, Bravo-Shugerman M, Terasaki PI: Kidney preservation for transportation: initial perfusion and 30 hours ice storage. Lancet 2: 1219, 1969.
4. Stuart FP, Veith FJ, Crawford RE: Brain death laws and patterns of consent to remove organs for transplantation from the United States and 28 other countries. Transpl 4: 238, 1981.
5. Sophie LR, Sulloway JC, Sorock G, Volek P, Merkel FK: Intensive care nurses' perceptions of cadaver organ procurement. Heart Lung 12(3): 261, 1983.
6. Merkel FK, Seim SK, Haynes KM, Volek PJ: The role of the community hospital in kidney transplantation. Comprehensive Therapy 4: 65, 1978.
7. Anderson OS, Jonasson O, Merkel FK: 'En bloc' transplantation of pediatric kidneys into adult patients. Arch Surg 108: 35, 1974.
8. Seim SK, Maisel KE, Merkel FK: The effect of length of preservation on renal transplant survival. Surg Gynecol Obstet 145: 705, 1977.
9. Rolles K, Calne RY, McMaster P: Technique of organ removal and fate of kidney grafts from liver donors. Transpl 28: 44, 1979.
10. Shaw BW, Hakula T, Rosenthal JT, Iwatsuki S, Broznick B, Starzl TE: Combination donor hepatectomy and nephrectomy and early functional results of allografts. Surg Gynecol Obstet 155: 321.
11. Merkel FK, Poticha SM, Nudelmann EJ, Colwell JA, Bergan JJ: Pancreas transplantation in man: I the donor and recipient operations. Arch Surg 103: 205, 1971.
12. Merkel FK, Straus AK, Anderson O, Barnett A: Microvascular techniques for polar artery reconstruction in kidney transplants. Surgery 79: 253, 1976.
13. Squifflet JP, Pisson Y, Gianello P: Safe preservation of human renal cadaver transplants by Euro-Collins solution up to 50 hours. Transpl Proc 13: 693, 1981.
14. Merkel FK, Seim SK, Haynes KM, Volek PJ: Relevant factors for worldwide sharing of kidneys. Transpl Proc 11: 1472, 1979.

# 11. Procurement of kidneys from non heart beating donors

T.J.M. RUERS, J.P.A.M. VROEMEN, J.A. VAN DER VLIET and G. KOOTSTRA

## Introduction

In the development of donor kidney procurement in the Netherlands two improvements can be noticed (Fig. 1). The first is the introduction of reimbursement of the procurement costs in 1974. The second is the appointment of transplant coordinators in the years 1978–1982. Nowadays five transplant coordinators are employed in the Netherlands. From 1974 to 1982 the yearly number of harvested kidneys was doubled (1). Since 1982, however, the number of harvested kidneys, mostly from heart beating cadaveric donors, has not increased. Presently 22 kidneys are retrieved per million inhabitants per year. The estimated need for the Netherlands is about 32 kidneys per million inhabitants per year (2). One of the possibilities to improve the supply of cadaveric kidneys for transplantation is to harvest kidneys from *non-* heartbeating donors (NHB).

Until recently the only source of cadaveric donor organs were the heart-beating braindead patients. From these donors kidneys can be harvested with short warm ischaemic periods, under elective surgical conditions. Patients with circulatory arrest were not considered for organ donation.

In 1975 Garcia Rinaldi (3) described a method for *in situ* cold preservation (ISP) of kidneys, that allowed the procurement of kidneys from these previously unsuitable donors. For this purpose the double balloon triple lumen (DBTL) catheter was designed. By flushing cold Eurocollins through this catheter, the kidneys can be cooled *in situ* within a few minutes. Once the kidneys have been cooled, metabolism is slowed down and subsequently elective nephrectomy can be performed.

In experimental as well as in clinical studies (3) it has been demonstrated that this technique is satisfactory for *in situ* renal preservation prior to nephrectomy. Recent reports by Garvin *et al.* (4), Van der Vliet (5) and Vroemen (6) confirm the suitability of this method for kidney retrieval.

In January 1981 facilities for this procedure were implemented in our institution. In January 1983 the ISP method was introduced in regional hospitals as well. Since 1981 30% of the donor kidneys in our area were retrieved from NHB donors using ISP.

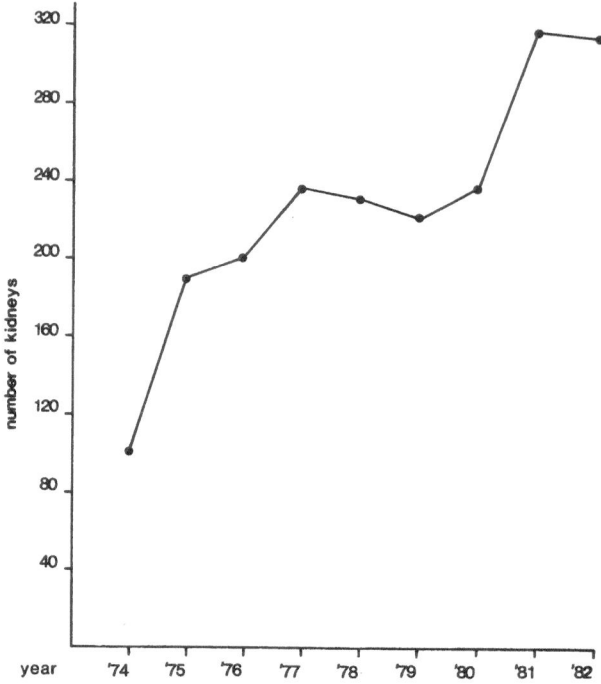

*Fig. 1.* Number of cadaver kidneys harvested in the Netherlands.

In this paper the possibilities and the problems we encountered with ISP are outlined and discussed.

## Materials and methods

*DBTL catheter.* The catheter is designed to selectively perfuse that part of aorta where the renal arteries take their origin. By means of two balloons the abdominal aorta is blocked at the bifurcation and at the level of the diaphragm, confining the infusion of Eurocollins to the area in between. In this way simultaneous perfusion of both renal arteries and any additional renal artery (Fig. 2) is obtained. In this study we used the DBTL catheter distributed by Warne Surgical Products.

*Method of insertion.* As soon as there is an indication for ISP we resume or start cardiac massage and artificial ventilation in order to provide the kidneys with oxygenated blood. The groin of the donor is disinfected and sterile drapes are applied. The required instruments are available in a sterile set in the emergency ward and at the intensive care station. A longitudinal incision is made over the femoral vessels from approximately 5 cm above to 10 cm below the inguinal

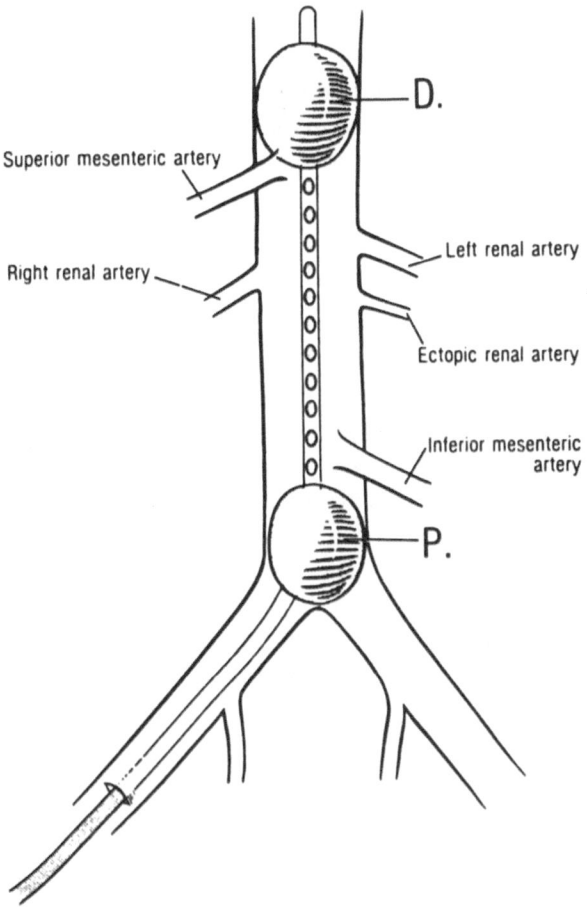

Superior mesenteric artery

D.

Left renal artery

Right renal artery

Ectopic renal artery

Inferior mesenteric artery

P.

*Fig. 2.* Diagnostic representation of the double balloon-triple-lumen catheter when inserted into the abdominal aorta.

ligament. The femoral artery is identified, and arteriotomy is performed. The DBTL catheter is inserted into the abdominal aorta as far as possible. The lower balloon (proximal) is inflated with 10–20 ml of sterile saline and the catheter is pulled back till it hooks on the bifurcation of the aorta. The diaphragmatic balloon (distal) is then inflated with 10–20 ml sterile saline. The segment of the aorta which is isolated includes the superior mesenteric artery, the renal arteries and the inferior mesenteric artery. Cold (4°C) Eurocollins solution is infused in the isolated segment of the aorta. An initial flow rate of approximately 150 ml/min is necessary to cool the kidneys. After 4000 ml, the infusion rate can be reduced. An additional phlebotomy of the femoral vein and introduction of an outflow catheter into the caval vein will improve the perfusion of the kidneys. The donor nephrectomy can now be scheduled.

*Preservation methods.* In this study two methods for long-term preservation of the organs were arbitrarily used. One group of kidneys was preserved by pulsatile perfusion on the Gambro preservation machine. Flow characteristics and LDH levels in the perfusate were studied in order to asses viability of the kidneys as described by Belzer and Kountz and Baxby and Johnson (7, 8, 9). The second group of kidneys was preserved by simple cold storage.

## Legal aspects

In the Netherlands it is mandatory to obtain permission for organ donation from relatives and in case of unnatural death also from legal authorities. If the patient is carrying a donor card, relatives consent is still necessary for donor nephrectomy but the ISP procedure can be started. If relatives cannot be found in time, donor nephrectomy is cancelled. If the patient is not carrying a donor card we always ask for relatives consent before inserting the DBTL catheters. Permission for organ donation from legal authorities can be asked after ISP has started. The incidence of refusal by relatives from NHB donors is higher compared to heart beating donors. An explanation could be that in case of a non-heart-beating donor the relatives are too abruptly confronted with the death of a family member and the request for organ donation.

## Donors

ISP was successfully performed in 12 patients with circulatory arrest. Two groups of NHB donors could be distinguished. The first group consisted of 8 patients who succumbed to cardiac arrest due to myocardial disease of multi trauma. These patients were often seen after a considerable period of circulatory arrest. The second group consisted of 4 patients who had been declared braindead, but developed circulatory arrest prior to the scheduled nephrectomy.

First warm ischemic time (WIT) defined as time lapse between cessation of circulation of the donor and the start of perfusion with Eurocollins, ranged from one minute to 80 min (mean: 32 minutes) (Table 1). Hypotensive periods before circulatory arrest ranged from a few minutes to $2\frac{1}{2}$ h. The age of the patients ranged from 11 years to 60 years with a mean value of 38 years.

In three patients ISP was attempted in vain. In two cases insertion of the catheter was impossible because of atherosclerotic stenosis of both iliac arteries. In one case severe kinking of the distal aorta due to malformations of the lumbar vertebral column prevented insertion. In these three cases kidneys were not harvested, and are therefore not included in this study.

Machine preservation was used in 7 cases; cold storage in the remaining 5 cases. Kidneys were distributed by the Eurotransplant Foundation. Recipient selection was based on HLA A-B and Dr matching criteria.

*Table 1.* Donor data.

| | |
|---|---|
| Number: | 12 |
| Age: | 11–60 (mean 38 year) |
| First WIT: | 1 min–80 min, mean 32 minutes |
| Indication: | – 8 cases of cardiac arrest due to heart disease or multitrauma |
| | – 4 cases of braindead patients who developed circulatory arrest |
| Preservation method: | – Gambro perfusion machine in 7 cases (14 kidneys) |
| | – Cold storage in 5 cases (9 kidneys). |

## Results

The 12 donor nephrectomies after ISP resulted in 23 harvested kidneys. One kidney was not removed because it was severely damaged by blunt trauma. Out of the 23 kidneys, two kidneys (one pair) were discarded because viability testing during machine preservation revealed negative data. In two other kidneys shipped outside the Eurotransplant area, the local crossmatch turned out to be positive and there was no time left to select another recipient. The total number of kidneys that were transplanted amounts to 19 (Table 2).

Eight grafts showed immediate function. Five grafts showed delayed function. Delayed function was defined as requiring dialysis treatment for some time, followed by good function. Six kidneys never functioned. Of these non functioning kidneys three never functioned probably because of severe ischaemic damage. Two out of these three kidneys showed ATN at micropathological examination. These two kidneys were from a 50 year old donor, who suffered from

*Table 2.* Results ISP technique.

| Kidney function | Number of kidneys | Meant WIT donor | Mean highest post-transplant creatinine clearance. ml/min |
|---|---|---|---|
| Immediate function | 8 | 23 min | 65 ml/min |
| Delayed function | 5 | 40 min | 68 ml/min |
| Never function | | | |
| – ATN (one pair) cortical necrosis | 2 1 | 35 min | – |
| – other causes acute rejection arterial trombosis recipient death, CVA | 3 | 32 min | – |
| Total | 19 | | |

circulatory instability for some days before cardiac arrest occurred. In the third kidney histopathological examination showed cortical necrosis. The twin kidney was never transplanted because of a positive crossmatch.

In the remaining three kidneys other causes were apparent for non functioning, while the respective twin kidneys were functioning well. One graft was lost due to arterial thrombosis eight hours after transplantation. Another kidney had to be removed because of acute rejection. In the third, the recipient died from a cerebral haemorrhage three days after transplantation.

In conclusion 18 patients have or could have profited from the energy invested in 12 ISP donors.

Table 3 shows graft function related to first warm ischaemic time. If WIT was shorter than 25 min all grafts were viable. Delayed or non function was seen more frequently when WIT was beyond 25 min.

As mentioned we used two different methods of preservation. Table 4 shows the influence of preservation method. Kidneys discarded because of perfusion characteristics (2) or positive cross match (2) are not shown.

*Table 3.* First WIT and graft function.

| WIT donor | Immediate function | Delayed function | Never function |
|---|---|---|---|
| 1–25 min | 5 | 1 | 1 trombosis<br>1 acute rejection |
| 25–40 min | 1 | 2 | 2 ATN (pair) |
| over 40 min | 2 | 2 | 1 cortical necrosis<br>1 recipient death |

*Tabel 4.* Machine perfusion versus cold storage of ISP kidneys.

| | Number of transpl. kidneys | Mean WIT donor | Immediate function | Delayed function | Never function |
|---|---|---|---|---|---|
| Machine preservation | 12 | 34 min | 7 | 2 | 2 ATN (pair)<br>1 recipient death |
| Cold storage | 7 | 23 min | 1 | 3 | 1 cortical necrosis<br>1 acute rejection<br>1 trombosis |

## Discussion

Although the optimal donor continues to be the braindead patient, with an intact circulation, the ISP technique allows the harvesting of kidneys from donors previously considered unsuitable (Garvin (4), Van der Vliet (5), Vroemen (6)).

This study confirms that NHB donor kidneys can reach adequate function and that WIT up to 25 min is safe.

Insertion of the catheter and start of ISP takes 5–10 min. The decision to start the ISP procedure has to be taken as soon as possible after circulatory arrest has occurred.

Prompt action and direct availability of personnel and equipment is necessary. The instruments and preservation fluid should be permanently available in the emergency ward, and Intensive Care Units. The minor surgical procedure required for ISP can be performed by any surgical resident on call.

In order to guarantee that the therapeutic management of the potential donor is not adversely affected, our protocol demands the declaration of death by two independent physicians, who are not involved in organ retrieval for transplantation.

Several anatomical disorders may be responsible for the failure of ISP. In those cases emergency laparotomy and insertion of the catheter in the iliac vessels or the aorta can be considered. Technical problems such as rupture of one of the balloons and obstruction of venous outflow can be encountered. ISP may increase the risk of contamination of the kidneys or vessel injury during surgery (6, 10).

The time interval between the start of the perfusion and subsequent donor nephrectomy varied between 45 min and three hours in our study. In the literature no limit concerning the admissable duration of ISP has been given. However, we recommend ISP to be as short as possible.

For kidneys, that have not been subjected to prolonged periods of warm ischaemia, preservation results of simple cold storage are equal to continuous pulsatile perfusion (11–20). For ischaemically damaged kidneys this is not firmly established (5, 15, 17, 18, 20, 21, 22). We used both methods, but the data do not warrant conclusions concerning the choice of preservation method after ISP.

Since the introduction of the DBTL catheter in our organ procurement area, 30% of all available donor kidneys are harvested from NHB donors.

We feel that in view of the persistent shortage of donor kidneys inclusion of non-heart-beating donors in all harvesting programs is justified.

114

## References

1. Cohen B: Eurotransplant Annual Report 1980 and 1981, Leiden, The Netherlands.
2. Van der Vliet JA, Kootstra G: The transplant coordinator: an answer to the shortage of cadaveric donor kidneys? Neth J Surg 34: 1, 1982.
3. Garcia-Rinaldi R, Lefrak EA, Defore WW et al: In situ preservation of cadaver kidneys for transplantation. Ann Surg 182: 576, 1975.
4. Garvin PJ, Buttorf JD, Morgan R et al: In situ cold perfusion of kidneys for transplantation. Arch Surg 115: 180, 1980.
5. Van der Vliet JA, Slooff MJH, Rijkmans BG et al: Use of non-heart-beating donor kidneys for transplantation. Eur Surg Res 13: 354, 1981.
6. Vroemen JPAM, Van der Vliet JA, Kootstra G: The emergency in situ preservation of kidneys for transplantation. Neth Journ Surg 35: 2, 1983.
7. Belzer FO, Kountz SL: Preservation and transplantation of human cadaver kidneys. Ann Surg 172: 394, 1970.
8. Belzer FO: Renal preservation. N Engl J Med 291: 402, 1974.
9. Baxby K, Johnson RWG. Prediction of kidney viability before transplantation. Br J Surg 62: 810, 1975.
10. Van der Vliet JA, Kootstra G, Krom RAF: Cadaveric organ retrieval for transplantation. World J Surg 6: 478, 1982.
11. Barry JM, Farnsworth MA, Bennett WM: Human kidney preservation by flushing with intra-cellular solution and cold storage. Arch Surg 113: 830, 1978.
12. Squifflet JP, Pirson Y, Gianello P et al: Safe preservation of human renal cadaver transplants by Euro-Collins solution up to 50 hours. Transplant Proc 13: 693, 1981.
13. Barry JM, Lieberman S, Wickre C et al: Human kidney preservation by intracellular electrolyte flush followed by cold storage for over 24 hours. Transplantation 32: 485, 1981.
14. Barry JM, Metcalfe JB, Farnsworth MA et al. Comparison of intracellular flushing and cold storage to machine perfusion for human kidney preservation. J Urol 123: 14, 1980.
15. Opelz G, Terasaki PI. Advantage of cold storage over machine perfusion for preservation of cadaver kidneys. Transplantation 33: 64, 1982.
16. Marchall VC: Renal preservation prior to transplantation. Transplantation 30: 165, 1980.
17. Collins GM, Halasz NA. Clinical comparison of methods for cadaveric kidney preservation. J Surg Res 24: 396, 1978.
18. Slooff MJH, Van der Wijk J, Rijkmans BG et al: Machine perfusion versus cold storage for preservation of kidneys before transplantation. Arch Chir Neerl 30: 84, 1978.
19. Belzer FO, Southard JH. The future of kidney preservation. Transplantation 30: 161, 1980.
20. Van der Vliet JA, Vroemen JPAM, Cohen B et al: Preservation of cadaver kidneys; cold storage or machine perfusion? Arch Surg (in press).
21. Halasz NA, Collins GM: Forty-eight-hour kidney preservation. Arch Surg 111: 175, 1976.
22. Johnson RWG, Anderson M, Marley AR et al: Twenty-four-hour preservation of kidneys injured by prolonged warm ischaemia. Transplantation 13: 174, 1972.

# 12. Donor age in cadaveric renal transplantation

J.A. VAN DER VLIET, G.G. PERSIJN, B. COHEN and
G. KOOTSTRA

## 1. Introduction

The number of cadaveric kidneys available for transplantation continues to be insufficient in most parts of the world. The persistent shortage of donor kidneys is reflected by increasing waiting lists of patients with end-stage renal failure and prolonged waiting times for renal transplantation. Activation of donor procurement programmes is necessary in order to reduce the shortage of donor organs. The influence of donor age is important, because donor age limits directly affect the number of available kidneys. Adult cadaveric donors under 50 years of age are the preferred organs source in many transplant centers. In view of the insufficient number of available kidneys, it is essential to avoid waste of useful donor kidneys. However, transplantation of unsuitable donor kidneys should always be avoided. Therefore a study was performed to determine advisable upper and lower age limits for cadaveric kidney donors, to enable us to make optimal use of the organ donor potential.

## 2. Material and methods

From 1967 to 1981, 7339 cadaveric renal transplantations were performed in 39 centers cooperating in the Eurotransplant organisation. In 539 cases no donor age was reported; these were excluded from the study. In the remaining 6800 cases, 626 renal allografts were from pediatric donors, under 11 years of age, and 181 were from donors over 50 years of age. The transplantation results in these two groups were compared with those of a control series consisting of 5993 transplantations of kidneys from adult cadaveric donors, between the ages of 10 and 51, performed in the same period. The mean donor age was 6.8 years (range: 0–10) in the pediatric kidney group, 26.3 years (range: 11–50) in the adult kidney control group and 54.1 years (range: 51–70) in the advanced age kidney group. There were no differences in the mean recipient age, mean mismatch for HLA-A and B antigens, pretransplant bloodtransfusion history, retransplantation rate and mean preservation time among the different groups. The selection of all recip-

116

ients was uniform and based on HLA matching criteria.

Actuarial methods were used to compute graft survival. Graft function was measured as the highest postoperative creatinine clearance in the group of advanced age kidneys and in a subgroup of 74 transplantations of kidneys from donors under 3 years of age. In this subgroup 39 kidneys were transplanted as single units and 35 were en bloc transplantations of both kidneys from the same donor. The mean donor age in these groups was 20.3 months and 15.2 months, respectively.

Statistical analysis was done by means of log-rank of chi-square tests.

## 3. Results

The cumulative graft survival of the pediatric kidney group and that of the adult kidney control series are shown in Figure 1. At one, two and five years after transplantation the graft survival in the pediatric donor group was 57,4%, 49,9% and 40,6%, respectively. There was no significant difference (p <0.09) with the graft survival in the adult donor control series, which was 61.8% at one year, 55.1% at two and 43.3% at five years after transplantation.

The 1 year graft survival of the en bloc grafts and the single renal transplants from donors under 3 years of age was 56.2% and 50.5%, respectively. There was no significant difference (p <0.4). Figure 2 shows the graft function in these subgroups. The mean highest creatinine clearance of the functioning grafts was 72.4 ml/min. No difference in graft function was observed between the en bloc grafts and the single renal transplants.

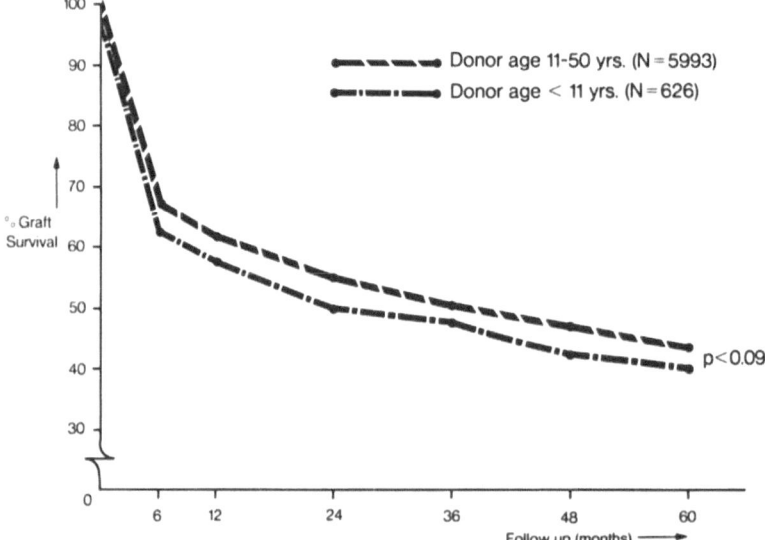

*Fig. 1.* Actuarial graft survival of the pediatric kidney group and the adult kidney control series.

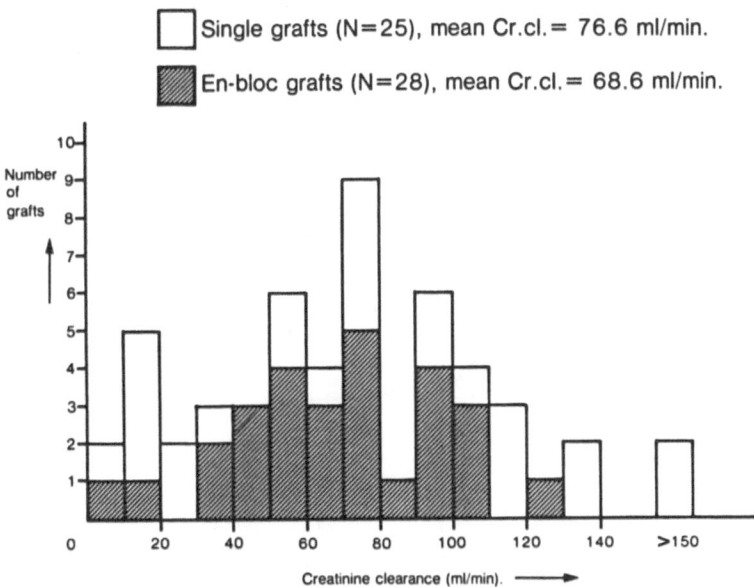

*Fig. 2.* Graft function of pediatric kidneys from cadaveric donors under 3 years of age.

Figure 3 shows the cumulative graft survival of the advanced age kidney group, compared to that of the adult kidney control series. The graft survival was 48.9%, 39.2% and 34.9% at one, two and five years after transplantation. The graft survival in the control series was significantly better (p <0.0002). This difference was partly due to the poor transplantation results in a subgroup of kidneys from donors of 60 years of age and above (n = 11). One year after transplantation the graft survival in this subgroup was 14.2%. The graft function analysis of the advanced age kidney group is shown in Figure 4. The mean highest creatinine clearance of the functioning grafts was 81.5 ml/min.

## 4. Discussion

Although cadaveric kidneys from pediatric donors are considered suitable for transplantation into pediatric recipients, they are relatively less often used for transplantation into adult recipients. Transplantation of pediatric kidneys into adult recipients is reported to result in poor graft survival caused by frequent vascular and urological postoperative complications (1–6) and damage to the grafts, inflicted at the time of the more difficult organ harvesting and preservation (4, 6, 7). It has also been suggested that pediatric kidneys have insufficient nephron mass to provide adequate graft function in adults (4, 5, 8). This study did not demonstrate a negative effect of pediatric donor age on renal allograft survival and its results are in accordance with other reports, which recommend

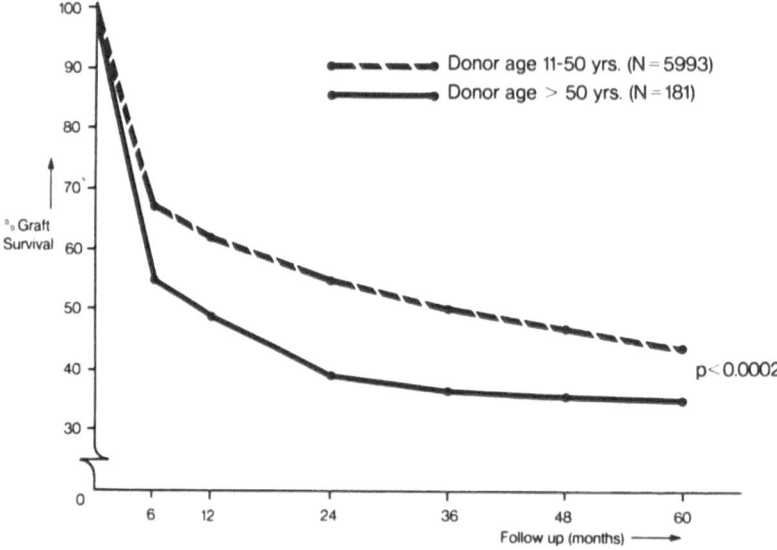

*Fig. 3.* Actuarial graft survival of the advanced age kidney group and the adult kidney control series.

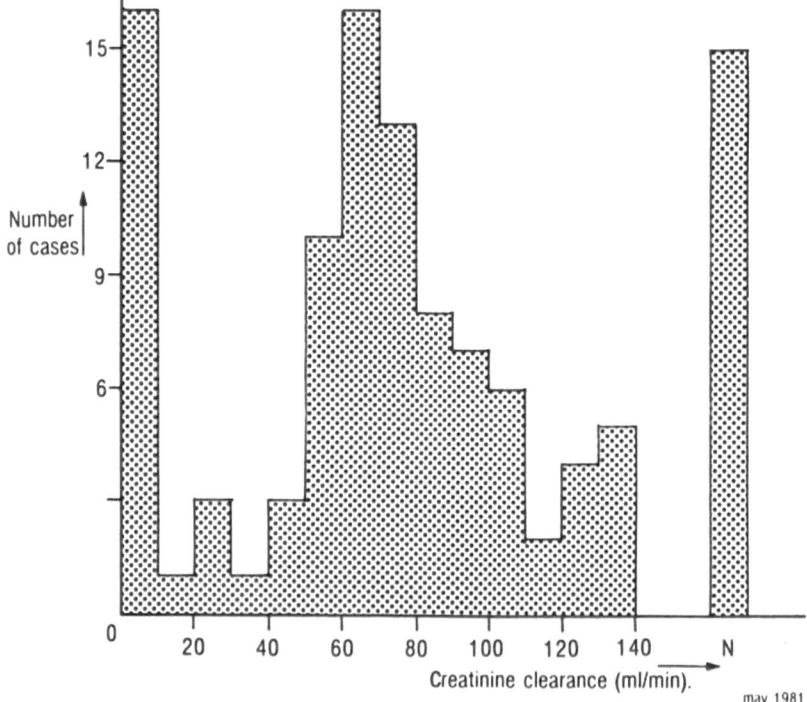

*Fig. 4.* Graft function of kidneys from elderly cadaveric donors. N = unspecified, indicated as 'normal'. Number of patients: 110.

the use of pediatric cadaver kidneys for transplantation in adult recipients (3, 6, 7, 9–12). The renal function of even the smallest pediatric allografts was satisfactory. En bloc transplantation of both kidneys from pediatric donors has been recommended in case of very small donor size (1, 4, 5, 8, 13–15). No beneficial effect of en bloc grafting could be demonstrated in this study. A disadvantage of the en bloc technique is that each donor provides or renal allograft for one recipient only. The advantage of a bigger nephron mass, more closely approximating the needs of the allograft recipient, offered by en bloc grafting, seems to be negated by early graft hypertrophy after transplantation (16–24). There seems to be no reason to propose a lower age limit for cadaveric kidney donors, as good results have been obtained even with transplantation of kidneys from anencephalic donors (4, 7, 13–16, 25). A recent report on the post mortem examinations of a large series of anencephalic newborns revealed a surprisingly low rate of anatomical abnormalities in their kidneys and urinary tracts (26).

Although effects of aging on renal function, renal haemodynamics and the histology of the human kidney have been extensively described no conclusions concerning the suitability for transplantation of the elderly kidney can be drawn from these reports (27–32). Of special interest are clinical studies of the compensatory renal hypertrophy following contralateral nephrectomy, which show that this mechanism is not impaired in older patients (33, 34). 'Experimental and clinical studies indicate that kidney response to temporary ischaemia is age independent (35, 36). The reluctance to transplant cadaveric kidneys from advanced age donors is mainly based on reports of a negative influence of progressing donor age on renal allograft survival (37, 38), although this finding is not confirmed in several other studies (9, 39–41). No reports have been made of decreased graft function in relation to increasing donor age and no adverse effect of the use of cadaveric kidneys from donors over 50 years of age on graft function could be demonstrated in this study. The graft survival in the group of advanced age donor kidneys was acceptable, but significantly decreased in comparison with the control series. Inferior results were obtained in a small subgroup of kidneys from donors over 60 years of age. Based on these observations it seems justified to advise an upper age limit of 60 years for cadaveric kidney donors.

As long as the amount of cadaveric donor kidneys for transplantation continues to be insufficient organ procurement activities must be intensified and attention must be paid to underdeveloped sources of usable donor kidneys (42, 43). This study has indicated that pediatric donors and advanced age donors up to 60 years of age can be valuable sources of cadaveric kidneys for transplantation.

## Acknowledgements

The material for this study was acquired by courtesy of all transplant centers cooperating in the Eurotransplant Foundation. The authors thank Ms. M. van den Berg for her secretarial assistance.

## References

1. Merkel MK, Ing TS, Ahmadian Y, Lewy P, Ambruster K, Oyama J, Sulieman JS, Belman AB, King LR: Transplantation in and of the young. J Urol 111: 679–686, 1974.
2. Managadze LG, Oesterwitz H, Scholtz D, May G, Mebel M: The use of pediatric cadaver kidneys in renal transplantation. Int Urol Nephrol 13: 95–104, 1981.
3. Fine RN, Brennan LP, Edelbrock HH, Riddell H, Stiles Q, Lieberman E: Use of pediatric cadaver kidneys for homotransplantation in children. JAMA 210: 477–484, 1969.
4. Meakins JL, Smith EJ, Alexander JW: En bloc transplantation of both kidneys from pediatric donors into adult patients. Surgery 71: 72–75, 1972.
5. Anderson OS, Jonasson O, Merkel FK: En bloc transplantation of pediatric kidneys into adult patients. Arch Surg 108: 35–37, 1974.
6. Kootstra G, West JC, Dryburgh P, Krom RAF, Putnam ChW, Weil R: Pediatric cadaver kidneys for transplantation. Surgery 83: 333–337, 1978.
7. Salvatierra O, Belzer FO: Pediatric cadaver kidneys. Arch Surg 110: 181–183, 1975.
8. Kinne DW, Spanos PK, McGrade-De Shazo M, Simmons RL, Najarian JS: Double renal transplants from pediatric donors to adult recipients. Am J Surg 127: 292–295, 1974.
9. Van Speybroeck J, Feduska N, Amend W, Vincenti F, Cochrum K, Salvatierra O: The influence of donor age on graft survival. Am J Surg 137: 374–377, 1979.
10. Boczko S, Tellis V, Veith FJ. Transplantation of children's kidneys into adult recipients: Surg Gyn Obstet 146: 387–390, 1978.
11. Glass RN, Stillman RM, Butt KMH, Kountz SL: Results of renal transplantation using pediatric cadaver donors. Surgery 85: 504–508, 1979.
12. Van der Vliet JA, Kootstra G, Tegzess AM, Meijer S, Slooff MJH, Krom RAF, Zwierstra RP: The use of pediatric cadaver kidneys for transplantation in adult recipients. Z Kinderchir 32 (2): 152–156, 1981.
13. Martin LW, Gonzalez LL, West CD, Swartz RA, Sutorius DJ: Homotransplantation of both kidneys from an anencephalic monster to a 17-pound boy with Eagle-Barrett syndrome. Surgery 66: 603–607, 1969.
14. Dreikorn K, Rohl L, Horsch R: The use of double renal transplants from pediatric cadaver donors. Br J Urol 49: 361–364, 1977.
15. Piza F: Zur Verwendung kindlicher Leichen für die homologe Nierentransplantation. Munch Med Wschr 50: 2286–2291, 1970.
16. Iitaka K, Martin LW, Cox JA, McEnery PT, West CD: Transplantation of cadaver kidneys from anencephalic donors. J Pediatr 93: 216–220, 1978.
17. Fine RN, Edelbrock HH, Brennan LP, Grushkin CM, Korsch BM, Riddell H, Stiles Q, Lieberman E: Cadaveric renal transplantation in children. Lancet I: 1087–1091, 1971.
18. Baden JP, Wolf GM, Sellers RD: The growth and development of transplanted neonatal canine kidneys. J Surg Res 14: 213–220, 1973.
19. Silber SJ: Renal transplantation between adults and children. JAMA 228: 1143–1145, 1974.
20. Shames D, Murphy JJ, Berkowitz H: Evidence for a humoral factor in unilaterally nephrec- tomised dogs stimulating renal growth in isolated canine kidneys. Surgery 79: 573–576, 1976.
21. Olivetti G, Anversa P, Melissari M, Loud AV: Morphometry of the renal corpuscle during

postnatal and compensatory hypertrophy. Kidney Int 17: 438–454, 1980.

22. Larsson L, Aperia A, Wilton P: Effect of normal development on compensatory renal growth. Kidney Int 18: 29–35, 1980.
23. Ingelfinger JR, Teele R, Treves S, Levey RH: Renal growth after transplantation: Infant kidney received by adolescent. Clin Nephrol 15: 28–32, 1981.
24. Herrin JT: Pediatric renal transplantation. Kidney Int 18: 519–529, 1980.
25. Kinnaert P, Persijn GG, Cohen B, Van Geertruyden J: Transplantation of kidneys from anencephalic donors. Transplant Proc: in press.
26. Spees EK, Clark GB, Smith MT: Are anencephalic neonates suitable as kidney and pancreas donors? Transplant Proc: in press.
27. Darmandy EM, Offer J, Woodhouse MA: The parameters of the aging kidney. J Pathol 109: 195–207, 1973.
28. Epstein M: Effects of aging on the kidney. Fed Proc 38: 168–172, 1979.
29. Friedman SA, Raizner AE, Rosen H, Solomon NA, Sy W: Functional defects in the aging kidney. Ann Int Med 76: 41–45, 1972.
30. Hollenberg NK, Adams DF, Solomon HS, Rashid A, Abrams HL, Merrill JP: Senescence and the renal vasculature in normal man. Circ Res 34: 309–316, 1974.
31. McLachlan MSF: The aging kidney. Lancet II: 143–146, 1978.
32. Boner G, Sherry J and Rieselbach RE. Hypertrophy of the normal human kidney following contralateral nephrectomy. Nephron 9: 364–370, 1972.
33. Takazakura E, Sawabu N, Handa A, Takada A, Shinoda A, Takeuchi J: Intrarenal vascular changes with age and disease. Kidney Int 2: 224–230, 1972.
34. Ekelund L, Göthlin J: Compensatory renal enlargement in older patients. Am J Roentgenol 127: 713–715, 1976.
35. Kunes J, Capek K, Stejskal J, Jelinek J: Age-dependent difference in kidney response to temporary ischaemia in the rat. Clin Sc Mol Med 55: 365–368, 1978.
36. Vroemen JPAM, Van der Vliet JA, Cohen B, Persijn GG, Lansbergen Q, Kootstra G: Warm and cold ischaemic time in cadaveric renal transplantation. Eur Surg Res: in press.
37. Darmandy EM. Transplantation and the aging kidney. Lancet II: 1046–1047, 1974.
38. Morling N, Ladefoged J, Lange P, Nerstrom B, Nielsen B, Staub-Nielsen L, Sorensen BL: Kidney transplantation and donor age. Tissue Antigens 6: 163–166, 1975.
39. Matas AJ, Simmons RL, Kjellstrand CM, Buselmeier TJ, Najarian JS: Transplantation of the aging kidney. Transplantation 21: 160–161, 1976.
40. Solheim BG, Thorsby E, Osbakk TA, Flatmark A, Enger E: Donor age and cumulative kidney graft survival. Tissue Antigens 7: 251–253, 1976.
41. Van der Vliet JA, Persijn GG, Kootstra G: Should the upper age limit for cadaveric kidney donors be changed? Proc Eur Dial Transplant Assoc 18: 439–445, 1981.
42. Van der Vliet JA, Cohen B, Vroemen JPAM, Ruers TJM, Kootstra G: Successful reorganisation of organ procurement in the Netherlands. Transplant Proc: in press.
43. Van der Vliet JA, Kootstra G, Krom RAF: Cadaveric organ retrieval for transplantation. World J Surg 6: 478–483, 1982.

# 13. Prolonged preservation of imported cadaveric grafts by ice cooling with Eurocollin's solution versus hypothermic pulsatile perfusion

GEORGE M. ABOUNA, M.S.A. KUMAR, ARTHUR G. WHITE, SALAH K. DADAH and O.S.G. SILVA

## Introduction

In transportation and sharing of organs between widely separated transplant centres, one of the most important criteria to be satisfied is that the kidney remains viable until it is revascularized in the recipient. Another less critical prerequisite is that the procedure of transportation and preservation be simple and in-expensive. Until recently most centres in North America have preferred to preserve kidneys and transport them by hypothermic perfusion using various machines as well as perfusates when ischemia time is expected to exceed 24 to 30 h (1, 2, 3). In many European centres however preservation in iced Eurocollin's solution is generally accepted for periods of 40 to 48 h (4, 5). In the transplant centre in Kuwait we have had the opportunity to utilise 33 kidneys that have been imported from United States and Europe and preserved for periods of 30 to 60 h by either machine perfusion or by simple cooling in Eurocollin's solution. We review herein an analysis of the performance of the first 30 kidneys which have been followed for periods of up to 26 months after transplantation.

## Criteria for acceptance of cadaveric grafts

Since cadaveric kidneys are not yet available in this part of the world we have become dependent upon kidneys offered to us from outside. Often this offer comes after the kidneys have been either rejected by the foreign centre because of some problem in the donor or in the graft (multiple arteries, surgical damage to the kidney or medical problems in the donor prior to death) or because no suitable local recipient can be found even after the kidney had been taken to several centres within the country of origin. Because of our desperate need for cadaveric kidneys our criteria for acceptance are less stringent than at most centres and many less than ideal grafts have been imported and used regardless of the cold ischemia time. However it is our policy not to accept any kidney which has a warm ischemia time of more than 15 min.

## Transportation and preservation of cadaveric grafts

Six of the 30 kidneys reviewed came from European centres (a distance of 5000 to 6000 km) and 24 from various centres within the U.S.A. (a distance of 8000 to 12000 km). The transportation time has been 16 to 26 h often employing the Concorde supersonic jet and at each end of the journey chartered aircrafts. The donors of these kidneys were 6 months to 62 years of age and the recipient age was 11 to 57 years. The HLA mismatch between donor and recipient was from 2 to 4 antigens (mean 2.45) (Table 1 and 2). Upon arrival a cross-match was carried out with several potential recipients before transplantation. Renal transplantation is then carried out using standard techniques except when multiple vessels are present when a variety of reconstructive vascular procedures were employed. During surgery all recipients followed a specified protocol with fluid infusion to a central venous pressure of 12 to 16 cm of water together with 20 grams of mannitol, 40 milligrams of Lasix and 1 gram of Methyl Prednisolone before graft revascularization. After transplantation graft function was monitored by urinary output, serum creatinine, creatinine clearance, radionuclide scanning and by ultrasonography.

In this series, 13 kidneys were preserved and transported by hypothermic perfusion and 17 kidneys by iced Eurocollin's solution. There was no significant difference between the two groups with regard to donor or recipient age, HLA mismatch or the frequency of other problems in the kidney or in the donor (Table 1 and 2).

The kidneys preserved by hypothermic perfusion had a mean total ischemic time of 51.3 h (44–60 h). 12 or 92% of these kidneys functioned within the first 24 h after transplantation and only one patient required four dialysis sessions (8%) before full recovery. This was the recipient of a kidney from a 62 year old donor preserved for 48 h. All kidneys in this group functioned at one month and 9 of these are currently functioning for two to 26 months. The remaining 4 grafts were lost to rejection at 2 to 7 months (Table 3). Nine of the kidneys from this group were preserved for periods greater than 50 h. All 9 kidneys had immediate diuresis and were functioning at one month, without requiring dialysis. At present 6 (66%) of these kidneys are currently functioning. The remaining 3 were lost to rejection.

The remaining 17 kidneys were transported in ice and transplanted after mean preservation period of 48 h (30–57 h). Fourteen of these kidneys functioned within 24 h (82%). Two kidneys required 1 to 3 dialyses before full function was resumed. One kidney never functioned due to histologically proven vascular rejection and was removed at one week. Discounting the latter kidney, the rate of dialysis in this group of kidneys was 12.5%. Fourteen of these 16 kidneys (85.5%) were functioning at one month and 9 (56%) are currently functioning at 2 to 18 months. There were 7 kidneys in this group which were preserved for a period greater than 50 h. Six of these kidneys (85.7%) had immediate diuresis and one

*Table 1.* Details of cadaveric kidneys transplanted after preservation and transportation by pulsatile perfusion.

| Tx. no. | Recip- ient age (sex) | Donor age | HLA mis- match | Problems in donor kidney | Total isch- aemic time (hours) | Immediate diuresis (Output in mls in 1st 24 h) | Function at 1 mon. | Current graft status |
|---|---|---|---|---|---|---|---|---|
| (41) | 42 (M) | 66 | 2 | Donor age 66 | 44 | None | Yes | Serum creatinine 1.9 mg% |
| (55) | 35 (F) | 63 | 4 | Donor age 63 | 60 | Yes (1400) | Yes | Graft rej. 6 weeks |
| (79) | 46 (M) | 37 | 3 | Diabetic donor damaged, 2 renal arteries | 46 | Yes (1665) | Yes | Serum creatinine 2.1 mg% |
| (80) | 42 (M) | 37 | 2 | Diabetic donor 2 damaged renal arteries | 52 | Yes (8000) | Yes | Serum creatinine 1.4 mg% |
| (90) | 43 (F) | 25 | 3 | 2 renal arteries | 44 | Yes (2000) | Yes | Graft rej. patient died at 2 months |
| (98) | 23 (F) | 4 | 3 | Decapsulated kidney. 3 renal arteries | 51 | Yes (1730) | Yes | Serum creatinine 1.5 mg% |
| (99) | 42 (M) | 4 | 3 | Decapsulated kidney 4 renal arteries | 54 | Yes (1225) | Yes | Serum creatinine 1.2 mg% |
| (100) | 25 (F) | 46 | 2 | Proteinuria + Bacteuria | 51 | Yes (2900) | Yes | Graft rej. patient died at 5 months |
| (101) | 45 (M) | 46 | 2 | Proteinuria + Bacteuria | 53 | Yes (5000) | Yes | Serum creatinine 1.2 mg% |
| (108) | 18 (F) | 17 | 3 | 3 renal arteries | 54 | Yes (1500) | Yes | Graft rej. 6 weeks |
| (112) | 22 (F) | 32 | 2 | None | 55 | Yes (1000) | Yes | Serum creatinine 0.6 mg% |
| (115) | 31 (M) | 20 | 3 | None | 52 | Yes (8000) | Yes | Serum creatinine 1.0 mg% |

*Table 2.* Details of cadaveric kidney transplanted after preservation and transportation in iced Eurocollin's solution.

| Tx. no. | Recip- ient age (sex) | Donor age | HLA mis- match | Problems in donor kidney | Total isch- aemic time (hours) | Immediate diuresis (Output in mls in 1st 24 h) | Function at 1 mon. | Current graft status |
|---------|------|-------|-------|--------|-------|---------|------|--------|
| (61) | 35 (F) | 60 | 3 | Donor age 60 devascularized ureter | 42 | Yes (2600) | Yes | Graft rej. 5 months |
| (68) | 34 (F) | 48 | 3 | None | 44 | Yes (2200) | Yes | Graft rej. 6 months |
| (76) | 34 (F) | 51 | 4 | Donor age 50 | 41 | None | Yes | Graft rej. 6 months |
| (104) | 55 (M) | 55 | 1 | Donor age 50 | 49 | No, hyper acute rej. | No | Graft neph- rectomy |
| (106) | 45 (M) | 34 | 3 | None | 47 | Yes (3000) | Yes | Graft rej. 3 months |
| (110) | 32 (M) | 17 | 2 | None | 47 | Yes (2100) | Yes | Serum creatinine 0.9 mg% |
| (113) | 27 (F) | 19 | 2 | None | 55 | Yes (1880) | Yes | Serum creatinine 0.7 mg% |
| (116) | 15 (M) | 37 | 3 | 2 renal arteries damaged renal vein. | 57 | None | Yes | Serum creatinine 0.8 mg% |
| (117) | 35 (F) | 37 | 3 | 2 renal arteries | 55 | Yes (1600) | Yes | Serum creatinine 2.5 mg% |
| (119) | 18 (F) | 13 | 4 | None | 30 | Yes (2990) | Yes | Graft rej. patient died at 2 months |
| (121) | 49 (M) | 18 | 2 | None | 54 | Yes (3500) | Yes | Serum creatinine 1.2 mg% |
| (122) | 30 (F) | 15 | 2 | None | 50 | Yes (1450) | Yes | Graft rej. 2 months |
| (123) | 30 (F) | 15 | 2 | Lacerated renal vein | 51 | Yes (5000) | Yes | Graft rej. 2 months |
| (125) | 47 (M) | 3 | 3 | Donor age 3 | 53 | Yes (4200) | Yes | Graft rej. 3 months |
| (127) | 13 (M) | 47 | 2 | None | 47 | Yes (1200) | Yes | Serum creatinine 1.2 mg% |
| (128) | 50 (M) | 47 | 3 | Devascu- larized ureter | 47 | Yes (500+) (Ureteric Fistula) | Yes | Serum creatinine 1.1 mg% |
| (131) | 31 (F) | 6 months | 2 | Donor age 6 months | 40 | Yes (1600) | Yes | Serum creatinine 1.2 mg% |

*Table 3.* Cadaver donor transplantation in Kuwait. Methods of organ preservation and graft function results.

| Method | No. | Mean ischaemic time (hours) | Immediate diuresis | Functioning at 2 weeks | Functioning at 1 month | Dialysis rate |
|--------|-----|------------------------------|---------------------|-------------------------|-------------------------|----------------|
| Machine | 13 | 51.3 (44–60) | 12 (92%) | 13 | 13 | 8% |
| Ice | 16* | 48 (30–57) | 14 (82%) | 16 | 14 | 12.5% |

* One graft was hyperacutely rejected and is not included.

required temporary dialysis. All 7 kidneys functioned at one month and four are currently functioning at 2 to 7 months after transplantation, but the other three kidneys were rejected at 2 to 4 months, (Fig. 1, Fig.2).

When kidney function at 24 h, 2 weeks and 1 month are compared between the ice preserved and the machine preserved kidneys there is no statistically significant difference (Table 3). Actuarial graft survival of machine preserved and ice preserved kidneys at 3 months, 6 months and one year are shown in Figure 1. Although the machine preserved kidneys have a slightly higher survival rate than the ice preserved kidneys the difference between the two is not statistically significant. The apparent difference was due only to the fact that more kidneys preserved in ice were rejected than those preserved with machine perfusion. In neither group of kidneys did we encounter grafts that never functioned due to ischemic injury or to technical failure. Four patients were lost in the whole series from complications of immunosuppression and 26 or 86.6% are currently alive.

### Discussion

It has been stated that preservation of kidneys by machine perfusion is much more successful when the cold ischemia time is greater than 30 h or when the warm ischemia time is greater than 20 min. (1, 6, 7). In addition, it is considered possible to determine the viability of the kidney when it is preserved by hypothermic perfusion from a study of its perfusion characteristics. Although there is a great deal of merit in this position, such a contention was based historically on earlier experiments with canine kidney preservation by ice cooling in Eurocollin's solution and when human cadaveric grafts had to be harvested under less than ideal conditions and with prolonged warm ischemia time (7, 8, 9, 10).

More recently, several reports have shown that ice preservation with hyperosmolar/intra-cellulartype flush out solutions is effective for safe preservation of human cadaveric kidneys for 40 to 48 h and with an incidence of acute tubular necrosis (ATN) very similar to kidneys preserved by hypothermic perfusion (2, 4,

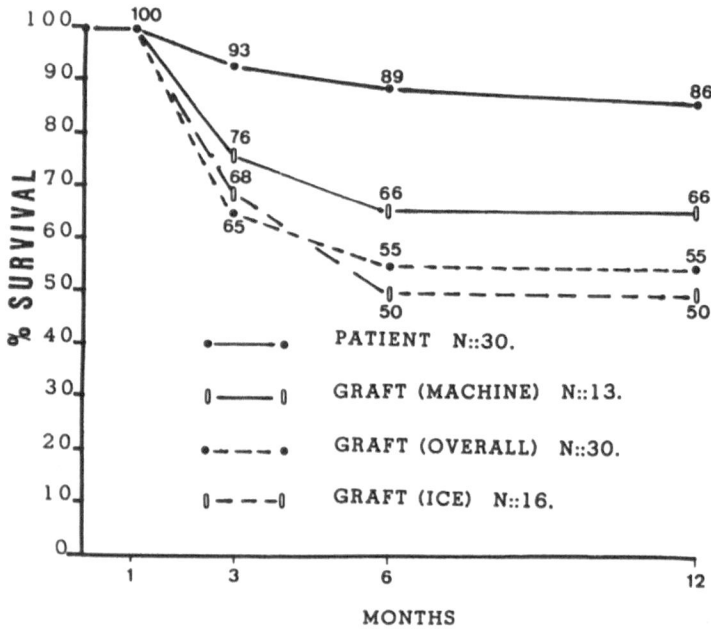

*Fig. 1.* Actuarial patient and graft survival for cadaveric kidneys preserved by ice and by pulsatile perfusion. Note: Graft function is similar regardless of the method of preservation.

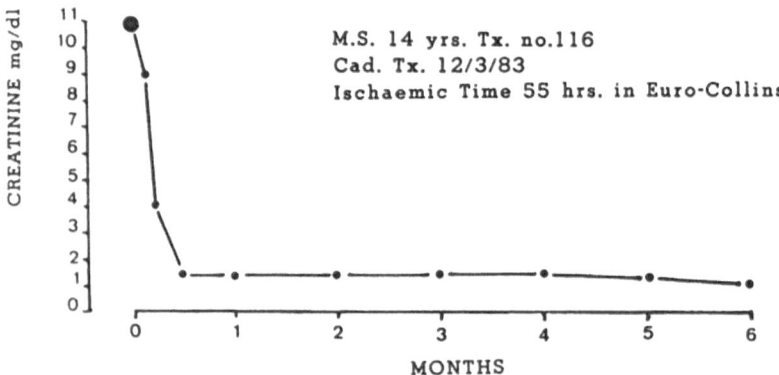

*Fig. 2.* Course of patient who received a cadaver kidney imported from U.S.A. after 55 h of preservation on Eurocollin's solution.

11, 12). Squifflet reported good function after 45 to 50 h preservation in Eurocollin's solution in 22 cadaveric grafts and in 1 kidney after 51 h of preservation, with a dialysis rate of 19%. Vaughn reported similar results for preservation of upto 48 h but with a higher incidence of ATN for ice preserved kidneys (40%) than for machine preserved kidneys (32%). Some workers have reported sporadic grafts successfully preserved for about 50 h with temporary dialysis support (4, 12). Experimentally it has been possible to preserve canine kidneys for 72–96 h by Collin's solution providing the ischemia time is less than 20 min (13). Our own observations indicate that human cadaveric kidneys can be safely preserved by simple cooling and with a dialysis rate and early function comparable to that of kidneys preserved by machines. The observations made on the 7 cadaveric grafts preserved for more than 50 h is particularly significant and recently we have had another three grafts preserved for similar periods with good early function. It is also important to note that some of these cadaveric grafts had been on a machine for several hours before they were transported after flushing with Eurocollin's solution. Although the numbers are small it is nevertheless clear that preservation by simple cooling can be as effective as preservation by perfusion machines with regard to the need for dialysis and early function of the grafts. There are obviously important logistic and economic advantages in being able to preserve human cadaveric kidneys by a simple and relatively inexpensive technique. When kidneys had to be transported on a machine with one technician and occupying two first class seats on an airliner the cost of cadaveric renal transplantation was quite prohibitive. Since we changed our policy to accepting kidneys preserved in ice, the method of transportation has become very much simpler and the costs have been reduced by more than 50%.

While we can confidently recommend that human cadaveric kidneys can be preserved in Eurocollin's solution for periods of 48 to 57 h with low and acceptable rate of post-transplant dialysis, we do so only for kidneys that are harvested under optimum conditions of the donor and with warm ischemia time of less than 10 to 15 min. Clearly if the warm ischemia time is prolonged or the agonal period of the donor is lengthy, ice preservation may not be adequate. Such a situation is probably the only indication for placing the kidneys on the perfusion machine since there is much experimental and clinical evidence that the energy reserves of an ischemically damaged kidney can be restored after a period of perfusion and oxygenation (14).

In conclusion we have shown that human cadaveric kidneys can be safely preserved and transported in iced Eurocollin's solution over distances of some 12000 km and be safely transplanted after a total ischemia time of upto 57 h, with 85% of these kidneys showing immediate diuresis and early function. When the warm ischemia time is less than 10 min preservation and transportation by hypothermic perfusion gives no additional benefit. It is cumbersome and very expensive and under these circumstances it is quite unwarranted. Preservation and transportation of kidneys in ice makes intercontinental sharing of grafts simple, practical, safe and inexpensive and should be more widely used.

130

## References

1. Belzer FO, Southard JH: The Future of Kidney Preservation. Transplantation 30: 161, 1980.
2. Vaughn WM, Mendez-Picon G, Humphries AL, Spees EK: Method of Preservation is not a determinant of graft outcome in Kidney Transplantation by Southeast Organ Procurement Foundation Institutions. Transplantation 32: 490, 1981.
3. Belzer FO, Hoffman RM, Southard JH: Aerobic and Anaerobic Perfusion of Canine kidneys with a new perfusate In: Organ Preservation. (Pegg DE, Iacohon IA, Halasz NA eds) MTP Press, Boston, 1982, p 253.
4. Squifflet JP, Pirson Y, Gianello P, Van Cangh P, Alexandre GP: Safe Preservation of Human Renal Cadaver Transplants by Eurocollin's solution upto 50 hours. Transplantation Proceedings 13: 693, 1981.
5. Van der Vliet JA, Vroemen JPA, Cohen B, Kootstra G: Comparison of Cadaver Kidney Preservation Methods in Eurotransplant International Congress on Organ Procurement, Maastricht, Holland, 1983 (Abstract).
6. Marshal VC: Renal Preservation Prior to Transplantation.Transplantation 30: 165, 1980.
7. Johnson RMG: Kidney Preservation by continous Perfusion In: Organ Preservation (Pegg DE, Jacobson IA, Halasz NA eds). MTP Press, Boston, p 215, 1982.
8. Collins GM, Bravo-Shugerman MB, Terasaki PI: Kidney Preservation for Transplantation by initial perfusion and 30 hour ice storage. Lancet 1: 219, 1969.
9. Halasz NA, Collins GM: Forty-eight Hour Kidney Preservation - A Comparison of Flushing and Ice Storage with Perfusion. Arch Surg 111: 175, 1976.
10. Watkins GM, Prentiss NA, Couch NP: Successful 24 hour kidney preservation using Hypothermic/Hyperosmolar/Intracellulor Washout Solution. Transplantation 21: 417, 1971.
11. Opelz G, Terasaki PI: Advantage of Cold Storage over Machine Perfusion of cadaver kidneys. Transplantation 33: 64, 1982.
12. Barry JM, Farnsworth MA, Bennett WM: Human Kidney Preservation by Flushing with intracellular Solution and Cold Storage. Arch Surg 113: 830, 1978.
13. Dreborn K, Horsch R, Rohl L: 48–96 Hour Preservation of Canine Kidneys by initial perfusion and Hypothermic storage using Euro-collin's solution. Eur Urol 6: 221, 1980.
14. Pegg DE, Wusteman MC, Foreman J: Metabolism of Normal and Ischemically Injured Rabbit Kidneys during perfusion for 48 hours at 10°C. Transplantation 32: 437, 1981.

# 14. A new approach to prolonged kidney preservation

G. KOOTSTRA, B.G. RIJKMANS and W.A. BUURMAN

## 1. Introduction

Nowadays, 48 h are available in clinical kidney transplantation, for matching and transportation of kidneys. Preservation, by either cold storage or hypothermic perfusion, permits these 48 h, sometimes with damage to kidney function, which is usually reversible within a few days. There are some reports in literature (1, 2) where preservation times over 48 h, and up to 90 h are mentioned. Nevertheless, transplant surgeons prefer to transplant a kidney within 48 h, and more time is seldom needed. Only when extended preservation times up to one week (intermediate term) are realized, will new immunological techniques intended to improve the results of clinical kidney transplantation and world-wide sharing of kidneys, necessary to reduce wastage of kidneys, become reality. Therefore research in the field of kidney preservation continues in several laboratories over the world.

We have introduced a new model of normothermic blood perfusion along with standard cold perfusion (3). The results are promising and might provide insight into the mechanism of failure of intermediate term kidney preservation on machines. Eventually, the new method might point the way along which intermediate term preservation in the clinical situation can be reached.

This chapter will compile the data from literature on experimental work on intermediate term kidney preservation and describes our model of normothermic blood perfusion in detail.

## 2. Literature on intermediate term kidney preservation

All work on experimental kidney preservation has been performed in the dog model. Intermediate term preservation has not been reached with the cold storage method: the maximum preservation time with cold storage in the dog model is 72 h. It is of interest that in the human situation several reports (1, 2) are now available which mention over 72 h in the human situation, leading to the assumption that the experimental dog models are a safe tool for the clinical situation.

In experimental kidney preservation the best results have been obtained with hypothermic continuous perfusion.

The longest preservation time so far has been reached by Cohen and Johnson (4), who preserved ten dog kidneys for 8 days (Table 1). Two out of the ten had life-sustaining function, the remaining eight died of uremia. Woods (5) succeeded in two experiments to preserve one kidney for 7 days, Liu (6) had three successes out of five, Cohen (7) two out of five and Ozaki (8) had no life-sustaining kidney out of four cases. In total, there are reports on 16 kidneys, preserved for 7 days. Only six were life-sustaining, i.e. an overall success rate of 38%.

Six day preservation experiments have been published by our group (9). After

*Table 1.* Results of experimental hypothermic continuous perfusion reported by several authors.

| Author | No. of days | Type of machine | Perfusate | Survivors out of total number |
|---|---|---|---|---|
| Cohen (4) GL, Johnson RWG | 8 | Modified Belzer | Plasma protein fraction phosphate buffer added frusemide premedication | 2 out of 10 |
| Woods (5) JE | 7 | Belzer type machine | Belzer plasma high dose steroids added | 1 out of 2 |
| Liu (6) WP et al. | 7 | Travenol Viacell | Human plasma protein fraction | 3 out of 5 |
| Cohen (7) GL et al. | 7 | Modified Belzer | Plasma protein fraction | 2 out of 5 |
| Ozaki (8) A et al. | 7 | Senko Machine (non-pulsatile roller pump, membrane oxygenator) | Modified Belzer's plasma (Amino acid solution in stead of mannitol) | 0 out of 4 |
| Rijkmans (10) BG et al. (controlgroup) | 6 | Gambro | Kabi® albumin | 1 out of 6 |
| Cohen (7) GL et al. | 5 | Modified Belzer | Plasma protein fraction | 13 out of 27 |
| Ozaki (8) A et al. | 5 | see above | see above | 2 out of 4 |
| Toledo-Pereyra (11) LH | 5 | Mox 100 | Fibrinogen free Belzer's plasma (Silica gel fraction) | 0 out of 8 2 out of 8 |

hypothermic perfusion only one out of six dogs survived with poor kidney function.

Five day preservation has been studied by Ozaki (8) (two out of nine dogs had life-sustaining function) and Cohen and Johnson (7), who obtained in 13 out of 27 experiments, life-sustaining function. Toledo-Pereyra (10) obtained two surviving dogs out of 16. It seems that in a 5 day preservation model less then half of the experiments will result in successful preservation.

Four day preservation experiments have a higher success rate. We (9, 11) have published life-sustaining function in six out of six experiments in the four day preservation setting.

The before mentioned 8, 7, 6, 5 and 4 day preservation studies were all realized with mechanical perfusion techniques. Nearly all groups used different machines and perfusates (Table 1). It seems unlikely that changes either in the machine or in the perfusate will improve results: 4 day hypothermic perfusion can be performed with a close to 100% success rate, while results of longer preservation are less consistent. Successful preservation for 7 or 8 days appeared to be an exception; the results were unpredictable and irreproducible!

We studied the effect of a normothermic blood perfusion halfway during the period of hypothermic preservation. We assume that after 4 days hypothermic preservation, a kidney is 'exhausted' which will lead to irreversible damage.

Just before complete exhaustion the kidney is recharged like a battery by a normothermic blood perfusion. It was supposed that a recharged kidney can sustain another period of cold ischaemia.

## 3. Previous work on the model

In the first study we developed an *ex vivo* perfusion system. Halfway through the preservation period the kidney was perfused extracorporally on the donor dog during 4 h. This was effective in reducing the mean serum creatinine peak after 4 days kidney preservation (3). Then we proved the *ex vivo* perfusion to work in a 6 day setting: in the control group without *ex vivo* perfusion there was one survivor out of six dogs, while in the *ex vivo* perfused group five out of six dogs had life-sustaining function (9, 11).

The ideal time for the *ex vivo* perfusion was studied and it turned out that the beneficial effect was reached at a three hours perfusion time (12). In this group six out of six kidneys survived with good kidney function. The next important step was the construction of a heart-lung machine that could replace the donor dog in the *ex vivo* perfusion. A roller pump with bubble oxygenerator was unsuccessful in providing the beneficial effect (unpublished data) and a cylinder film oxygenator and Dale Schuster-type pump resulted in three out of eight life-sustaining kidneys (13). This result was considered inadequate and a new machine was constructed. It combined the Dale Schuster-type pump with a membrane oxygenator. The results with this machine are reported in this chapter.

## 4. Heart-lung machine and experimental setting

A hydraulic balloon pump (Dale Schuster-type) (Fig.1) with two light valves delivered a pulsatile flow at a fixed rate of 120 strokes per minute. The mean perfusion pressure was maintained at 100 mm Hg. The blood was oxygenated in a membrane oxygenator (Kolobow 400 2A, Scimed, Minneapolis, MN.) by air to which 20% $O_2$ and 5% $CO_2$ was added to maintain an oxygen saturation of the blood of about 95% and a pH of 7.4. The oxygenated blood passed through a single-layer nylon filter of 200 $\mu$m pore size. In the organ chamber, made of PVC (RV 500–1, Scimed, Minneapolis, MN.) the blood flowed freely out of the renal vein and was collected together with the blood leaking from the vessels of the capsule. The blood/gas interface was limited to a few square centimeters just beneath the kidney. From the organ chamber the blood was sucked into the venous reservoir which was also made from PVC (RV 500–1, Scimed, Minneapolis, MN.). All connections were made of silicone tubing. The whole circuit except the organ chamber was placed in a thermostatic water bath (38° C). At the start of the perfusion 20 ml of a solution containing 0.21 g sodium carbonate, 0.75 g glucose and 200 $\mu$g carbacholamine was added per liter blood perfusate. During the last 5 min of the 3 h blood perfusion, 20 ml mannitol solution (20 g/ 100 ml) was added to the perfusate.

The heart-lung machine was primed with fresh alloblood (10 ml/g kidney weight). The blood donor dog was anaesthetised with nembutal, and treated with 400 IU heparin/kg body weight and 1 g amoxicilline. The carotid artery of the donor dog

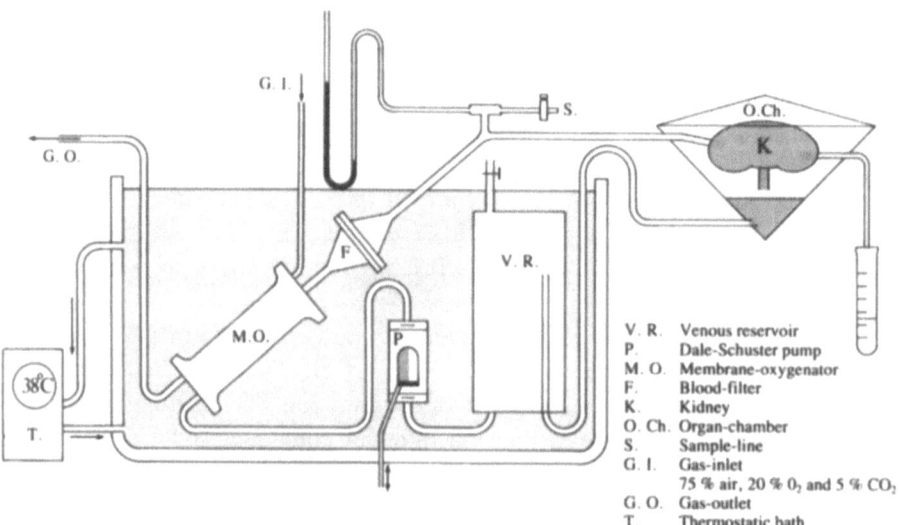

| | |
|---|---|
| V. R. | Venous reservoir |
| P. | Dale-Schuster pump |
| M. O. | Membrane-oxygenator |
| F. | Blood-filter |
| K. | Kidney |
| O. Ch. | Organ-chamber |
| S. | Sample-line |
| G. I. | Gas-inlet |
| | 75 % air, 20 % $O_2$ and 5 % $CO_2$ |
| G. O. | Gas-outlet |
| T. | Thermostatic bath |

*Fig. 1.* Scheme of the heart-lung machine for the normothermic blood perfusion. Halfway the six day preservation period the kidneys of the experimental group were perfused in the heart-lung machine with heparinized alloblood during 3 h.

was cannulated and the venous reservoir of the heart-lung circuit was filled rapidly. The perfusion of the preserved kidney started within two minutes after priming of the circuit.

*Control group.* In the control group of 8 dogs the kidneys were preserved for 6 days by hypothermic perfusion in a Gambro machine (Lund, Sweden) using a Kabi[R] albumin perfusate at 5–7° C. The composition of the perfusate has been reported previously[10]. After one hour hypothermic perfusion the perfusate pressure was adjusted to 20 mm Hg.

*Experimental group.* In the experimental group of 11 dogs the hypothermic perfusion of the kidneys was identical to the control group. However, on the third day of the preservation period the kidneys were perfused in the heart-lung machine with blood at 38° C. After 3 h blood perfusion the kidneys were flushed with Eurocollins at 4° C and perfused in the Gambro machine with the same perfusate for the rest of the 6 day preservation period. In the control and in the experimental group the kidneys were tested for life-sustaining function by transplantation to the neck of the donor dog and immediate contralateral nephrectomy.

## 5. Results

*Survival and function after implantation.* In the blood perfused group all kidneys regained normal colour upon revascularisation and produced urine immediately. Nine out of eleven dogs of the blood perfused group survived in healthy condition. Two dogs had to be sacrificed at respectively day 3 and 7 after implantation because of wound dehiscence and urine leakage respectively. The serum creatinine of these two dogs followed the pattern of the others in the experimental group, compatible with functional recovery. In the blood perfused group the mean serum creatinine concentration returned to normal within 2 weeks after implantation and had a maximum value of 533 µmol/l on day 2 (range 279–885 µmol/l) (Fig. 2).

In the control group with continuous hypothermic perfusion the kidneys also regained their normal colour upon revascularisation. However, the urine production was low. In the control group only one out of eight dogs survived; the others died uremic within 5 days. The only survivor reached a maximum serum creatinine concentration of 1080 µmol/l on day 5 (Fig. 2).

*Histology.* At autopsy the kidneys were sliced and fixed in formalin. Sections of 4 µm were stained with hematoxylin and eosin. Severe tubular damage and many casts were observed in the no life-sustaining kidneys of the control group (Fig. 3). Dispersed tubular regeneration was seen. The glomeruli and blood vessels had a normal aspect.

136

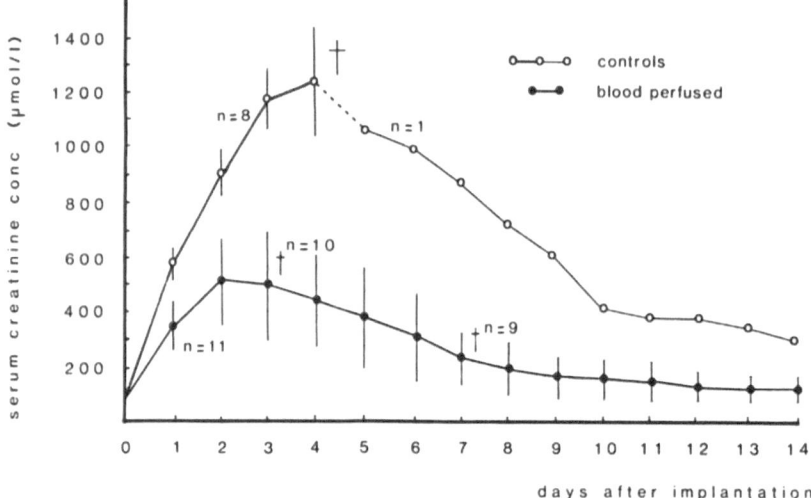

*Fig. 2.* Serum creatinine concentration after autotransplantation of 6 days preserved kidneys in contralateral nephrectomized dogs. Mean values ± S.D. are given. In the control group with hypothermic perfusion only, one out of 8 dogs survived. In the intermediate blood perfused group 9 out of 11 dogs survived. Two dogs had to be sacrified for technical reasons at respectively day 3 and 7 after implantation.

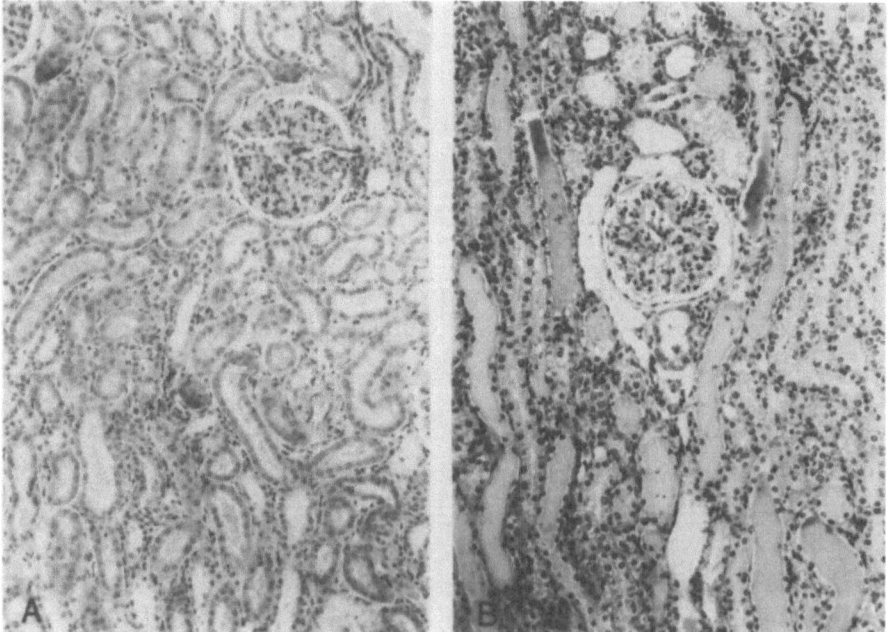

*Fig. 3.* (A) 7 days after implantation one dog of the blood perfused group had to be sacrificed because of urine leakage. Histological sections showed no signs of severe tubular damage. (B) In the control group, with hypothermic perfusion only, biopsies were taken after uremic death. Severe tubular damage and casts were observed. In both groups the glomeruli and blood vessels had a normal aspect.

In the blood perfused group two dogs had to be sacrificed for technical reasons as mentioned above at respectively 3 and 7 days after implantation. Their kidneys showed normal glomeruli and blood vessels. Signs of severe tubular damage were not seen in both kidneys (Fig. 3). In both kidneys only a few casts were observed. At autopsy 3 weeks after implantation the kidneys of the perfused group showed normal morphology, however all kidneys contained neutrophils in the pyelum and interstitium.

## 6. Discussion

In this study the preservation time of dog kidneys could be extended successfully up to 6 days, by 3 h blood perfusion in a heart-lung machine halfway during the hypothermic preservation period.

In a consecutive series, nine out of eleven kidneys showed life sustaining function after 6 days preservation. Unfortunately two dogs had to be sacrificed for technical failures, but provided tissue for histological investigation. In the control group only one out of eight dogs survived.

In the blood perfused group the serum creatinine levels after implantation were similar to or even lower than those reported by other authors after 3 days hypothermic perfusion (14).

Histological examination of the blood perfused kidneys at autopsy 3 weeks after implantation showed normal architecture. However, the light microscopic evaluation was influenced by signs of pyelonephritis: a commonly observed complication of ureterocutaneostomy after implantation in the neck (15, 16). The histology of the kidneys from the two technical failures in the blood perfused group allowed interpretation of the beneficial effect of the normothermic isolated perfusion, since it could be compared with the histology of the control group, in which the animals died at about the same time after implantation. In contrast to data reported by other authors (7, 8) the histological sections of both groups showed normal glomeruli and vessels. Signs of endothelial damage leading to intravascular coagulation and fibrin thrombi in the glomular capillaries have not been observed. This socalled 'perfusion nephropathy' following hypothermic continuous perfusion has been described by several authors (17, 18). It has been suggested that perfusion nephropathy can be prevented by low perfusion pressure in hypothermic perfusion (19) as applied in our experiments. The kidneys of the control group showed severe tubular damage, many casts were observed. In the perfused group, however, relatively well preserved tubules were observed in the kidneys of the two cases with technical failure.

Although the exact mechanism of the beneficial effect of the blood perfusion on the kidneys remains so far unknown, the histological data suggest a recovery of tubular cells during the blood perfusion at normothermia.

From this study it can be concluded that it is possible to prevent preservation damage by 3 h normothermic isolated blood perfusion after which the organ can be preserved for another 3 days. Furthermore, by using an artificial perfusate it would be possible to find out which factors are responsible for the beneficial effect of the intermediate perfusion. This might also contribute to the development of improved hypothermic preservation techniques.

Finally, the good results of these 6 day preservation experiments suggest that the application of alternating hypothermic and normothermic perfusion might enable intermediate kidney preservation in the clinical situation.

## References

1. Abouna GM, Kumar AS, White AG, Daddah S, Omer OF, Samhan M, Kusma G, John P, Soubky AS, Abbas AR, Kremer G: Experience with imported human cadaveric kidneys having unusual problems and transplanted after 30–60 hours of preservation. Transplant Proceed 16: 61, 1984.
2. Squifflet JP, Pirson Y, Gianello P, Van Caugh P, Alexandre GPJ: Safe preservation of human renal cadaver transplants by Euro-Collins solution up to 50 hours. Transplant Proc 13: 693–696, 1981.
3. Kootstra G, Van der Wijk J, Rijkmans BG: A New device towards intermediate term kidney preservation. An experimental study. (Suppl) Scand J Urol Nephrol 54: 86–89, 1980.
4. Cohen GL, Johnson RWG: Perfusate Buffering for 8–day canine kidney storage. Proc Eur Soc Art Org VII: 235–239, 1980.
5. Woods JE: Successful Three-to-Seven-Day Preservation of Canine Kidneys. Arch Surg 102: 614–617, 1971.
6. Liu WP, Humphries AL, Russell R, Stoddard LD, Garcia LA, Serkes KD: Three- and seven-day perfusion of dog kidneys with human plasma protein fraction IV–4. Surgical Forum 24: 316–318, 1973.
7. Cohen GL, Ballardie FW, Mainwaring A, Johnson RWG: Lysosomal enzyme release during successful 5–, 7– and 8–day canine kidney storage. In: Organ Preservation. Basic and Applied Aspects. (Pegg DE, Jacobsen IA, Halasz NA eds). MTP Press Ltd, Lancaster-Boston The Hague, 1982, p 249–253.
8. Ozaki A, Fukao K, Sano M, Okamura T, Iwasaki Y: Five-day preservation of canine kidneys using a preservation machine. In: Organ Preservation. Basic and Applied Aspects. (Pegg DE, Jacobsen IA, Halasz NA eds). MTP Press Ltd, Lancaster-Boston-The Hague, 1982, p 245–249.
9. Rijkmans BG, Van der Wijk J, Donker AJM, Slooff MJH, Kootstra G: Functional studies in 6 days successful preserved canine kidneys. J Urol 127: 163–165, 1982.
10. Toledo-Pereyra LH, Condie RM, Malmberg R, Simmons RL, Najarian JS: A fibrinogen-free plasma perfusate for preservation of kidneys for one hundred and twenty hours. Surg Gyn Obst 138: 901–906, 1974.
11. Van der Wijk J, Slooff MJH, Rijkmans BG, Kootstra G: Successful 96 and 144 hour experimental kidney preservation: a combination of standard machine preservation and newly developed normothermic ex-vivo perfusion. Cryobiology 17: 473–477, 1980.
12. Van der Wijk J, Rijkmans BG, Kootstra G: Six day kidney preservation in a canine model. Influence of a 1 to 4 hr ex-vivo perfusion interval. Transplantation 35 (5): 408–411, 1983.
13. Rijkmans BG, Kootstra G, Van der Wijk J, Nizet A: In: Organ Preservation. Basic and Applied Aspects. (Pegg DE, Jacobsen IA, Halasz NA eds). MTP Press Ltd, Lancaster-Boston-The Hague, 1982, p 267–272.
14. Abouna GM, Lim F, Cook JS, Grubb W, Craig SS, Seible HR, Hume DM: Three-day canine

kidney preservation. Surgery 71: 436–444, 1972.

15. Van der Wijk J, Rijkmans BG, Kootstra G: Light microscopic findings in intermediate term preservation. In: Organ Preservation. Basic and Applied Aspects. (Pegg DE, Jacobsen IA, Halasz NA eds). MTP Press Ltd, Lancaster-Boston-The Hague, 1982, p 239–243.

16. Lapchinsky AG: Recent results of experimental transplantation of preserved limbs and kidneys and possible use of this technique in clinical practice. Ann NY Acad Sci 87: 539–571, 1960.

17. Spector D, Limas C, Frost JL, Zachary JB, Stenoff S, Williams GM, Rolley RT, Sadler JH: Perfusion nephropathy in human transplants. N Engl J Med 295: 1217–1221, 1976.

18. Hill GS, Light JA, Perloff LJ: Perfusion-related injury in renal transplantation. Surgery 79: 440–447, 1976.

19. Cerra FB, Raza S, Andres GA, Siegel JH: The endothelial damage of pulsatile renal preservation and its relationship to perfusion pressure and colloid osmotic pressure. Surgery 81: 534–541, 1977.

# 15. The upper arm A-V fistula for chronic hemodialysis: long term followup

FUAD JOSEPH DAGHER

## Introduction

Most surgeons dealing with vascular accesses for chronic hemodialysis agree that the surgically constructed A-V fistula at the wrist is the procedure of choice in the new dialysis patient when adequate vessels are still available (1). However, major problems arise when adequate vessels at these conventional sites become unavailable (2).

As an alternative, a good number of surgeons employ one type or another of the available synthetic prosthetic vascular grafts which carry a high incidence of complications such as venous outflow obstruction and graft infection. However, instead of vascular prosthetic grafts, we have preferred the use of the patient's own basilic vein in the upper arm and the brachial artery in the anticubital space as previously reported (3) (4), a technic which we first used in July 1974 and which we refer to as 'the upper arm A-V fistula'.

## Procedure

The portion of the basilic vein used for this access lies for its most part in the upper arm. From a point just below the anticubital space this vein passes anterior to the medial epicondyle of the humerus and enters the medial bicipital groove of the upper arm. A little below the junction of the middle and lower one third of the upper arm this vein perforates the deep fascia and ascends medial to the brachial artery before entering the axilla. In order to obtain sufficient length, this vein is freed from 2–4 cm distal to the anticubital space. Dissection of the vein is carried out through two separate incisions, one along the medial bicipital groove and the other in the lower one third of the upper arm curved towards the anticubital space through which the brachial artery can be dissected.

All tributaries to the basilic vein must be suture ligated with non-absorbable vascular sutures to avoid serious bleeding from the arterialized vein. Some of these vein tributaries may be so wide-based and of such short length as to require closure with running vascular sutures rather than suture ligatures.

There are two nerves that run close to the vein; the medial cutaneous nerve of the fore arm spirals along the anterior surface of the basilic vein, and the median nerve which courses between the brachial artery and the basilic vein in the middle third of the upper arm. Care should be taken to protect both nerves from damage.

When the proper length of the vein is free, it is divided, then delivered through the upper incision and drawn through a subcutaneous tunnel along the anterior aspect of the upper arm. A 1.0 to 1.2 cm arteriovenous anastomosis of the spatulated distal vein to the adjacent brachial artery is carried out in the anticubital space. Prior to the anastomosis it must be ascertained that there is no torsion of the vein during its subcutaneous transposition. This operation is usually carried out under axillary block anesthesia supplemented at times by General Anaesthesia.

**Patient load and results**

Since 1974, 176 upper arm fistulas were performed in 167 patients ranging in age between 16 and 73 yrs. There were 77 males and 90 females. All except two patients had at least two of the more conventional procedures and at times three or more other procedures performed prior to consideration of the upper arm fistula.

A minimum of ten days to two weeks is allowed to pass before the newly created fistula is used. Most patients are dialyzed two times and in a few others three times per week using 14 or 15 gauge needles.

At the end of eight years, 123 of 176 upper arm fistulas are still patent and functional in maintaining chronic hemodialysis making the eight years functional patency and survival 70%. Most fistulas lost are lost in the first and second years as demonstrated by the 6 and 12 months patency rates of 83 and 75%.

Operative complications and complications encountered during dialysis are minimal as demonstrated in Table 1. Embolization to the fingers and symptomatic vascular steal each occurred in less than one percent. Pseudo aneurysms at the site of repeated punctures occurred in less than three percent of the patients. These pseudoaneurysms are easily excised under local anesthesia without compromising the continuity and patency of the conduit. Thrombosis of the conduit and superficial infection of the incision each occurred in 3.5% of the patients. However, in both of these complications, patency of the conduit was not affected and the conduit successfully declotted. In slightly over five percent of the fistulas, there was spontaneous thrombosis within six to eight months of their creation. All patients here demonstrated redness and tenderness along the course of the superficially located vein, associated with erythema, warmth and local tenderness. Biopsy of these thrombosed veins revealed thickening of the vein wall and the presence of non-specific inflammatory process. There was one death in this

*Table 1.* Upper arm A-V fistula complications.

|  | % |
|---|---|
| Digital embolization | 0.57 |
| Vascular steal | 0.57 |
| Pseudo aneurysm | 2.27 |
| Thrombosis, caused by repeated punctures at same site | 3.40 |
| Superficial wound infection | 3.40 |
| Spontaneous thrombosis/phlebitis | 5.68 |
| Hemorrhage/M.I./death | 0.57 |

series, a 73 year old black male who developed severe infection of the incision on the third postoperative day. This was managed by open drainage and treatment with systemic organ specific antibiotic; however, the patient bled massively from a side branch of the arterialized vein due to the loss of a ligature on a side branch of the vein. As a result of hypotension the patient developed acute myocardial infarction and died.

During dialysis, flow measurements within the fistula revealed flows of over 600 ml/min.

### Discussion

The above results demonstrate that this described upper arm fistula in which the transposed basilic vein is sutured to the side of the brachial artery is one of the most reliable and dependable secondary hemoaccess procedures for chronic hemodialysis reported to date. Our own data (5) and those of Le Gerfo (6) reflect considerably better results than those obtained with bovine or with PTFE grafts. Long term patency rates of PTFE grafts as vascular accesses are not impressive despite a good and acceptable one and two years patency rate (7).

Furthermore, the upper arm fistula with the transposed basilic vein compares favorably well with the more standard radial- cephalic fistula at the wrist; the latter has a reported one year patency rate of 90% (8). Both fistulas have lots in common; they both utilize the patient's own autologous vein using a single vascular anastomosis while keeping the proximal end of the vein in continuity with a larger venous channel, in this case the axillary vein in the upper arm avoiding a veno-venous anastomosis and its common complication of stenosis.

We believe that the long term functional patency rate of this vascular access of 70% appears to be among the best if not the best reported to date. This is partly due to the use of the patient's own autologous vein which is kept in continuity with a larger vein, a single vascular anastomosis and a high flow rate of blood from the brachial artery into the basilic vein.

The complications reported are minimal and by no means inherent to this type of vascular access. While serious infections remain to lead the complications of accesses using prosthetic grafts (9) none of the patients with this type of fistula experienced infections of the access while on dialysis. Minor superficial infections of the surgical incision were encountered in three patients in the immediate postoperative period, but they were all successfully managed using local cleaning and organism specific antibiotics.

Distal embolization can result from any surgically created arteriovenous fistula whether or not autologous or prosthetic material have been used. Fibrin deposition and platelets thrombi at the site of anastomosis are potential sources of microemboli.

Shunting of significant blood flow away from the fore arm, severe enough to cause hand ischemia can theoretically occur in any type of arteriovenous communication in the upper extremity, specifically when the A-V anastomosis is large. When patients with this problem appear to be markedly symptomatic and indeed bothered by this problem, surgical revision to reduce the actual size of the anastomosis may be necessary.

High output failure while occasionally encountered with large A-V fistulas at any anatomic site, is not noted in the present series. In addition to increased cardiac output, other contributing factors include severe anemia, commonly present in these patients, fluid over loading, hypertension and preexisting heart disease.

Based on the above experience, we believe that the above described upper arm fistula, utilizing the end of the transposed basilic vein sutured to the brachial artery is the most reliable of the secondary hemoaccesses. Its advantages include the use of the patient's own autologous vein, maintaining proximal anatomic venous continuity with the axillary vein, its ease of performance and the use of a single vascular anastomosis, providing a superficially located, long and easily accessible conduit with long term functional patency rate.

## References

1. Brescia MJ, Cimino JE, Appel K, Hurwich BJ: Chronic hemodialysis using venepuncture and surgically created arteriovenous fistula. N Eng J Med 275: 1089, 1966.
2. Merill RH: Review of vascular access. Dial Transplant 6: 22, 1977.
3. Dagher FJ, Gelber RL, Ramos EJ, Sadler J: Basilic Vein to brachial artery fistula: A new access for chronic hemodialysis South Med J 69: 1438, 1976.
4. Dagher FJ, Gelber RL, Ramos EJ, Sadler J: The use of the basilic vein and brachial artery as an A-V fistula for long term hemodialysis. J Surg Res 20: 373, 1976.
5. Dagher FJ, Gelber R, Reed W: Basilic vein to brachial artery. Arteriovenous fistula for long term hemodialysis: A five year followup. Proc Dialysis Transplant forum No 1: 126–128, 1980.
6. Logerfo FW, Menzoean JO, Kumak DJ, Idelson BA: Transposed basilic vein brachial arteriovenous fistula. A reliable secondary access procedure. Arch Surg 113: 1008, 1978.
7. Anderson CB, Etheredge EE, Gregorio AS: One hundred polytetrafuoroethylene vascular access grafts. Dial Transplant 9: 237, 1980.

8. Kinnaert P, Vereerstraeten P, Toussaint C, Van Geertruyden J: Nine years experience with internal arteriovenous fistula for hemodialysis. Br J Surg 64: 242, 1977.
9. Bhat DJ, Tellis VA, Kahlberg WI, Driscoll B, Veith F: Management of sepsis involved expanded polytetrafluoroethylene grafts for hemodialysis access. Surg 87: 445, 1980.

# 16. Permanent vascular access for haemodialysis: the Kuwait experience

S.K. DADAH, M. SAMHAN, O.F. OMAR and G.M. ABOUNA

## Introduction

Renal replacement therapy in the form of dialysis and renal transplantation are widely accepted as the treatment of end stage renal disease while acute dialysis is a life saving procedure. Since the establishment of the Organ Transplantation programme in Kuwait in March 1979 all acute and permanent vascular accesses for haemodialysis and permanent intra-peritoneal catheters for intermittent and ambulatory peritoneal dialysis have been performed by the same team.

Historically long term haemodialysis was first made possible by the development in 1960 of the Scribner external plastic shunt (1) but this suffered from infective and arterio-venous thrombotic complications. In 1966 the Brescia-Cimino fistula was described (2) but this too had its limitations and a substantial number of patients were not suitable for this form of access because of inadequate peripheral vessels and thus prompted the search for a variety of secondary procedures. The autogenous saphenous vein graft (3) is successful initially but is restricted by complications and a short life. 1972 saw the introduction of the bovine heterograft (4) and in 1975 the PTFE (GORETEX) synthetic vascular graft became available commercially) (5).

In Kuwait, as elswhere, the Brescia-Cimino fistula remains the primary procedure and the bovine heterograft and Goretex conduits are used when the construction of a primary fistula is impossible of the fistula has failed.

## Patients and methods

Two hundred and twenty patients between the ages of 12 and 65 years were given primary or secondary accesses. There were 136 males and 84 females and the distribution of accesses in relation to age and sex is summerised in Table 1.

The accesses were constructed under local anaesthesia by infiltration with 1% or 2% xylocaine and valium sedation. The A-V fistulae were normally performed at the wrist, the radial artery and the cephalic vein being mobilised for 5 cm and a 2 cm wide side to side anastomiosis of the artery and vein was carried out using a 6°

*Table 1.* Distribution of accesses in relation to sex and age range.

| Type of access | Males | Females | Age years | Total No. | % |
|---|---|---|---|---|---|
| Brescia-Cimino fistula | 117 | 44 | (12–73) | 161 | (73) |
| Bovine heterograft | 12 | 25 | (13–56) | 37 | (17) |
| Goretex graft | 7 | 15 | (18–70) | 22 | (10) |
| Total | 136 | 84 | (12–73) | 220 | (100) |

prolene suture. In most patients the distal end of the vein was ligated thus creating an end to side fistula. Seventy-one patients had a side to side fistula and 90 end to side. The arterio-venous fistulae were allowed to mature for 2–4 weeks before use, when all the oedema had subsided and the wound healed.

Of 59 vascular grafts, 37 were bovine heterografts and 22 were Goretex conduits. Nine of these vascular grafts were placed in the forearm between the radial artery at the wrist and the antecubital vein and 49 grafts were in the upper arm between the brachial artery at the elbow and the axillary vein at the entrance to the axilla. One bovine graft was placed in the thigh. Irrespective of the site, all grafts were straight, 10–16 cm long, subcutaneously placed and easily accessible for puncture and haemodialysis. The graft diameter varied between 5–8 mm depending on the size of the patients vessels. All accesses were periodically assessed for patency and complications over a period of 1–4 years.

### Results

The cumulative patency rates for all types of access are shown in Figure 1 and demonstrate the superiority of the primary A-V fistula over the bovine and Goretex grafts. Division of the primary A-V fistula into side to side and end to side reveals a marked difference in patency ($p = .01$). The end to side anastomosis had a 3 year patency of 95% whereas the side to side, 71%. Furthermore, as would be expected, the end to side had fewer complications. Table 2, summarises the early and late complications in all the types of accesses with subdivision into the location of the access. The major cause of access failure whatever the type of access was late clotting and this was the main factor influencing the difference in patency rate between the end to side and the side to side A-V fistulae. The blood flow obtained for all the vascular accesses was 200–300 mls. per minute when connected to the dialysis machine and it was adequate for haemodialysis.

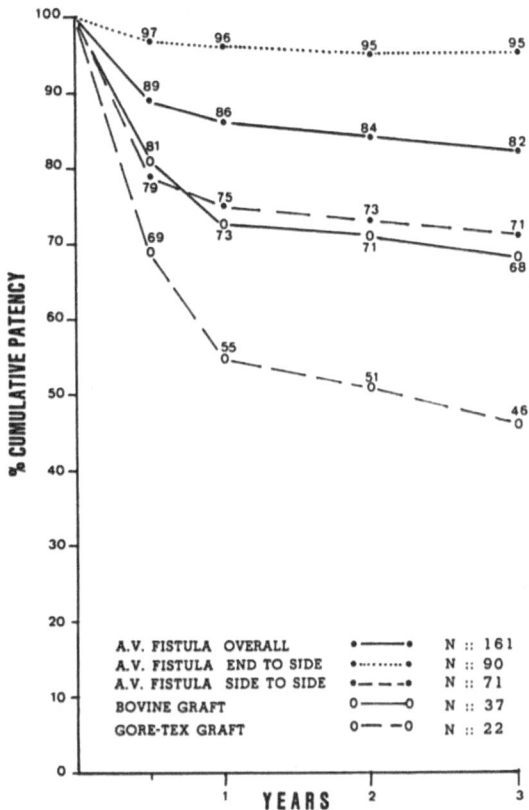

*Fig. 1.* Cumulative patency rates in the different accesses.

## Discussion

Of the 220 vascular accesses reported here, 161 (73%) were the Brescia-Cimino arteriovenous fistula (2). Our overall cumulative patency rate for this type of access was 82% at 3 years and is comparable to the patency rate reported by others. Limet and Lejeune (6), Cohn and Solit (7) and Zerbino *et al.* (8) have found cumulative patency rates of 82%, 88% and 89% respectively at 3 years. Other workers have had less success. Kinnaert *et al.* (9) report 72%, Haimov *et al.* (10) 66% and Higgins *et al.* (11) 29% at 3 years. From our experience it is apparent that the type of anastomosis used for the fistula can greatly influence the patency. The side to side A-V fistula had a 3 year patency of 71% whereas the end to side A-V fistula had a patency of 95% at the same period. The difference was statistically significant (p <.01). Differences depending on the type of ana-stomosis have been recorded by others. Kinnaert *et al.* (9) have reported 88% patency for side to side radio cephalilic A-V fistulas at the wrist and 78% for the end to side fistula at the wrist. However, for the end to side fistula in the mid forearm they found 100% survival. Haimov (12) reported that the end to side fistula was preferable because of retrograde arterialisation at the end of the vein which frequently caused swelling and discomfort. Also our findings (Table 2) show a greater incidence of complications in the side to side A-V fistulae compared to end to side. Sixteen out of 71 fistulas (23%) were lost as a result of 'late clotting', but only 2 out of 90 (2%) end to side had this complication. Bovine heterografts were constructed in 37 patients with a cumulative patency rate at 3 years of 68%. This is the same as that reported by Butler *et al.* (13) and superior to the findings of Owens (14) of 50% and Morgan (15) of 25% at 3 years. The major cause of failure of our bovine heterografts was again 'late clotting' with 4 deaths (Table 2). Twenty-two patients received Goretex PTFE grafts and the 3 year patency rate was only 46% with 6 deaths. The 2 years patency rate was 51% which was considerably less than that reported by Chatterjee (16) of 84% and by Anderson (17) of 73%. However, Morgan *et al.* (15) reported a patency rate of only 33%. Although our results indicate superior access and patient survival in those with A-V fistulas, it should be emphasised that the patient groups are not

*Table 2.* Complications of the different types of accesses.

| Type of access | No. | Early (surgical) | | | Late (due to haemodialysis) | | | | | Total fail-ures |
|---|---|---|---|---|---|---|---|---|---|---|
| | | Clot-ting | Hae-ma-toma | Infec-tion | Clot-ting | Oede-ma | Vari-ces | Aneur-ysm | Infec-tion | |
| Cimino-Bresico fistula | | | | | | | | | | |
| 1. End to side | 90 | 3 | – | – | 2 | – | – | 1 | – | 5 |
| 2. Side to side | 71 | 5 | – | – | 16 | – | 3 | 1 | – | 21 |
| Total | 161 | 8 | – | – | 18 | – | 3 | 2 | – | 26 |
| Bovine hetero grafts | | | | | | | | | | |
| 1. Upper arm | 33 | 2 | 2 | – | 8 | 2 | 1 | 2 | – | 10 |
| 2. Forearm | 3 | 1 | – | – | – | – | – | – | – | 1 |
| 3. Lower limb | 1 | – | – | – | – | – | – | – | – | – |
| Total | 37 | 3 | 2 | – | 8 | 2 | 1 | 2 | – | 11 |
| Gore-tex grafts | | | | | | | | | | |
| 1. Upper arm | 16 | 2 | – | – | 7 | 1 | 1 | 1 | 1 | 9 |
| 2. Fore arm | 6 | 1 | – | – | 2 | – | – | – | 1 | 3 |
| Total | 22 | 3 | – | – | 9 | 1 | 1 | 1 | 2 | 12 |

N.B. Deaths were counted as late clotting.

strictly comparable. Those patients with A-V grafts were not suitable for the construction of an A-V fistula and are therefore 'selected'. This selection procedure, based on the suitability of the blood vessels might also select for risk factors which lead to poorer patient and graft survival.

In conclusion, our study indicates that the Cimino-Brescia A-V fistula is the primary procedure of choice for patency and patient survival. Our results further indicate a greatly improved patency rate in the end to side compared to the side to side fistulas. In the secondary procedures the bovine heterograft was superior to the Goretex PTFE graft for patency and patient survival.

## References

1. Quinton WE, Dillard DH, Scribner BH: Cannulation of blood vessels for prolonged dialysis. Transactions of the American Society for Artificial Internal Organs 6: 104–109, 1960.
2. Brescia MJ, Cimino JE, Appel K, Hurirch BJ: Chronic Haemodialysis using venepuncture and a surgically created Arteriovenous fistula. N Engl of Med 275: 1089–1092, 1966.
3. May J, Tiller D, Johnson J, Stewart J, Shiel AGR: Saphenous vein arteriovenous fistula in Regular dialysis treatment. N Engl of Med 280: 770, 1969.
4. Chinitz JL, Yokoyama T, Bower R, Swartz C: Self sealing prosthesis for arteriovenous fistula in man. Transactions of the American Soc for Artificial Internal Organs 18: 452–455, 1972.
5. Jerkins A Mcl: Gore-Tex: A new Prosthesis for vascular access. B Med J 2: 280, 1976.
6. Limet RR, Lejeune GN: Evaluation of 110 sub-cutaneous arteriovenous fistulae in 100 chronically haemodialysed patients. J Cardiovasc Surg (Torino) 15: 573–576, 1974.
7. Cohn HE, Solit RW: Arteriovenous fistulas for Chronic haemodialysis. Surg Clin North Am 53: 673–84, 1973.
8. Zerbino VR, Tice DA, Katz LA, Nidus BD: A 6 year clinical experience with arteriovenous fistulas and bypasses for haemodialysis. Surgery 76(6): 1018–23, 1974.
9. Kinnaert P, Vereerstraeten P, Toussaint C, Geertruyden J Van: Nine years experience with internal arterio venous fistulas for haemodialysis; a study of some factors influencing the results. Br J Surg 64: 242–246, 1977.
10. Haimov M, Burrows L, Casey JD, Schupak E: Problems of vascular access for haemodialysis - Experience with 214 Patients. Proc Eur Dial Transp Assoc 173–178, 1972.
11. Higgins MR, Grace M, Bettcher KB, Silverberg DS, Dossetor JB: Blood access in haemodialysis. Clin Nephrol 6(5): 473–77, 1976.
12. Haimov M: Vascular access for Haemodialysis. Surg Gyn Obst 141: 619–625, 1975.
13. Butler HG, Baker LD, Johnson JM: Vascular access for chronic haemodialysis. Polytetrafluoroethylene (P.T.F.E.) versus bovine heterograft. Am J Surg 134(6): 791–93, 1977.
14. Owens ML, Stabile BE, Gahr JA, Wilson SE: Vascular grafts for haemodialysis; an evaluation of sites and materials. Dialysis Transplantation 8(5): 521–30, 1979.
15. Morgan AP, Dammin GJ, Lajans JM: Failure Modes in Secondary Vascular Access for Haemodialysis. ASAIO Journal 1: 44–52, 1978.
16. Chatterjee SN: Use of Gore-Tex grafts as vascular access procedure for chronic haemodialysis. Abstract of a paper submitted to the European Society for Artificial Organs, Eight Annual Meeting, Copenhagen, 1981.
17. Anderson CB, Sicard GA, Etheredge EE: Bovine Carotid Artery and expanded polytetrafluoroethylene grafts for haemodialysis vascular access. J Surg Res 29: 184–188, 1980.

# 17. Current status of renal transplantation

JAMES CERILLI

## Introduction

This paper is designed to present an overview of the current status of clinical renal transplantation. Not all aspects of transplantation will be covered because of the complexity of the issue, but it is hoped that the salient points of the discipline, emphasizing the newer aspects of renal transplantation, will be in enough detail to provide a useful synopis of the topic.

## Indications

In the absence of specific contraindications, all patients with end stage renal disease (ESRD) who are under the age of 60 should be transplanted (1). The transplantation of patients with diabetic nephropathy is occurring with increasing frequency and is the most common cause of ESRD in some transplant centers (2, 3). Chronic glomerulonephritis is still a very common cause of ESRD requiring transplantation. A variety of other diseases including chronic phylonephritis, congenital anomalies, polycystic kidneys, lupus nephritis, cystinosis, and more recently patients with oxalosis are suitable for transplantation (4, 5, 6, 7, 8, 9, 10). Transplantation is suitable for all ages. I have successfully transplanted two infants (5 kg and 9 kg) over 10 years ago. One is now 10 years posttransplant and is doing very well; the second had two recurrences of her original disease (hemolytic uremia), ultimately going back on dialysis 11 years posttransplant. Thus, the very young age group is suitable for transplantation (11, 12). Some older patients, even with associated vascular disease, can be suitable candidates, as evidenced by the successful simultaneous performance of a renal transplant and abdominal aneurysmectomy. There are, however, specific contraindications to transplantation. Patients over the age of 65 or with a non-cured malignancy are best treated with dialysis because of the shortage of kidneys and because patients with malignancy have a limited life expectancy (1). Patients who have survived two years without evidence of recurrent renal cell carcinoma have a high probability of cure and do become transplant candidates (13). Patients with active systemic infection or very severe vascular disease are poor transplant candidates (1).

### Immunological contraindications

Immunological contraindications to transplantation are changing rapidly. ABO incompatibility was once an absolute contraindication to transplantation, but it is now possible to cross the ABO barrier using appropriate immunological manipulation (14). A positive lymphocytotoxicity crossmatch to donor T cells was previously an absolute contraindication. However, if the recent sera is negative and the only positive sera is older than one year, then the patient can be transplanted with an expected graft success of about 50% (15). If a patient has had two prior transplants that have both been rejected within the first six months, this patient is best treated with hemodialysis if standard immunosuppressive techniques are used.

The timing of transplantation is important. The diabetic and young child should be transplanted as early as possible. The young child should be transplanted prior to his requiring dialysis to avoid imposing the psychological and medical morbidity of dialysis (16). Although most transplant surgeons prefer to wait until such immunological diseases as lupus nephritis are inactive, there is little evidence that this is important. All other patients are transplanted when stable on dialysis and a kidney is available (1).

### Organ source

The use of heterografts, i.e. cross-species transplantation, was abandoned because of the uniform failure rate. Increasing utilization has been made of kidneys obtained from cadaver donors. These donors usually have neurologic head injury with approximately normal renal function (creatinine >3mg%) at the time of death. They are usually less than 60 years of age and older than $2\frac{1}{2}$ years of age. Systemic infection should be absent although local infections such as pneumonia, urinary tract infections and meningitis do not exclude a given donor. Malignancy excludes a donor, except central nervous system malignancy becauce of the risk of transmitting the cancer cells with the transplanted kidney. It is preferable that warm ischemia be less than 20 min following death and most donors are declared dead on the basis of 'brain death'. Brain death is an accepted methodology for determining death in the presence of a functioning heart thus maintaining reasonably adequate perfusion of the kidney. It is defined in most centers as the presence of fixed, dilated pupils, no spontaneous respirations, no central reflexes, relative normothermia, minimal to absent barbiturate levels and 'flat' EEGs. New techniques such as intracranial pressure monitoring and cerebral arteriography are being evaluated but neither have gained widespread acceptance because of cost, complexity and potential risk to the donor (17, 18).

There are two current methods of preservation that are widely utilized. The first is pulsatile perfusion of the kidney on a pump oxygenator at 6–10° C using such solutions as cryoprecipitated plasma or a plasma-like solution. Twenty-four to forty-eight hours of storage is easily obtained if a good kidney is utilized. The perfusion characteristics, i.e. the flow and mean and diastolic pressures, provide an index as to the likelihood of acute tubular necrosis in the recipient. Another technique that is becoming more widely applied is cold storage in which the kidney is flushed with an intracellular-like solution, i.e. Collins or Sacks at 4° C and stored sterilely on ice. This method is equally effective as perfusion for preservation up to 24 h but it is not adequate for storage after 36–48 h. However, excellent storage can be obtained up to 24–36 h simply with cold storage and good donor procurement techniques (19, 20, 21).

**Living-related donors**

Living-related donors are associated with optimal graft survival and this is the major justification for their utilization. Donors should be at least 18 years of age and preferably under 55 years of age. Donor evaluation involved a medical evaluation as well as a variety of immunological tests. The most important immunological test to determine donor/recipient antigen compatibility is the mixed lymphocyte culture. A mixed lymphocyte culture (MLC) is performed by culturing together the recipient's and donor's lymphocytes and quantitating the blastogenic response of the recipient's lymphocytes to the donor antigens. In patients who are 'low responders', graft survival rates approximate 90% inspite of HLA disparity. Patients who are MLC positive (high responders) even though they are related have graft survival rates with current immunosuppression techniques, (namely Imuran, Prednisone and ALG), of 55–60% (22).

**Role of sensitization**

The importance of sensitization as a factor in transplantation outcome is undergoing change. The significance of a positive lymphocytotoxicity crossmatch once thought to uniformly lead to rejection has now been modified. When the crossmatch with current recipient sera is positive to donor T cells, transplantation with the donor is not indicated. Thoracic duct fistula, the use of F(AB)$_2$ fragments, anti-thymocyte globulin (ALG) or other immunologic manipulations have not made possible the successful transplantation across a positive T cell crossmatch with fresh sera. Nevertheless, if the crossmatch is positive only with sera over a year old, successful transplantation has been reported providing the fresh sera exhibits no cytotoxicity to donor T lymphocytes. A high percentage of sensitization to a random lymphocyte panel was once thought to be associated with lower graft survival. If the patient has a negative crossmatch with a specific donor the concomitant presence of a high degree of sensitization to a random panel does not adversely affect graft survival (23). Most patients become sensitized through prior transplantation but certainly pregnancy and particularly blood transfusions will also cause sensitization. A few develop antibodies to HLA antigens in the absence of these etiologies.

**Modulation of the immune response**

After transplantation it is still necessary to modulate the immune response in order to prevent graft rejection. Currently, all patients are treated with Imuran (Azathioprine) and must stay on this drug indefinitely. Discontinuing Imuran even in well matched patient/donor combinations ultimately leads to graft rejection. Imuran is associated with leukopenia and some hepatic toxicity, but it is a safe drug in experienced hands. Its maintenance dosage is approximately 1–2 $\frac{1}{2}$ mg/kilo and its dosage is not increased during acute rejection episodes. A second immunosuppressive drug is Cytoxan (cyclophosphamide), which can induce sterility and occasionally bladder cancer when used for prolonged periods. Some patients, particularly those with significant proteinuria, appear to improve when changed to cytoxan. Steroids are still necessary following transplantation. However, they are used in much lower maintenance doses, i.e. 10–20 mg/day of prednisone or prednisone equivalents, than in the past. Although steroids are the most widely used therapy for rejection episodes, ATG is recently being used more frequently. A typical antirejection course of steroids would be 500 to 1,000 mg qd × 3 days followed by 250 to 500mg qd × 3. However, this is often varied depending upon the aggressiveness of the rejection. The toxic effects of steroids, particularly opportunistic infections, are seen much less frequently than in the past. Steroid-induced hypertension, diabetes and aseptic necrosis, particularly of the femoral head, still occur. ATG is produced by injecting human thymocytes into animals. It is usually given intravenously for 10–15 days in doses of 10–15 mg/kilo/day and can delay the onset of rejection episodes when used prophylactically and can reverse acute rejection episodes when used therepeutically. It has a relatively low toxicity, which is manifested by leukopenia and by thrombocytopenia (24, 25). Other techniques have been used to modulate the immune response. Splenectomy in cadaveric transplantation appears to improve graft survival about 10–15% but a similar improvement can also be obtained with ATG (26). Splenectomy incurs an increased risk of infection in children unless long term antibiotics are used. Splenectomy also permits higher doses of Imuran in patients with leukopenia secondary to hypersplenism. Graft irradiation may slightly delay the onset of rejection but does not increase overall graft survival. The use of pretransplant thoracic duct fistula has been abandoned because of expense, a high complication rate and its logistical complexity (27). Plasma exchange or plasmaleukophoresis appears to be a promising new technique, particularly in patients who may be resistant to standard antirejection therapy (28, 29). However, the data is still inconclusive. Anticoagulation, particularly Persantin, with or without aspirin, has been shown to be beneficial in cardiac transplantation, but its usefulness in renal transplantation is still uncertain (30).

## New immunosuppressives

### Cyclosporin A

One of the major advances in the last two or three years has been the utilization of Cyclosporin A as an immunosuppressant drug. Cyclosporin A (CSA), unlike traditional immunosuppressive regimens, appears to be specific in that CSA induces tolerance to alloantigens. Apparently without impairing B cells, CSA alters the early stages of T cell activation. The induction of the cytotoxic effector arm of the immune response is inhibited, while CSA permits the activation of suppressor cells (31). This drug has improved one year graft survivals in cadaveric transplantation at the University of Minnesota and University of Pittsburgh to over 80%. Cyclosporin A is nephrotoxic and its dosage must be carefully monitored by the use of renal biopsy and blood levels of the drug. It is probably best administered with steroids. Due to its nephrotoxicity as well as its cost, it will possibly be used short term posttransplant, ultimately converting the patient to Imuran. In several recipients cyclosporin has resulted in the development of a lymphoma, but this is probably dose-related (32, 33).

### Monoclonal antibody

The development of the hybridoma technique in 1975 has opened a new realm of possible clinical transplant immunology. A number of monoclonal antibodies (MCAB) specific for markers differentiating subpopulations of lymphocytes have been identified. MCAB are of high specificity and would, potentially, serve as useful immunosuppressive agents. The MCAB to T cells have been used clinically in man (34). The MCAB, OKT3 has been found to be a potent immunosuppressant, but two problems must be overcome before MCAB can be utilized as a therapeutic agent; namely, antigenic modulation and immunization. The mechanism for the loss of antigen remains unknown. The loss of cell surface antigen induced by MCAB permits the cell to eventually escape immunosuppression. Another problem with the use of MCAB to date is the development of anti-murine antibody by the recipient. The development of detectable levels of human anti-murine antibody now limits the usefulness of murine MCAB as a therapeutic agent.

As the problems with MCAB are overcome. MCAB 's would theoretically have advantage over ATG as a specific clinical immunosuppressive agent since MCAB could be selected which only react to cell populations relevant to allograft rejection and leave other immune systems intact.

*Transfusions*

Probably the most important recent development in transplantation has been the application, pretransplant, of donor specific blood transfusions (DST) in living-related donors. In donor/recipient combinations that are MLC positive, the recipient receives three transfusions from the donor approximately two weeks apart. Using fresh blood approximately 30–35% of the recipients become sensitized to the donor (35). This sensitization can be decreased by giving the recipient Imuran at the time of the transfusions (36) or by using stored blood (37). The mechanism of this improved graft survival is postulated to be the induction of a population of suppressor cells that are specifically targeted to the antigens in the donor and not by selecting out high responders as previously thought (38). With this technique, graft survivals of 90–95% in MLC positive combinations are being recorded by many centers. In my experience in 26 patients with living-related MLC positive donors that underwent donor specific transfusions, 10 patients became sensitized (38%). The remaining 16 (100%) have functioning grafts for a minimum of 18 months posttransplant.

The use of pretransplant blood transfusions in cadaver transplantations has not yielded as clear a beneficial effect as the use of donor specific transfusions in living-related donors. Several centers have reported improved graft survival by giving 1–20 transfusions pre-transplant to the recipient. However, some centers have also reported no beneficial effect. Terasaki has reported a 70% graft survival at 6 months in patients receiving more than 20 transfusions as compared to 40% graft survival at 6 months in patients with no transfusions (39). The National Institute of Health's study showed a 1 year graft survival in the transfused population of 52% as compared to a 36% graft survival with no transfusions. Neither of the previous studies have shown any beneficial effect of peri-operative transfusions, i.e. given at the time of surgery. Similarly, Belzer reported a 72% graft survival rate in transfused patients compared with a 52% graft survival in patients not being transfused or receiving transfusions prior to surgery. Thus, it is becoming increasingly clear that > 5 non-specific blood transfusions do improve graft survival to a modest degree in cadaveric transplantation.

## Improving results

The results of transplantation have improved significantly over the last several years. This is illustrated by an analysis of my results at Ohio State University broken down into categories based upon the time of their transplant. For the 12 year period prior to 1977 with cadaveric donors, there was a 40% overall mortality rate, with a one year graft survival of approximately 30%. In patients transplanted after 1977, the 1 year mortality rate was 3% with a 1 year graft survival of 57%. With living-related donors prior to 1977, patient mortality rate was 15% with a 78% overall graft survival. After 1977, the mortality rate fell to 6% with an overall graft survival of 74%. From 1980 to 1982, the 1 year graft survival with living-related donors was 92% in 48 patients. Only 8% of the grafts during this two year period rejected. Patients received a kidney from a living-related donor if they were MLC negative with their donor. If they were MLC positive, they received donor specific transfusions from their potential donor prior to transplantation. Thus, a patient with a MLC negative living-related donor should undergo immediate transplantation using low dose immunosuppression. If the patient has a MLC positive donor, he should undergo donor specific transfusions. If sensitization occurs, the patient should be placed on a waiting list for a cadaveric kidney. If sensitization does not occur, transplantation should be performed approximately 4–8 weeks after the last transfusion using low dose immunosuppression. Either Imuran should be given at the time of transfusions or stored blood used instead of fresh blood to minimize the incidence of sensitization. Transplantation can now be offered to a non-selected recipient pool with a mortality risk of less than 3% to the patient. This should be compared to the overall results with hemodialysis in many centers. The mortality rate on hemodialysis inmost series is approximately 6–8% per year in patients under the age of 55 even when those patients who have been on dialysis less than 3 months are excluded. In a study of 307 patients on hemodialysis who were less than 55 years of age, there was a 30% mortality at 24 months at Ohio State University. The mortality rate decreases in the subsequent two year period but nevertheless the overall mortality clearly exceeds that of transplantation. While it is difficult to get comparable patient groups (i.e. transplant vs. dialysis), it is becoming increasingly apparent that the risk to the life of the patient with transplantation is less than it is on hemodialysis. In addition, several studies have shown that rehabilitation is much better with transplantation than with any form of dialysis. Lastly, the overall cost of transplantation is less than any type of dialysis, making it possible to treat more patients with the same resources (40, 41, 42).

*In summary,* the results of transplantation have improved dramatically in the last 2–3 years, yielding markedly diminished mortality rates, improved graft survival, particularly with living-related donors using donor specific transfusion protocols and the advent of Cyclosporin for cadaveric transplantation. In addition, rehabiliation rates are improved and costs are lower utilizing transplantation as a methodology for treating end stage renal disease. Therefore, patients with end stage renal disease, particularly those that are less than 55 years of age, transplantation is the optimal method and most cost effective form of therapy.

# References

1. Hamburger T, Cosnier J, Bach J, Kreis H: Renal transplantation theory and practice. Williams and Wilkins, Baltimore 1981.
2. Sutherland DER, Fryd D, Morrow CE et al: Renal transplantation in the diabetic patient. Transplant Proc 15: 1110–1113, 1983.
3. Najarian JS, Sutherland DER, Simmons RL et al: Ten year experience with renal transplantation in juvenile onset diabetics. Annals of Surg 190: 487–499, 1979.
4. Sanfilippo FP, Vaughn WK, Peters TG et al: Transplantation for polycytic kidney disease. Transplantation 36: 54–59, 1983.
5. Salvatierra O, Wolfson M, Cochrum K et al: End stage polycystic kidney disease: Management by renal transplantation and selective use of preliminary nephrectomy. J of Urol 115: 5–7, 1976.
6. Longlois RP, O'Regan S, Pelletier M, Robitaille P: Kidney transplantation in uremic children with cystinosis. Nephron 28: 273–275, 1981.
7. Malekzadeh MH, Neustein HB, Schneider JA et al: Cadaver renal transplantation in children with cystinosis. Am J Med 63: 525–533, 1977.
8. Yakub YN, Freeman RB, Pabico RC: Renal transplatation in systemic lupus erythematosis. Nephron 27: 197–201, 1981.
9. Amend WJC, Vincent F, Feduska NJ et al: Recurrent systemic lupus erythematosis involving renal allografts. Annals of Int Med 94: 444–448, 1981.
10. Bohannon LL, Norman DJ, Barry J, Bennett WM: Cadaveric renal transplantation in a patient with primary hyperoxaluria. Transplantation 36: 114–115, 1983.
11. Lum CT, Fryd DS, Polta TA, Najarian JS: Results of kidney transplantation in the young child. Transplantation 34: 167–171, 1982.
12. Potter DE, Holliday MA, Piel CF et al: Treatment of end-stage renal disease in children: A 15 year experience. Kidney International 18: 103–109, 1980.
13. Spees EK, Light JA, Smith EJ, Mostofi FK, Oakes DD: Transplantation in patients with a history of renal cell carcinoma: Long term results and clinical considerations. Surgery 91: 282–287, 1982.
14. Alexander GPJ, DeBruyer M, Moriau M et al: ABO incompatible living donor kidney allografts presented at American Society of Transplant Surgeons, June 2–3, 1983, Chicago.
15. Cardello CJ, Falk JA, Peters P, Nicholson J, Harding M: Do repeated blood transfusions prevent successful transplantation in highly sensitized potential transplant recipient. Transplant Proc 14: 359–360, 1982.
16. Gradus D, Ettenger RB: Renal transplantation in children. Ped Clin of North Am 29: 1013–1038, 1982.
17. Kaste M, Palo J: Criteria of brain death and removal of cadaveric organs. Annals of Clin Res 13: 313–317, 1981.
18. Luksza AR: Brain dead kidney donor: Selection, care and administration. Br Med J 1: 1316–1319, 1979.
19. Belzer FO, Hoffman RM, Southard JH: Kidney preservation. Surg Clin of North Am 58: 261–271, 1978.
20. Belzer FO, Southard JH: The future of kidney preservation. Transplantation 30: 161–165, 1980.
21. Marshall VC: Renal preservation prior to transplantation. Transplant 30: 165–166, 1980.
22. Cerilli J, Williams MA, Newhouse YG, Fesperman DP: The correlation of tissue typing, mixed lymphocyte culture and related donor renal allograft survival. Transplantation 26: 218–220, 1978.
23. Feduska NJ, Amend WJ, Vincenti F et al: Graft survival with high levels of cytotoxic antibodies. Transplant Proc 13: 73–80, 1981.
24. Chatterjee SN: Immunosuppressive drugs used in clinical renal transplantation. Supplement to Urol 9: 52–60, 1977.
25. Starzl TE, Rosenthal JT, Hakala TR et al: Steps in immunosuppression for renal transplantation. Kidney International 23: S60–S65, 1983.

26. Mozes MF, Spigos DG, Thomas PH et al: Antilymphocyte globulin (ALG) and splenectomy or partial splenic embolization (PSE): Evidence for a synergistic beneficial effect on cadaver renal allograft survival. Transplant Proc 15: 613–616, 1983.

27. Starzl TE, Weil R, Koep LJ et al: Thoracic duct fistula and renal transplantation. Annal Surg 190: 474–486, 1979.

28. Alijani MR, Pechan BW, Darr F et al: Treatment of steroid-resistant renal allograft rejection with plasmaleukopheresis. Transplant Proc 15: 1063–1066, 1983.

29. Gurland HJ, Blumenstein M, Lysaght MJ et al: Plasmapheresis in renal transplantation. Kidney Internat 23: 582–584, 1983.

30. Czervionko RL, Smith JB, Fry GL et al: Inhibition of prostacyclin by treatment of endothelium with aspirin. J Clin Invest 63: 1089–1092, 1979.

31. Wagner H: Cyclosporin A: Mechanism of action. Transplant Proc 15: 523–526, 1983.

32. Ferguson RM, Rynasiewicz JJ, Sutherland DER et al: Cyclosporin A in renal transplantation: A prospective randomized trial. Surg 92: 175–182, 1982.

33. Thiru S, Henderson RG, Hamilton DV et al: Cyclosporin in cadaveric organ transplantation. Lancet 282: 934–936, 1981.

34. Cosimi AB, Colvin RB, Burton Rc et al: Use of monoclonal antibodies to t cell subsets for immunologic monitoring and treatment in recipients of renal allografts. NEJM 305: 308–314, 1981.

35. Salvatierra O, Vincenti F, Amend W et al: Deliberate donor-specific blood transfusions prior to living related renal transplantation: A new approach. Annals of Surg 192: 543–552, 1980.

36. Anderson CB, Sicard GA, Etheredge EE: Pretreatment of renal allograft recipients with azathioprine and donor-specific blood products. Surgery 92: 315–321, 1982.

37. Light JA, Metz SJ, Oddernino: Donor specific transfusion with minimal sensitization. Transplant Proc 15: 917–923, 1983.

38. van Rood JJ: Pretransplant blood transfusion: Sure! But how and why. Transplant Proc 15: 915–916, 1983.

39. Opelz G, Terasaki PI: Dominant effect of transfusions on kidney graft survival. Transplantation 29: 153–158, 1980.

40. Standards Committee of the American Society of Transplant Surgeons. Current results and expectations of renal transplantation. JAMA 246: 1330–1331, 1981.

41. Vollmer WM, Wahl PW, Blagg CR: Survival with dialysis and transplantation in patients with end stage renal disease. NEJM 308: 1553–1558, 1983.

42. Krakauer H, Grauman JS, McMullan MR, Creede CC: The recent experience in the treatment of end stage renal disese by dialysis and transplantation. NEJM 308: 1558–1563, 1983.

# 18. The living donor for kidney transplantation: a review of 100 consecutive donors

P. JOHN, M.S.A. KUMAR, M. SAMHAN and G.M. ABOUNA

## Introduction

The use of living related donors for transplantation was first carried out in Boston and in Paris in the early 1950's (1). Most of these transplants were between monozygotic twins and this procedure proved highly successful and the final results gave satisfaction to both donor and recipient as well as the whole family.

Since that time many thousands of kidneys have been transplanted between family members and in a small number of cases between unrelated individuals as well. In Kuwait the renal transplantation programme was established in March 1979 and by October 1983 nearly 120 patients received kidneys that were donated by their living relatives and another 30 patients were given imported cadaveric grafts. Because of the non-availability of cadaveric organs in this country, due to social and cultural reasons, renal transplantation has been dependent largely on living donors. This review outlines the problems, the effects and the results in the first 100 living donors who gave kidneys to their relatives and who have been followed up for periods of 4–54 months after nephrectomy.

## Patients and methods

All living donors were adults of legal age (over 18 years) who had volunteered to give a kidney to a relative. 95 of these donors were genetically related to the recipient but in 5 they were only related by marriage. Some of the relevant details on these donors are given in Table 1. There were 55 males and 45 females. 62% were siblings, 21% were parents and 9% were offsprings. There were 3 distant relatives. Donor selection was based first on immunological criteria and when possible the best matched donor with lowest reaction in mixed lymphocyte culture was selected if more than one donor was available. However, in many cases there was only one volunteer donor and apart from ABO compatibility and negative cross match, HLA typing was of little consequence. After the immunological selection was completed, the donors were interviewed by members of the transplant team in order to be satisfied that the donation was freely given and

*Table 1.* Data on 100 living donors.

| Donors | No. |
|---|---|
| Male | 55 |
| Female | 45 |
| Total | 100 |
| HLA identical | 18 |
| No HLA mismatch | 18 |
| One HLA mismatch | 31 |
| Two of more mismatch | 33 |
| Total | 100 |
| Parents | 21 |
| Siblings | 62 |
| Offsprings | 9 |
| Spouses | 5 |
| Others (uncle, nephew, cousin) | 3 |
| Total | 100 |

that the donor understood the possible danger of the operation and the possible future consequences of nephrectomy. If the donor was still willing to proceed with the operation after this interview, he was then admitted to the hospital for full medical evaluation. The medical criteria used in our programme for accepting a donor for transplantation are that he or she should be in normal health, normotensive, euglycaemic and with normal renal function (Table 2). The age distribution of the donors in this series is shown in Table 3. Although it was our protocol not to accept any patient over the age of 60, several patients who were too anxious to donate a kidney for their relatives did not reveal their right age and it turned out that at least 3 of them were well over the age of 60 (Table 3).

The medical evaluation consisted of full history and physical examination, haemogram, biochemical profile, chest X-ray and ECG, measurement of blood pressure, fasting blood sugar and 2 h post prandial sugar level. Renal function studies including routine examination of the urine, microscopy and culture of urine, blood urea, serum creatinine and 24 h creatinine clearance were assessed on at least 3 different occasions. The urine was also cultured on 2–3 occasions. When these investigations were satisfactory, the patient then underwent an intravenous pyelogram, and if this was normal, a renal angiogram was carried out. When all the data was obtained, another interview was held with the patient at which he was informed that he is a suitable and acceptable donor and he was given another opportunity to reconsider his decision. At the same time donor and recipient were reviewed by a transplantation committee which meets weekly when the final decision was made and the operation was scheduled. Before the transplant operation the donor was admitted to the hospital and on the day before surgery, the procedure was again explained. Prior to surgery an intravenous line was inserted for administration of intravenous fluids in an attempt to prevent dehydration and oliguria. The operation was carried out under endotracheal general anaesthesia with the patient lying on one side in the kidney position. Nephrectomy was carried out through an extraserous approach through the bed of the 11th rib. Whenever possible a right nephrectomy was carried out in the female in view of the higher susceptibility of this kidney for developing problems during pregnancy. Also whenever possible the kidney with a single artery was chosen but in several cases there were bilateral renal arteries in which case the left kidney was removed.

During operation, a catheter was also inserted in order to monitor renal function before and immediately after operation. The patient was given high fluid intake and mannitol to maintain good urine flow. Meticulous and gentle nephrectomy was carried out and after cooling with Collin's solution the kidney was given to the recipient team. The catheter was removed the next day when the patient was fully alert and a urine culture was obtained. All wounds were closed by the subcuticular technique without drainage. Within 48 h, the patients were fully ambulant and they were discharged from hospital as soon as the wound was healed and according to their home situation. During their hospital stay regular measurements were made of urinary output, renal function and blood pressure. Following discharge, the patient was seen as an outpatient at intervals for a period

Table 2. Criteria for evaluation and acceptance of living donors.

1. Satisfactory immunological criteria of ABO, HLA and MLR
2. Donor age above 18 years
3. Normal renal function, blood pressure and blood sugar on at least three occasions
4. Donor is free from all medical diseases and disabilities
5. Donor well motivated, is freely willing to donate a kidney
6. Donor is psychologically stable and is of sound mind
7. The donation is freely made and there is no financial transaction between donor and recipient
8. Donor is a blood relative of the recipient or, in specific cases, is related through marriage
9. After due explanation of possible consequences an informed consent is obtained

Table 3. Age range of 100 living donors.

| Age range in years | No. |
|---|---|
| 18–30 | 54 |
| 31–40 | 24 |
| 41–50 | 15 |
| 51–60 | 4 |
| 60 and over | 3 |
| Total | 100 |

of 3–6 months when renal function was assessed and a final IVP taken. Those patients who live in Kuwait were seen subsequently but those who came to Kuwait for transplantation from other countries of the Middle East were followed up by their own doctors after their discharge.

## Results

All patients left hospital after a period of 8–21 days (mean 11 days). There was minimal morbidity and post-operational complications in 11 patients. These are detailed in Table 4. All complications responded satisfactorily to treatment. Intraoperative blood transfusion was used in only one case as a result of accidental avulsion of renal artery pedicle after nephrectomy. Another three patients received blood after surgery, for anemia. In this series, the left kidney was removed in 64% of the patients and right in 36%. Angiography in the donor before nephrectomy showed multiple renal arteries in 8 patients and in 5 of these the condition was bilateral. Since many angiograms were not selective, in almost all of these patients some of the smaller multiple arteries were missed and accurate diagnosis was only made at operation. Table 5 gives details of these cases together with the surgical procedure used and the subsequent results in the recipients. One donor was found to have an aneurysm arising from one of the intra-renal branches of the renal artery. After nephrectomy and cooling the aneurysm was removed using microvascular technique before transplantation into the recipient. Four donors were found to have benign cysts in one kidney and of course this side was chosen for nephrectomy. Three of these were diagnosed pre-operatively by IVP and/or angiography but the fourth was diagnosed at operation. In all cases biopsy was taken and frozen section examination obtained before proceeding. In several recipients with polycystic renal disease, members of the family were investigated for donation. In our earlier experience no CT scanning was available and when all the investigations were negative and the donor was over 30 years of age, donor nephrectomy was proceed with. Before the kidney was removed, a renal biopsy was taken and subjected to frozen section examination. In one case, son to father, the biopsy was positive when all other investigations were negative and the operation was not carried out. The recipient has since received a cadaveric transplant which is functioning normally for nearly two years. During the past two years we have employed the C.T.scan very frequently and in 3 families in which it has been employed, it has proved accurate (Table 6).

Evaluation of the patients post operatively and at 4 months after nephrectomy has shown no significant change in the blood pressure or the serum creatinine from the preoperative value (Table 7). IVP examination has shown appreciable hypertrophy of the remaining kidney within 2–3 months after nephrectomy.

Five of the forty-five women who donated their kidneys have gone through

*Table 4.* Post-operative complications after donor nephrectomy.

| Complications | No. |
|---|---|
| Intraoperative avulsion of renal artery | 1 (1%) |
| Wound infection/haematoma | 2 (2%) |
| Chest infection/atelectasis | 3 (3%) |
| Bacturia | 4 (4%) |
| DVT | 1 (1%) |
| Total | 11 (11%) |

*Table 5.* Multiple vessels in the kidneys of donors on angiography and at operation.

| Donor no. | Kidney used | No. of arteries on angiography | No. of arteries during surgery | No. of arteries in the contra lateral kidney (angiography) | Result in recipient |
|---|---|---|---|---|---|
| 9 | Left | 1 | 2 | 1 | Good graft function Normotensive |
| 34 | Left | 1 | 2 | 1 | Good graft function Normotensive |
| 44 | Right | 1 | 2 | 2 | Good graft function Normotensive |
| 60 | Right | 1 | 2 | 2 | Good graft function |
| 86 | Right | 1 | 2 | 2 | Good graft function |
| 90 | Left | 2 | 3 | 2 | One artery thrombosed Mild hypertension well controlled Renal function good |
| 93 | Left | 1 | 2 | 1 | Good graft function |
| 105 | Left | 2 | 3 | 2 | Good graft function |

168

Table 6. Simple cysts in the kidney of donors on I.V.P. and at operation.

| Donor no. | Donor kidney used | Radiological findings (IVP & Angiography) | Findings during surgery | Surgical procedure for the cyst | Histology |
|---|---|---|---|---|---|
| 2 | Right | Small cyst in the lower pole of right kidney. Left kidney-normal | Small cyst 1 cm in diameter at the lower pole of kidney | Excision & biopsy | Simple cyst - no evidence of malignancy |
| 33 | Right | Small cyst in the lower pole of right kidney. Left kidney-normal | Small cyst 2 cms in diameter at the lower pole of kidney | Excision & biopsy | Simple cyst - no evidence of malignancy |
| 56 | Left | IVP - normal findings Angiography shows small cyst in left kidney Right kidney-normal | Small cyst 1 cm in diameter at the upper pole of kidney | Excision & biopsy | Simple cyst - no evidence of malignancy |
| 82 | Right | IVP & angiography - normal findings | Small cyst 1 cm in diameter at the lower pole of right kidney | Excision & biopsy | Simple cyst - no evidence of malignancy |

Table 7. Blood pressure and serum creatinine of living donors before and after nephrectomy.

| | Before nephrectomy | One week after nephrectomy before discharge | 3 months after nephrectomy |
|---|---|---|---|
| Mean serum Creatinine (mg%) | 1.0 (0.7–1.3) | 1.2 (0.8–1.4) | 1.2 (0.9–1.5) |
| Mean blood Pressure (mm of Hg) | 117/75 (110/70–134/80) | 125/75 (110/70–140/80) | 125/75 (120/70–140/80) |

several successful pregnancies. Of the 5 non-related donors 4 were wife to husband and the other was husband to wife. All of these have continued to do well and one of them has given birth to a healthy infant.

All donors returned to their original occupation within one month after nephrectomy. There have been no long term morbidity during the period of follow-up. After transplantation all kidneys functioned immediately but some grafts were subsequently rejected at 2–26 months after grafting but both patient and graft survival remains high. At present the actuarial graft survival rates for these 100 kidneys is 91, 89, 88 and 87% at 1, 2, 3 and 4 years after transplantation. In addition to helping the recipient, most donors and their families benefited emotionally from the act of donation; the donors feeling proud with high self-esteem and family members becoming closer together than before operation.

## Discussion

Since the advent of Renal Transplantation some 35 years ago, it has been repeatedly shown that survival of kidney grafts is best when the kidney comes from a living related donor (2, 3). However, since nephrectomy is a major surgical procedure with inherent risks and complications of any operation, removal of a kidney from a healthy volunteer donor naturally carries certain moral, social and legal implications. For this reason the use of living related donors is not universally accepted, it is controversial in some centers and it is not practised at all in few others. In those countries where cadaveric grafts are becoming plentiful, it is argued that the use of living donors should become less common. However, in those countries of the world such as the Middle East where cadaveric organs are not yet available, the use of living related donors for transplantation is the only practical alternative. Fortunately, there is now a considerable volume of data which shows that the risk of nephrectomy to the donor is extremely small and the morbidity minimal (4, 5).

It was for these reasons and particularly for the fact that the results of renal transplantation from living donors are superior to those obtained from cadavers, that the transplantation programme in Kuwait has relied mainly on living donors and only recently has used cadaveric kidneys imported from United States and Europe. In this controversial situation the real issue becomes that of ensuring that the living donor is sufficiently protected by taking every possible, medical, legal and social precautions to eliminate mortality and reduce possible morbidity of this procedure. It is also important to ensure, by every means possible, that the decision to donate has been given freely and voluntarily and with informed consent.

The protocol used in our centre, such as those used in other major centres, has been carefully planned and it is rigorous enough to ensure the protection of the interests of the donor. Indeed, during the course of the development of the transplantation programme in Kuwait, many more donors presented themselves with motives other than those of charity and were turned down. We have also turned down sibling and offspring donors below the age of 18 who came forward to donate a kidney in order to help a loved relative. In our series, 83% of the donors were either siblings or parents and while every attempt was made to obtain a fully matched donor, this was only possible in about 18% of the cases. There is a small preponderance of male donors over female donors and this may be due to the fact that in several instances female donors were not allowed to proceed with the operation because of pressure from their husbands. The use of spouses as donors was used in a few cases in our programme because we were convinced that the motivation to donate was made out of charity and love for the recipient.

There was no mortality in this small series of donors and this is in keeping with several other reported series (5). However, donor mortality has been reported but the incidence is extremely small (4). The incidence of post-operative complications and morbidity in our series (11%) is less than that reported in other larger series which has varied from 17–28% (4, 5). All donors left hospital within a short time after nephrectomy and within one month they were all back in their former occupation. However, subsequently some donors requested a change of occupation to lighter work but in all cases the donor continued to enjoy full and normal life. Five of the female donors have gone through several normal pregnancies. We have not seen any long term sequelae of nephrectomy although our follow-up period is relatively short and does not extend beyond five years. However, in a recent report by Weiland and others (5) from the Minnesota Transplantation Team where 628 living related donors were reviewed, long term sequelae were seen in about 17% of patients that had been followed up for periods of up to 14 years. The most important of these was the development of moderate to severe hypertension in 5.7% of the patients, an incidence which is probably comparable to that of the general population of the same age group. While we preferred the use of young healthy individuals, we did use rather inadvertently, several patients who were older than 60 years of age. All these patients did well and had no specific complications. In a report from Boston Transplant Team, Bennett reported that 10% of their living donors were older than 60 years of age and the maximum age was 80(4).

In the evaluation of the living donors, extreme care is taken to eliminate any abnormalities which will make nephrectomy unsuitable or will compromise the health of the donor. In our series 8 donors were found to have multiple renal arteries and in most of these the diagnosis was not made by angiography but at the operating table. We believe this can be avoided, if selective angiography, with adequate precautions, is carried out during donor evaluation. Other abnormalities such as solitary cyst and even polycystic disease were discovered during the preoperative evaluation. Four patients had single cysts and obviously the kidney bearing the cyst was used. In all cases the cysts proved benign and there were no complications. Our follow up of the patients after nephrectomy has shown that within a short time normal renal function is restored by the usual compensatory hypertrophy of the other kidney thus maintaining normal serum creatinine. There was no change in the blood pressure and there was no proteinurea in any of the patients during the period of follow-up. Our operative procedure employs an extra serous subcostal incision in all cases, full hydration of the donor and a gentle technique. As a result of this every kidney that was removed functioned with immediate diuresis. There were no serious intraoperative complications in these patients and only one patient required intraoperative blood transfusion during nephrectomy. We have employed intraoperative catheterization in order to monitor the blood volume and the renal function and we have not found this to cause increase in the incidence of bacteriuria or renal infection providing that the catheter is removed within 24 h.

While donating a kidney for transplantation is a definite sacrifice by a healthy donor, this major sacrifice and loss to the donor is not without gain. Not only is the recipient given a second lease of life and enabled to live normally once again but in our experience there were many psychological benefits to the donor himself. Many of our donors expressed the feeling of satisfaction, of pride and of heightened self-esteem following the act of donation and in a few cases, who were at first doubtful to donate, came forward after nephrectomy to express definite regret for their behaviour since the problems following nephrectomy were so minor and the results so gratifying. We also noticed that the act of donation of one member of the family to another brought enormous happiness and helped strengthen the family ties which in some cases had been strained by misunderstandings and past feuds. Similar psychological benefits have been reported by others (7). When a kidney rejected in a few patients after transplantation, there was a feeling of regret and sometimes of guilt on the part of the donor.

While the use of living donors for transplantation is likely to decrease in the future because of the greater availability of cadaveric organs and because of the improvement in the results of those grafts with the use of Cyclosporin, we believe that even under those circumstances there is still a place for living donor transplantation particularly in the circumstances where the use of a perfect match is necessary and in those parts of the world, such as the Middle East, where cadaveric organs are not yet available. Our experience in living donor transplantation herein reported is gratifying and encouraging, and until cadaveric organs become freely available in this part of the world we intend to continue to use living donors for our patients employing the same rigorous criteria for selection and for the intraoperative and post operative management.

## References

1. Murray JE: Reminiscences on Renal Transplantation. In: Organ Transplantation (Chatterjee SN ed). John Wright, PSG Inc, Boston, 1982, p 1.
2. Najarian JS, Van Hook EJ, Simmons RL: Kidney Transplants from Distant Relatives. Am Jr Surg Vol 135 No 3, p 362–66, March, 1972.
3. The 12th report of the ACS/NIH. Human Renal Transplant Registry JAMA 233: 787, 1975.
4. Bennett AH, Harrison JH: Experience with Living Familial donors. Surg Gynec Obstet 139: 894, 1974.
5. Weiland D, Sutherland DER, Chavers B, Simmons RL, Ascher N, Najarian JS: Information on 628 Living related donors at a single institution with 1–19 years follow-up. American Society of Transplant Surgeons. 9th Annual Meeting, June 1983 (Abstract).
6. Bernstein DM, Simmons RG: The adolescent Kidney donor - The right to give. Arm J Psychiat 131: 1339, 1974.
7. Fellner CH, Marchall JB: Twelve Kidney Donors. JAMA 206: 2703, 1968.

# 19. Kidney transplantation in diabetic recipients: factors leading to improved results

D.E.R. SUTHERLAND, D.S. FRYD, C.E. MORROW, F.C. GOETZ, R.M. FERGUSON, R.L. SIMMONS and J.S. NAJARIAN

## Introduction

Diabetic nephro-sclerosis in the United States has been the primary cause of death in 50% of patients with Type 1 diabetes. Diabetic nephropathy is now responsible for 25% of all new cases referred to transplant units in the United States (1). Average patient survival of diabetic patients maintained on dialysis is 60–70% at 2 years and this represents on improvement on the results obtained in the early 1970's where only 25% of the patients were alive at 2 years (2). The results of maintaining diabetics on dialysis have improved tremendously (3) and this has also been paralleled by an improved survival after renal transplantation. It has been considered that the diabetic patient is a high risk patient for dialysis or transplantation but this is only in relation to the non-diabetic patient who receives the same treatment. It is important to consider what is the best treatment for the individual patient. Particularly since diabetic patients do better with renal transplantation then if they are maintained on dialysis. However, elderly patients tended to do better on dialysis rather than transplantation (in the pre-Cyclosporin era) and this group are therefore 'high risk' for transplantation.

This contribution describes our experiences at Minnesota with renal transplantation in diabetic patients from 1968 to 1981.

## Patients and methods

During this period 1294 primary renal transplants were performed in patients over 2 years old. Four hundred and seventy patients with Type 1 diabetes received primary renal allografts thus representing 36% of the total number. Of the 470 patients, 173 received cadaver kidneys (37%), 196 HLA non-identical kidneys (42%), 91 HLA identical sibling grafts (19%) and 10 were recipients of kidneys from distant relatives (2%) or unrelated living donors. Immunosuppression consisted of azathioprine, prednisone and anti-lymphocyte globulin and later some patients were given Cyclosporin A and low dose prednisone (1). Obviously, because of the extended period of study (13 years) there were changes in the

immunosuppressive management of patients. These changes included splenectomy or no splenectomy, deliberate blood transfusion and the introduction of
Cyclosporin A.

Actuarial analysis of patient survival at 4 years in the diabetic patients was 68%
and in non-diabetic patients was 80%. Corresponding graft survival figures were
62% in diabetics and 67% in non-diabetics. The donor source obviously affected
the graft survival. HLA identical siblings donors gave 4 year actuarial graft
survival in diabetics of 84% and in non-diabetics of 91%. Non-identical relatives
in diabetics the graft survival was 61% and non-diabetics 68% while in cadavers
the survival was 56% for diabetics and 58% in non-diabetics. Overall the 4 year
graft survival rate was upto 7% better in the non-diabetics depending on the
donor source utilised. The date reported in our study is comparable to that
reported by other U.S. centers in which diabetic recipients of related and cadaver
donors had graft survivals of 69% and 58% respectively (4). Improved patient
survival rate in diabetics may of course be related to better control of hyper-
glycaemia (4).

## Discussion

These results of renal transplantation in uraemic diabetics illustrate that both
patient and graft survival are similar to non-diabetics. Therefore these patients
should not be considered as high risk candidates. In addition to better patient
survival compared to dialysis, transplantation results in a large measure of
rehabilitation but of course there may be a recurrence of diabetic nephropathy
and a progression of vascular disease.

Since the advent of kidney transplantation and dialysis the diabetic patient is
living much longer and the progress of vascular disease results in a significant
number of patients requiring amputation, 14.5% of our diabetic transplant recipients have required amputation of a leg, foot, toe, hand or finger. In fact there
appears to be 3 subgroups of transplanted diabetic patients - those that die early
and never get amputated, those that survive long enough to require amputation,
and those that do not have a progression of vascular disease and do not need
amputation.

In conclusion we believe that the treatment of diabetic and non-diabetic
recipients should be similar. Once end stage renal failure occurs, the patient
should be evaluated and transplanted as soon as feasible. The patient and graft
survival rates in uremic diabetic patients have improved and they should no
longer be considered as high risk for graft loss or patient death in relation to non-
diabetics.

# References

1. Kjellstrand CM, Avram MM, Blagg CR, Friedman EA, Salviettera O, Simmons RL, Williams GM, Terasaki P: Panel Conference. Cadaver Transplantation versus Haemodialysis. Trans Am Soc Artif Intern Organs 26: 611–624, 1980.
2. Kjellstrand CM, Simmons RL, Goetz FC, Buselmeir TJ, Shideman JR, Von Hartitzsch B, Najarian JS: Renal Transplantation in Patients with Insulin dependent diabetes. Lancet 2: 4–8, 1973.
3. Kjellstrand CM, Compty CM, Shapiro FL. In: Diabetic Renal Retinal Syndrome. Prevention and Management (ed. 2) (Friedman EA, L'Esperance SA Jr eds) and Stratton, New York, 1982.
4. Standards Committee of the American Society of Transplant Surgeons: JAMA 246: 133, 1981.
5. Barbosa J, Menth L, Eaton J, Sutherland D, Freier EF, Najarian JS: Long term, ambulatory, subcutaneous insulin infusion versus multiple daily injections in brittle diabetic patients. Diabetes Care 4: 269–274, 1981.

# 20. Fungal infections in 135 renal transplantations

M. HABERAL, Z. ONER, N. YULAG, H. GULAY and N. BILGIN

## Introduction

Kidney transplantation has proven to be an effective method of treatment for chronic kidney disease. Despite improved surgical technique and a better understanding of immunosuppression, serious complications still exist. Some of these complications are immunosuppression related, and the remainder can be counted as actual complications, as reported from various different centers (1, 2, 10). Among these, the ones with a high morbidity and mortality rate are infectious complications as a result of bacterial, fungal, viral and protozoan agents. The effects of these agents on immunosuppressed patients have been well documented (3, 4, 5, 10).

In our studies we found that fungal infections were the most difficult to treat and unresponsive to medication. As a result of this difficulty, the morbidity and the mortality rate in these patients was high.

## Material and methods

From November 1975 to September 1982, 135 kidney transplantations were performed at our center. Of these, 118 (87,4%) were living related donor transplants, and 17 (12.6%) were from cadaver donors. Forty one of the 135 transplanted patients displayed symptoms of infection: 22 (16.3%) bacterial, 10 (7.4%) fungal, and 9 (6.6%) viral (clinical diagnosis of herpes simplex) (Fig. 1). Nine of the 10 patients developed fungal infections early in the post operative period (18 to 92 days), and one patient after two years. Of the ten fungal infected patients, 3 were male and 7 female, between the ages of 14 to 33 years.

Immunosuppressive treatment for these patients consisted of azathioprine, prednisone, and methyl prednisolone was used during rejection. All of the patients were on antibiotic therapy (carbenicillin, keflin, bactrim, ampicillin and gentamicin) due to unrelated infections at least 10 days prior to the diagnosis of fungal infection (Table 1).

With the exception of 2 patients, all received 1 to 6 gms. of steroids. Three

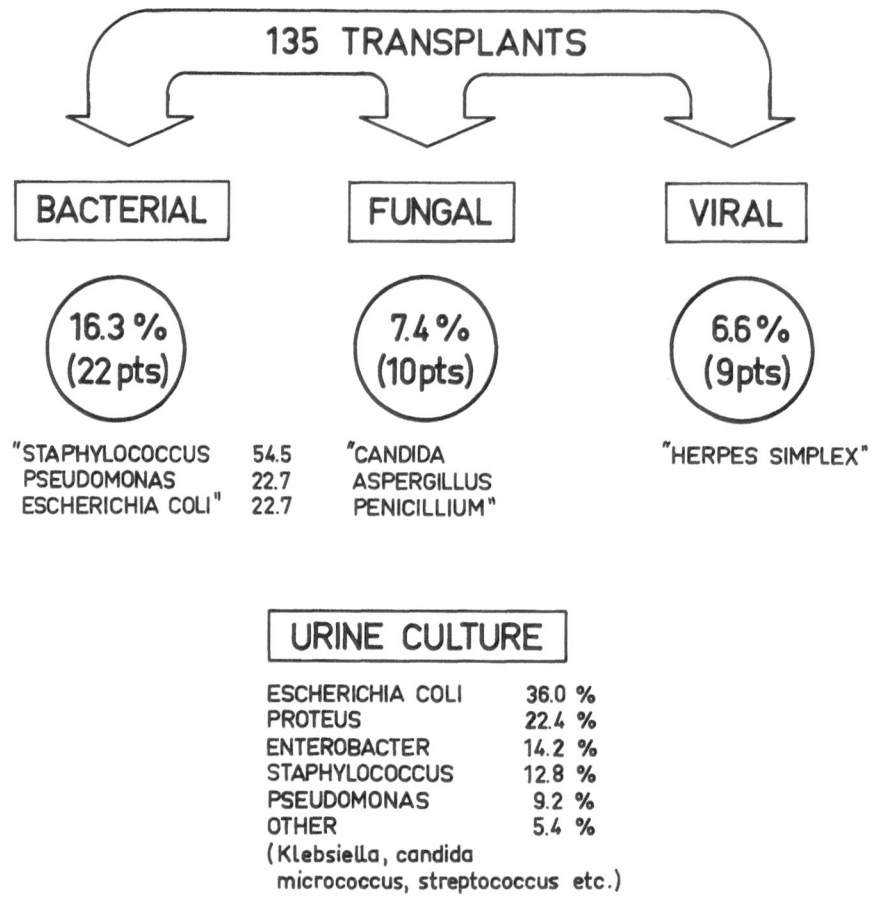

*Fig. 1.* Complication of infections in 135 kidney transplants.

patients had normal kidney function (Table 1). Fungal infection diagnosed in these 10 living related transplanted patients were as follows: 6 patients *Candida,* 3 patients *Aspergillus,* and 1 *Penicillium* (Table 2).

**Results**

Five of the 10 patients died as a result of fungal infections. Two of the 5 patients died due to *Aspergillus* infections immediately after diagnosis. Two patients with *Candida* refused treatment and were released against medical advice. One *Candida* patient was treated with amphotercin B, with no response and died 15 days later. In the last 3 patients immunosuppressive therapy was decreased and discontinued by the time of diagnosis. The reason for a high dose of steroids was that 2 patients showed signs of chronic rejection, 1 patient acute rejection, and the

*Table 1.* Analyses of 10 patients with fungal infections.

| Case No. | Immunosuppression[a] | | Antibiotic[a] | Kidney functions[b] | Rate of immuno-suppression | Treatment of fungal infections | Results |
|---|---|---|---|---|---|---|---|
| | Steroid | Azathioprine | | | | | |
| 1 | 6 gm | 1 gm | Gentamicin Carbenicillin | Acute rejection | No change | None | Died |
| 2 | 1 gm | 1 gm | Keflin Gentamicin Carbenicilin | Normal | Decreased and discontinued | Amphotericin B | Died |
| 3 | 4 gm | 0.5 gm | Gentamicin | Normal | No change | None | Died |
| 4 | 3 gm | 1 gm | Gentamicin Bactrim | Chronic rejection | Discontinued | None[c] | Died |
| 5 | 3 gm | 1 gm | Gentamicin Ampicillin | Chronic rejection | Discontinued | None | Died |
| 6 | 100 gm | 1.5 gm | Bactrim | Chronic rejection | Discontinued | Amphotericin B | Graft nephrectomy |
| 7 | 3.250 gm | 1gm | Gentamicin | Normal | Decreased and discontinued | Amphotericin B | Graft nephrectomy |
| 8 | 3.250 gm | 0.5 gm | Bactrim Gentamicin | Chronic rejection | Discontinued | Amphotericin B | Graft nephrectomy |
| 9 | 250 gm | 0.5 gm | Ampicillin | Chronic rejection | Discontinued | None | Graft nephrectomy |
| 10 | 3.250 gm | 0.5 gm | Gentamicin Ampicillin | Chronic rejection | Discontinued | None | Graft nephrectomy |

[a] 10 days prior to diagnosis.
[b] At the time of diagnosis.
[c] Patients refused treatment.

*Table 2.* Fungal infections and their diagnoses.

| Fungus | No of patients | diagnoses | |
|--------|----------------|-----------|---|
| Candida | 6 | Blood | 1 |
| | | Urine | 3 |
| | | Sputum | 3 |
| | | Stool | 1 |
| Aspergillus | 3 | Peritoneum | 2 |
| | | Wound | 1 |
| Penicillium | 1 | Sputum | 1 |

remaining 2 received high steroids in the early post transplantation stage.

Of the 5 remaining living patients, 2 received high steroids because of chronic rejection, 1 patient was given a high dose due to showing symptoms of rejection, and 2 were receiving the required amount of steroids. All patients were on antibiotics for various other infections. At the time of fungal infection diagnosis, the patient's immunosuppression was decreased and discontinued. Three patients were treated by amphotericin B.

Discontinuation of immunosuppression resulted in graft failure, therefore graft nephrectomies were performed on all 5 patients and they were placed on haemodialysis.

## Discussion

Successful and life saving kidney transplantations are being performed in our center as well as in many others, but the problem of infections still present a life threatening situation. There are many factors contributing to the subject of fungal infections, including the general and metabolic condition of the patient prior to transplantation, the side effects of aggressive immunosuppressive therapy, antibiotic therapy due to other types of infection and the environment to which the patient is exposed to at home after being released (3, 4, 8).

In our series, the analyses of 10 patients that had 100% follow-ups showed that the majority of fungus infections occur in the first 90 days (early post transplantation), with a high rate of mortality. This statement has been confirmed by Ahern *et al.* (2), Anderson *et al.* (3), and Rifkind *et al.* (4).

In our series the majority of this type of infection were seen more often in women, which is in contrast with Rifkind *et al.* (4).

It is our belief that sex is not a contributing factor in fungal infections, but kidney dysfunction and high dose steroid therapy due to rejection, may be contributing factors in fungal infections, as also shown by Rifkind *et al.* (6), Bach *et al.* (7) and Lobo *et al.* (9).

Of our 5 surviving patients with kidney dysfunction, high steroid therapy and antibiotic treatment due to bacterial infections were discontinued when fungal infection was diagnosed, immunosuppressive therapy stopped, and amphotericin B treatment was started. Even though the patients lost their grafts and graft nephrectomies were performed, the most rewarding result was saving the patient's life. Our studies confirm that any combination of kidney dysfunction, the presence of concomitant bacterial infection, the use of antibiotics and high dose steroid therapy can be predisposing factors to fungal infections.

We therefore recommend that the immunosuppression therapy be utilized with extreme care for the prophylaxis of fungal infection.

## Summary

Since November 1975 to September 1982, 10 fungal infections were encountered in 135 transplant patients, with the majority of infections occurring in the first 90 days after transplantation.

Our experience showed that during the post-transplantation follow-up, the use of antibiotics and aggressive immunosuppressive therapy can be predisposing factors to fungal infections, which may lead to a high mortality rate.

Therefore, with the patient's well being in mind, the above therapies should be utilized with extreme care.

## References

1. Chatterjee SN: Complications of renal transplantation. Manual of renal transplantation, SN Chatterjee, Springer Verlag, New York, Heidelberg, Berlin, 1979.
2. Ahern MJ, Comite H, Andriole VT: Infectious complications associated with renal transplantation: an analysis of risk factors. Yale J Biol and Med 54: 513, 1978.
3. Anderson RJ, Schafer LA et al: Infectious risk factors in the immunosuppressed host. Amer J Med 54: 453, 1973.
4. Rifkind D, Marchioro TL et al: Systemic fungal infections complicating renal transplantation and immunosuppressive therapy. Amer J Med 43: 28, 1967.
5. Unalmiser S, Haberal M et al: Strongyloidiasis in kidney transplantation. Hacettepe Bullt Med Surg 10: 95, 1977.
6. Rifkind D, Marchioro TL et al: Infectious diseases associated with renal homotransplantation. JAMA 189: 398, 1964.
7. Bach MC, Adler JL et al: Influence of rejection therapy on fungal and nocardial infections in renal transplant recipients. Lancet 27: 180, January, 1973.
8. Finkelstein FO, Black HR: Risk factor analysis in renal transplantation: Guidelines for the management of the transplant recipient. Amer J Med Scin 267: 159, 1974.
9. Lobo PI, Rudolf LE, Krieger JN: Wound infections in renal transplant recipients. A complication of urinary tract infections during allograft malfunction. Surg 92: 491, 1982.
10. Brynger H, Bitter-Suermann H et al: Complications after renal transplantation. In: Renal Transplantation, Lars Gelin Gotab, Kungalv, Stockholm, 1976. p 113.

# 21. Bilateral renal transplantation: effect on pelvic hemodynamics and sexual function in male patients

FUAD J. DAGHER, ADAM BILLET and LUIS QUERAL

## Introduction

Approximately 50% of male patients with chronic renal failure treated by hemo-dialysis complain of sexual dysfunction of some degree or another (1). While successful renal transplantation improves sexual performance of a large number of these patients, close to 30% continue to experience poor sexual function. Further, and in the event a second contralateral transplant procedure is performed, the rate of impotence increaces once again to 50% or more (2). It is suggested that this increase might be due to vascular insufficiency resulting from ligation of both internal iliac arteries (3).

In this chapter an attempt is made to identify such patients using questionnaires and personal interviews, to assess pelvic hemodynamics using a penile/brachial pressure index and to correlate sexual function with pelvic hemodynamics, internal iliac artery patency and age.

## Patient load and results

Comprising this study group are patients who received at least two bilateral kidney transplants from 1975 to 1979. Of 36 patients identified, 24 were geographically accessible and consented to participate in the study. Their ages ranged between 19 and 53 years with a mean of 33 years.

Impairment or unimpairment of sexual function was based on detailed sexual histories obtained by personal interviews and questionnaires. Patients with unimpaired sexual function are those that are regularly able to achieve and maintain an erection that would allow sexual intercourse. Patients with impaired sexual function are divided into two groups: Those with total impotence, i.e. with complete loss of erections and those with partial impotence. The latter group are in turn divided into two categories; those with inadequate tumescence to permit pentration and those with adequate tumescence but with insufficient duration to permit satisfactory intercourse. Patency or occlusion of each internal iliac artery was noted after reviewing the operative record and patients records, and when in doubt with an arteriography.

A penile/brachial blood pressure index (PBI) was calculated for each patient by dividing the penile systolic blood pressure by the brachial systolic blood pressure. These PBI results are analyzed for age, number of patent iliac arteries and correlated with sexual dysfunction. The statistical significance of each finding was determined by the student t-test and chi-square binary matrix analysis.

A total of 52 kidney transplants were performed on the 24 patients evaluated. Each of 21 patients received two transplants, two patients received three transplants each and one patient received four transplants. At the time the study was conducted seven patients had already rejected their kidneys and were on chronic hemodialysis.

Fifteen of the 24 patients had bilateral internal iliac artery occlusion, most commonly as a result of using both internal iliac arteries in an end to end fashion. Other causes include atherosclerosis, post nephrectomy ligation of the artery and severe infection. Nine of these 15 patients with bilateral internal iliac artery occlusion reported impaired sexual function (60%).

Of the total 24 patients, eleven patients (46%) reported impaired sexual function and 13 had no impairment. Two of the 11 patients with impaired sexual function had at least one patent internal iliac artery each, but had other sources of dysfunction such as psychogenic factors. In the remaining 9 patients, both internal iliac arteries were occluded and in four of these the PBIs were less than 0.70 which is consistent with vasculogenic impotence. One of these four patients regained full sexual potency following revascularization procedure in which a vein bypass was performed between the external iliac and the remaining stump of the ligated internal iliac artery (4). Of the remaining five patients, and despite higher PBIs than 0.7, four were on chronic hemodialysis which could explain their sexual impairment and one patient had no discernible cause.

The PBI correlated very well with the status of sexual function and with patency of internal iliac artery. In general those patients with higher PBI and at least one patent internal iliac artery had better sexual function. Further, differences in PBI between patients younger than and those older than 32 years of age were statistically significant.

### Discussion

Based on the above results we believe that patients with bilateral renal transplants in whom both internal iliac arteries are occluded have a high rate of sexual impotence, i.e. 60%.

The PBI has been shown to be an effective and accurate method of measuring blood flow to the pelvis (5, 6) and to the phallus. In the present study, the calculated penile brachial pressure index was used to evaluate vascular insufficiency to the pelvis and, hence, impotence of a vascular etiology. Using a cut off index of 0.70, it was noted that blood flow to the phallus was significantly lower in patients with bilateral internal iliac artery ligation than in those with one artery patent (p <0.001). There was also a definite correlation between the level of PBI, the status of sexual function and patency of the internal iliac arteries.

Because not all patients with bilateral kidney transplants developed sexual impotence, each case had to be carefully evaluated. When evaluating data concerning sexual function to patients, several factors need to be considered. Data derived from personal interviews and questionnaires can be inaccurate specifically if the interviewer fails to establish good rapport with the patient, or if the patient fails to report honestly (7). Further, the variety of causes for impotence in the general population are numerous and varied. Of importance to proper sexual function are the endocrine, metabolic, neurologic and vascular systems (8). In addition, the renal transplant patient experiences changes that can affect many of these systems simultaneously which makes identification of a single specific cause of impotence rather difficult. Immunosuppressive medications which are taken by most kidney transplant patients can in more than one way cause endocrine and metabolic disorders (9), and as many as 45% of these patients take antihypertensive medications as well which may also be associated with impaired sexual function (10). Also psychologic and socioeconomic stresses may be severe and may seriously impair sexual function (11).

In addition to the above, age can play a role. As a rule sexual function declines with increasing age (12). We also have noted that the PBI decreases with increasing age regardless of internal iliac artery status. Of patients with bilateral internal iliac artery occlusion, those younger than 32 had significantly higher PBIs than those older than 32 years of age, suggesting that younger patients may compensate by developing collaterals with better pelvic perfusion (13).

Despite the numerous and extenuating factors in evaluating data on male impotence and in the light of the above data it is our belief that vascular insufficiency is an important component of sexual dysfunction in patients with bilateral renal transplantation in whom both internal iliac arteries are ligated. While second transplants performed on the opposite side adversely affect pelvic hemodynamics and sexual function, and in order to preserve direct blood flow to the pelvis, we recommend that, in patients undergoing second renal transplants, arterial continuity be in the form of end of renal artery to side of either common, external or even internal iliac arteries.

## References

1. Abrams HS, Hester LR, Sheridan WF, Epstein GM: Sexual functioning in patients with chronic renal failure. J Nerv Ment Dis 160: 220, 1975.
2. Brannen GE, Peters TG, Hambidge KM, Kumpe DA, Kempczinski RF, Schroter GP, Weil R: Impotence after kidney transplantation. Urology 15: 138, 1980.

3. Burns JR, Houttuin E, Gregory JG, Hawathem IS, Sullivan TR: Vascular induced erectile impotence in renal transplant recipients. J Urol 121: 721, 1979.

4. Billet A, Dagher FJ, Queral LA: Surgical Correction of vasculogenic impotence in a patient after bilateral renal transplantation. Surgery 91: 108–112, 1982.

5. Gaskell P: The importance of penile blood pressure in cases of impotence. CMA J 150: 1047, 1971.

6. Kempczinski RF: Role of vascular diagnostic laboratory in the evaluation of male impotence. Am J Surg 138: 278, 1979.

7. Levy NB: Sexual adjustment of maintenance hemodialysis and renal transplantation: National Survey by questionnaire: preliminary report. Transcrp Soc Artif Int organs 19: 138, 1973.

8. Weiss HD: The physiology in human penile erection. Ann Intern Med 76: 793, 1972.

9. Zadeh JA, Koutsaimanis KG, Roberts AP: The effect of maintenance hemodialysis and renal transplantation on plasma testosterone levels of male patients in chronic renal failure. Acta Endocrinol 80: 577, 1975.

10. Procci WR, Hoffman KI, Chatterjee SN: Persistent sexual dysfunction following renal transplantation. Dialysis and Transpl 7: 891, 1979.

11. Fielding JM: Psychiatric aspects of renal hemotransplantation. Aust NZ J Psychiat 6: 57, 1972.

12. Ruzbarsky V, Michal V: Morphologic changes in the arterial bed of the penis with aging: Relationship to the pathogenesis of aging. Invest Urol 15: 194, 1977.

13. Friedenberg MJ, Perez CA: Collateral circulation in aorto-ilio-femeral occlusive disease: As demonstrated by a unilateral percutaneous common femoral artery needle injection. Am J Roentg 94: 145, 1965.

# 22.  Renal replacement therapy in Kuwait

G. KUSMA, N.A. HILALI and G.M. ABOUNA

Renal replacement therapy namely haemodialysis, peritoneal dialysis and renal transplantation has become a well established procedure for the treatment of patients with end stage renal failure. Currently more than 60,000 patients are maintained on regular dialysis throughout the world (1). In the Arab world, there are a few dialysis centres reported in the registry of the European Dialysis and Transplant Association (2, 3).

In Kuwait the dialysis programme was begun in March 1976, with a few patients on haemodialysis in the Amiri Hospital. This programme has now developed into a major centre for treatment of patients with end stage renal failure by haemodialysis and peritoneal dialysis (both intermittent peritoneal and continuous ambulatory peritoneal dialysis). A second dialysis unit was established in 1982 in the Mubarak Al Kabeer Hospital with a few patients on peritoneal and hemodialysis. Renal transplantation was commenced in 1979, initially using only living related donors and later with imported cadaver kidneys as well (4).

During the last 5 years the number of patients admitted to the programme has increased rapidly (Fig. 1). In 1983 a total of 150 patients have been maintained on regular dialysis. Of the 150 patients, 115 on haemodialysis and 35 on peritoneal dialysis. Forty-eight percent of the patients are Kuwaiti and 52% non Kuwaiti. The majority of these non-Kuwaiti patients are Arabs (80%) from the neighbouring countries of Palestine, Egypt, Syria, Saudi Arabia, Yemen, Jordan and Iraq. The non Kuwaiti non Arab patients (20%) are from India, Pakistan and Thailand. Kuwait is a cosmopolitan country and only 44% of the pupulation are Kuwaiti nationals (5) and this is obviously reflected in the balance of patients on the dialysis programme.

The population of Kuwait is about 1.5 million and the number of patients on the dialysis programme is about 100 per million of population. This is similar to the incidence of patients on hospital dialysis in Europe (2). The number of patients admitted to the programme in 1983 was 48 per million of population. There is no age bar in accepting patients on dialysis in Kuwait and the patients' ages range between 5–70 years of age, the majority being adult patients between 21–50 years of age. Forty-five percent are male and 55% are female.

After commencing the dialysis programme in 1976 with 3 dialysis machines and

188

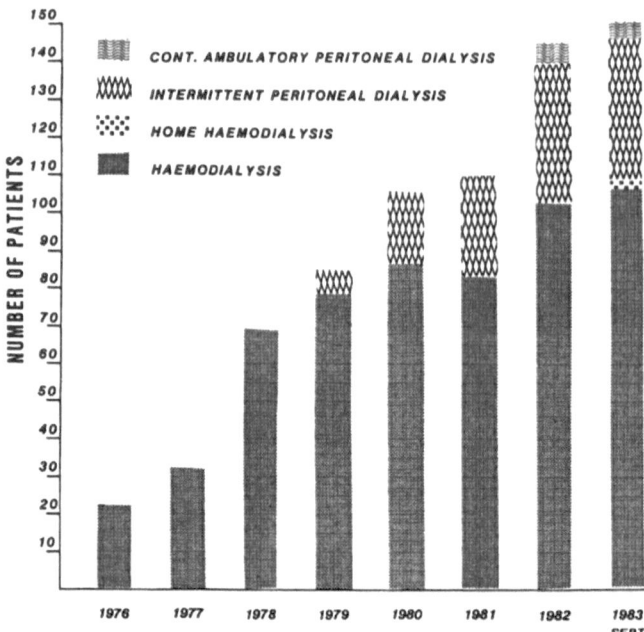

*Fig. 1.* Progressive increase of the patients accepted on dialysis programme at Amiri Hospital, Kuwait.

considering the rapid increase in patients being diagnosed and treated for end stage renal failure (Fig. 1), the Ministry of Public Health has expanded facilities for dialysis and there are now 13 machines at the Amiri Hospital dialysis centre and another 3 at the Mubarak Hospital. One of these machines is reserved for Hepatitis B surface antigen positive patients. In addition there are 5 peritoneal dialysis cyclers. All of these machines are functioning for 24 h with 3 shifts per day. The period of haemodialysis for the patients is 5 h, 2 or 3 sessions per week. The duration of peritoneal dialysis is one session of 24 h every 5 days, using 80 l of peritoneal dialysis fluid. Prior to taking any patient on to the regular dialysis programme a screening test for Hepatitis B surface antigen is performed. All patients accepted onto regular dialysis undergo a complete accessment in search of primary renal disease, are investigated as possible candidates for renal transplantation with tissue typing, lymphocytotoxic antibodies, cystography, barium meal and a bone X-ray and a search is made for a living related donor. Bilateral or unilateral nephrectomy for specific cases such as uncontrolled hypertension, pyelonephritis or ureteric reflux are carried out. Those who have no suitable or willing related donor are placed on the cadaver list.

The primary causes of renal disease are shown in Table 1. The major cause of renal failure is chronic glomerulo-nephritis, this occuring in 52% of the patients. Pyelonephritis occurs in 24% of the patients, 7% have polycystic kidneys, 3.5% have renal stone disease and 2.2% have diabetic nephropathy.

*Table 1.* Primary renal disease.

| | |
|---|---|
| Glomerulonephritis | 52% |
| Pyelonephritis | 24% |
| Poly-cystic kidney | 7.2% |
| Renal stone disease | 3.5% |
| Diabetic nephropathy | 2.2% |
| Medullary cystic disease | 2.2% |
| Obstructive uropathy | 1.5% |
| Interstitial nephritis | 0.7% |
| Hypertension | 0.7% |
| Uncertain | 6.2% |
| Total | 100% |

The mortality rate on dialysis prior to 1981 was very high, approximately 26% per year. In 1982 this mortality rate was reduced to 14.5% per year as a result of intensive patient education, good personnel training and early renal transplantation. The major cause of death on dialysis is hyperkalemia causing 60% of the deaths. The other main causes are pulmonary oedema 20% and cardiovascular problems (10%). These major factors were usually due to the non compliance of our patients as regard to medication, fluid intake and food restriction. The cost of hospital haemodialysis in Kuwait is about K.D.8000 (1 KD = US$ 3.5) per patient per year. It is similar to the cost of hospital haemodialysis in Europe (6, 7). The cost of dialysis is higher than the cost of renal transplantation which is about 5000 KD per patient.

Prior to starting renal transplantation in Kuwait, 10 patients had received kidney transplants in Europe. Since 1979, when kidney transplantation was initiated in Kuwait, all patients who are not contraindicated for transplantation and have a willing and suitable donor are referred for renal transplantation (4). Table 2 shows the number of patients referred from the Amiri hospital who were transplanted in the years 1979 to 1983. In 1981 the first imported cadaver kidney

*Table 2.* Patients transplanted in Kuwait from the Amiri Hospital Dialysis Centre.

| Year | Living donor | Cadaver | No. |
|---|---|---|---|
| 1979 | 11 | – | 11 |
| 1980 | 20 | – | 20 |
| 1981 | 20 | 2 | 22 |
| 1982 | 19 | 6 | 25 |
| Oct. 1983 | 15 | 13 | 28 |
| Total | 85 | 21 | 106 |

was transplanted and the number of these has steadily increased. By October 1983 the number of patients transplanted who were referred from the Amiri hospital dialysis centre was 106, 21 of these having received cadaveric kidneys. Figure 2 shows the parallel development of renal transplantation and the number of patients coming on to dialysis.

## Discussion

In Kuwait, medical care, including dialysis, is given freely by the State and since its inception in 1976 the programme has been given increasing support. In 1976 dialysis started with 20 patients. In 1979, intermittent peritoneal dialysis was started and in 1982 continuous ambulatory peritoneal dialysis commenced. In 1983, home dialysis was begun. There are now 120 patients being supported by dialysis. One hundred and thirteen of these are on hospital dialysis, 2 are on home dialysis, 3 on intermittent peritoneal dialysis and 2 on continuous ambulatory dialysis. The low number of patients on home haemodialysis is because this treatment is only advised for patients with a high level of education and with suitable accommodation. Thus 97% of dialysis treatment in Kuwait is confined to hospitals.

The number of patients on dialysis per million of population and the number of newly accepted patients are comparable to the figures in other European dialysis centres (2, 3).

An increasing number of elderly patients are being admitted on regular dialysis and this is also the experience in many European centres (1). The expected mortality rate on our dialysis programme for 1983 is 11% which is similar to the

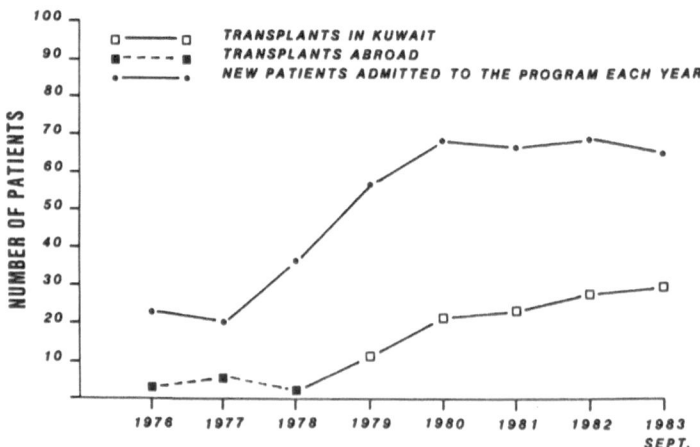

*Fig. 2.* The rise in number of new patients admitted on dialysis each year with a parallel increase in number of patients referred for transplantation in the same year.

mortality rate in Europe (2, 8). However, while in Kuwait the major cause of death in dialysis patients is hyperkalemia in Europe the cardiovascular and cerebrovascular causes are the most common (8). In view of the rapid progress of renal transplantation and considering the high patient and graft survival after transplantation, it has become our policy to refer all patients unless specifically contraindicated for renal transplantation. This policy is based on our own experience and that of others that renal transplantation gives higher patient survival and excellent rehabilitation, provides a better quality of life and it is a cheaper treatment than haemodialysis. As a consequence of this policy our current rate of transplantation is parallel to the numbers of patients admitted to the dialysis programme each year (Fig.2). Since the renal transplantation unit in Kuwait has become a referral centre for many Arab countries it is expected that the number of patients admitted to our dialysis programme will continue to increase and consequently a major dialysis centre is currently under construction in order to meet the demand.

## References

1. Gurland HJ, Brunner FP, Chantter C, Jacobs L, Sharar K, Selwood NH, Spies G, Wing AJ: Combined report on regular dialysis and transplantation in Europe VI, 1975. Proc EDTA 13.
2. Jacobs C, Broyer M, Brunner FP, Brynger H, Donckerwolck RA, Kramer P, Selweed NH, Wing AJ, Bloke PH: Combined report on regular dialysis and transplantation in Europe XI, 1980, Proc EDTA 18: 14, 1981.
3. Jacobs C, Broyer M, Brunner FP, Brynger H, Donckerwolck RA, Kramer P, Selwood NH, Wing AJ, Bloke PH: Combined Report on regular dialysis and transplantation in Europe XII, 1981, Proc EDTA 19: 14, 1982. .
4. Abouna GM, Kumar A, White A, Al Dadah S, Samhan M, John P, Kusma G, Bassiouny H: Kidney Transplantation Surgery in Kuwait the Results in the first 72 Recipients, Arab Journal of Medicine 1: 5, 1982.
5. Ministry of Public Health, Annual Health Agenda, Kuwait, 1982.
6. Hoffstein PA, Kruegerk K, Wincman RJ: Dialysis cost, Kidney Int 9: 286, 1976.
7. Stange PV, Summer AT: Predicting treatment costs and life expectancy for end stage renal disease. New England J Med 298: 372, 1978.
8. Degonlet P, Roulex JP, Aime F, Berger C, Block P, Goupy F, Legrain M: Programme Dialyse informatique, données épidémologiques, stratégies de dialyse et résultats biologiques. J.Uro-nephro 82–1001, 1976.

# 23. The development of renal transplantation programme in Kuwait and the results in the first 142 grafts

GEORGE M. ABOUNA, ARTHUR G. WHITE, M.S.A. KUMAR, S.K. DADAH and M. SAMHAN

## Development of the transplant programme

Renal Dialysis Therapy was introduced in Kuwait and other Arab Middle Eastern countries in the mid 1970's, but renal transplantation, as a well organized programme was not introduced until several years later. The State of Kuwait became one of the earliest countries in the Middle East to embark on the establishment of such a programme on a national and regional scale. Since established transplant programmes did not exist in the neighbouring Arab countries, it was envisaged that such a programme will most likely provide the required renal replacement therapy not only for Kuwait but also for some of its neighbours.

It was realised from the outset that in order for such a national and regional programme to be viable and successful, particularly in the environment of a developing country, it was necessary to ensure that several related hospital services and personnel become available at a sufficiently high standard, such as nursing, anaesthesia, and intensive care, nephrology and dialysis, radiology and radiotherapy, microbiology and infectious disease, immunology, organ function and preservation laboratories, in addition to surgery. After nearly one year of development and preparation, recruitment and training of personnel and the creation of a small nursing transplantation unit in one of the local hospitals, the first renal transplant was carried out in Kuwait in March 1979. In that year 9 more transplants were successfully carried out, all from living related donors. Since that time the renal transplant output has continued to increase very rapidly so that in 1982, 42 renal allografts were performed and another 50 have been carried out in the first nine months of 1983. By September 1983, 148 grafts have been carried out in 146 patients (Fig. 1). With this increase in the output, the transplantation facilities were also increased to the present capacity which consists of an eighteen-bed nursing unit in the teaching hospital with its own biochemical, haemotological and immunological laboratories. This unit has now become a referral centre for patients from the Arabian Gulf and many other countries of the Arab Middle East. Since Cadaveric organs are not yet available in this part of the world the programme was initially dependent upon living related donor grafts. How-

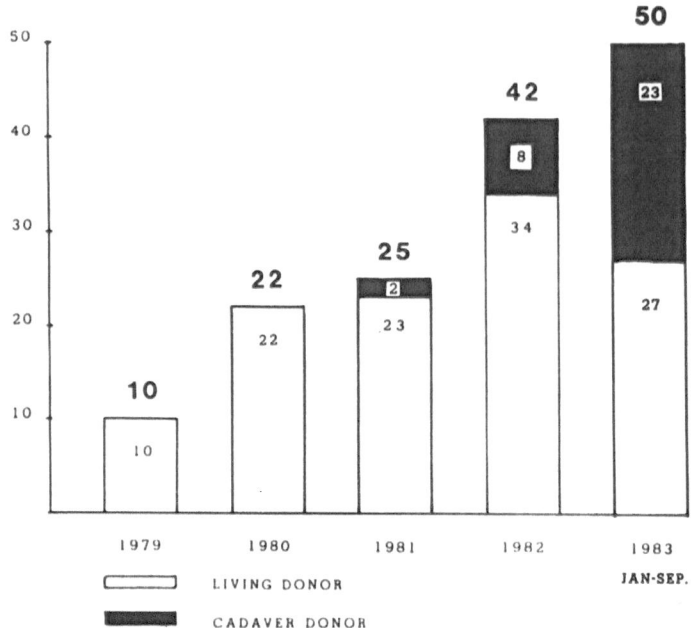

*Fig. 1.* The increase in the annual renal transplantation output in Kuwait, March 1979 – September 1983.

ever, during the past two years cadaveric organs have been imported from Europe and the United States and a small number of living non-related donors, (mostly husband and wife situation) have also been accepted.

In view of the nature of the population, the geographical location and the existing cultural and educational differences, several important observations have become possible particularly with regard to organization and the development of transplantation in a developing country, the effect of factors such as tissue typing, prolonged graft preservation, the use of less than optimal cadaveric grafts and the different methods of immunosuppression, on graft outcome. This review will outline our experience in the first one hundred forty-two renal grafts carried out in one hundred and forty patients.

## Patients and methods

From the beginning of the programme it was decided to accept all potential recipients for transplantation, providing they were free from infection and malignancy. All patients referred for transplantation locally or from outside the country are reviewed for acceptance on the programme by a transplantation committee made up of the transplant surgeons and nephrologists. Transplantation surgery, living donor nephrectomy and all post transplant care and follow up are carried out by the same transplant team within the transplantation unit according to specific protocols.

In the series to be reviewed 110 patients received 112 living donor grafts and another 30 patients received cadaveric grafts. Recipient's age varied between 6 and 56 years (Table 1). The indication for renal transplantation in this series were variable but the majority had chronic glomerulonephritis and some of the children had congenital renal diseases (Table 2). In addition to renal failure other high risk factors included age greater than 50 years, uncontrolled hypertension, diabetes, bladder neck obstruction, valvular disease of the heart, presence of hepatitis B associated antigen, maintenance on peritoneal dialysis, and multiple renal arteries in the donor (Table 3). The national origin of the recipients was also variable: 32% were Kuwaiti nationals, 42% were nationals of the other Middle Eastern and Asian countries living in Kuwait and 26% were patients referred specifically in Kuwait for transplantation from other countries of the Middle East and in some cases from North America. Donor recipient selection was based on medical and immunological criteria including ABO, HLA, MLC and direct cross match. Standard surgical technique was employed except where multiple arteries or damaged vessels were present when a variety of surgical reconstructive techniques had to be employed. Immunosuppression was with azathioprine and prednisone in most patients of the series. In 3 patients Cyclosporin A has been employed. Acute allograft rejections were treated with high pulse doses of methyl prednisolone initially. Later a prospective trial was carried out comparing two different anti-rejection therapies. In one group of 30 patients a standard

*Table 1.* Number of renal transplants and donor source. March 1979 – October 1983.

| | |
|---|---|
| Living related donor | 106 |
| Living non-related donor | 6 |
| Cadaveric donor | 30 |
| Total no. of grafts | 142 |
| Total no. of patients | 140 |

Sex: 91 M, 37 F; Age: 6–56 years

*Table 2.* Indications for transplantation.

| | |
|---|---|
| Chronic glomerulo nephritis | 102 |
| Chronic pyelonephritis/reflux | 21 |
| Diabetic nephropathy | 3 |
| Shunt (septic) nephritis | 1 |
| Bladder neck obstruction | 3 |
| Medullary cystic disease | 6 |
| Polycystic kidneys | 4 |
| Total no. of patients | 140 |

*Table 3.* Additional risk factors in renal transplant recipients present before transplantation.

| | |
|---|---|
| Uncontrolled hypertension | 21 |
| Prediabetic state | 5 |
| Hepatitis B antigenemia | 7 |
| V-P Shunt for hydrocephalus with concontrolled arcites | 1 |
| Diabetes | 3 |
| Severe renal osteodystrophy | 3 |
| Mitral & aortic valve incompetence | 1 |
| Bladder neck obstruction | 4 |
| Tuberculus adenitis | 4 |
| Chronic duodenal ulcer | 5 |
| Peritoneal dialysis | 19 |
| Multiple renal arteries in graft | 20 |

pulse dose of steroid was given for five to seven days while in the other group of 36 patients ALG infusion was given for ten to twelve days. These patients have now been followed up for nearly three years and the results of this study are reported in Part 2 section 6 of this volume.

**Living-donor transplantation**

The 112 living donor grafts of this series came from the following sources: 65 grafts were siblings, 24 parents, 12 offsprings, 5 distant relatives and 6 unrelated donors (spouses). Donor-recipient HLA matching showed HLA identity in 18, no HLA mismatch in 17, one antigen mismatch in 34 and 2 or more HLA mismatches in 43. Mixed lymphocyte culture reaction was carried out in 72 patients and 18 of these showed a negative reaction. The remainder showed varying degrees of positive stimulation (see Part 1 section 2).

Of the 110 recipients of living donor grafts 103 (93.6%) are alive for periods of 1 to 54 months after transplantation. Two patients died in the post operative period from septicemia and myocardial infarction. Five other patients died subsequently from unrelated causes or from complications of immunosuppression at 2 to 24 months after grafting. Ninety-eight of 112 grafts (87.5%) are currently functioning for the same period of the time. Causes of graft loss were; accelerated rejection which was seen in one HLA identical graft, acute and chronic rejection in 10 grafts at 1 to 3 months and another 3 functioning grafts were lost due to recipient death. Actuarial analysis gives a patient survival rate at 1, 2, 3, 4 and 5 years of 96, 95, 94, 94 and 94% and graft survival of 92, 90, 89, 89 and 89% respectively (Fig. 2). When the results were analysed according to the HLA matching no significant difference was seen regardless of the degree of mismatch. Likewise there was no significant difference in graft survival between those with negative and those with positive MLC reaction. (see Part 1, section 2).

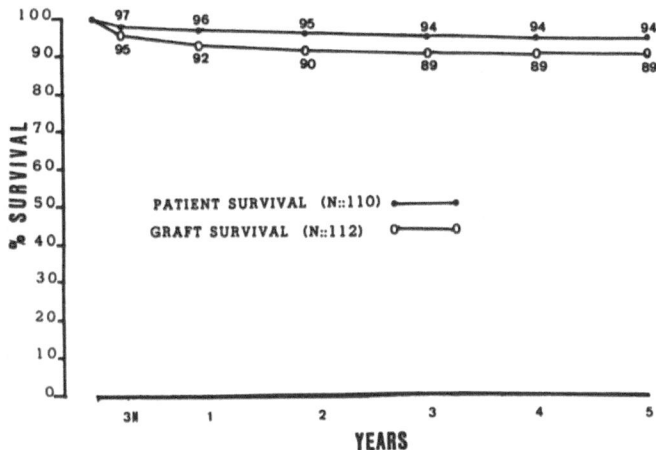

*Fig. 2.* Patient and graft survival in living donor transplantation in Kuwait.

Of the living non-related grafts all continue to have excellent function for periods of 3 months to 3 years, except in one instance a second graft, which was rejected by a highly sensitized recipient spouse.

## Cadaveric transplantation

Cadaveric kidneys were imported from Europe (6 grafts) and from the United States (24 grafts). Transportation of these kidneys was carried out across distances of 5 000 to 12 000 km and often employing the Supersonic Concorde and chartered aircrafts. In some cases cadaveric grafts were offered to Kuwait because no suitable recipients were available locally (usually blood group A, B or AB) but in many cases the reasons were the existence of some problems with the kidney and/or its donor or because of prolonged cold ischemia time. Such problems included donor age greater than 50 years or less than 4 years, multiple arteries, surgical damage during nephrectomy and medical problems in the donor (Table 4).

Thirteen kidneys were transported by machine perfusion and transplanted after ischemia time of 44 to 60 h. The remaining 17 kidneys came in iced Eurocollins solution and were transplanted after ischemia time of 30 to 57 h. In all cadaveric transplantations there was no possibility of selecting patients by HLA A & B or DR matching consequently the mean HLA antigen mismatch in this series of cadaveric grafts was 2.54 (1 to 4 antigens). After arrival of the kidney in Kuwait direct lymphocytotoxicity crossmatch was carried out with several potential recipients before transplantation. Twelve of the 13 grafts (91%) were preserved by machine preservation, and 14 of the 17 grafts (82%) preserved by Eurocollins solution (see Part 3, section 13). One kidney never functioned due to

Table 4. Problems existing in the imported cadaveric kidneys and/or their donors before despatch to Kuwait.

|  | No. |
|---|---|
| 1. Multiple vessels | 9 |
| 2. Surgical damage | |
| Decapsulation (4), Devascularized ureter (2), Divided renal artery at hilum (2), Lacerated main renal vein (2) | 10 |
| 3. Paediatric kidneys (<5 years) | 4 |
| 4. Donor age >50 years | 5 |
| 5. Infections | 5 |
| 6. Medical diseases | |
| Juvenile diabetes (2), Proteinurea (2), Hypertension (3) | 7 |

accelerated vascular rejection. Sixteen grafts are functioning at 1 to 26 months and the remaining 13 kidneys were rejected at 1 to 4 months. Four patients were lost due to pulmonary embolism, pneumonitis and sepsis. Twenty-six patients are alive for 2 to 26 months.

Actuarial analyses for patient and graft survival are shown in Figure 3. Four of the 5 kidneys from the donors older than 50 years have functioned for at least 5 months. No cadaveric kidneys were lost because of surgical injury occurring at the time of organ harvest. Two kidneys developed temporary urinary fistula because of vascular necrosis of the donor ureter but were successfully corrected by ureteroureteric anastomosis using the patient's own ureter. The 2 kidneys removed from an insulin dependent diabetic donor with nephrosclerosis have continued to function for more than 16 months and subsequent biopsy of the graft has shown reversal of previous diabetic lesion. Four of the 5 kidneys removed from donors aged 6 months to 4 years are functioning. Neither bacturia nor mild proteinurea in the donor during their terminal illness had any significant effect on graft outcome. (Table 5).

## Complications

There were relatively few non-infective complications in this series of patients. These are shown in Table 6. None of these complications resulted in the loss of patients or of the grafts. One patient has developed non-Hodgkin's Lymphoma and is receiving chemo/radiotherapy. There was a wide spectrum of infective complications which were largely the consequences of immunosuppression as shown in Table 7. One patient developed abscess of the left temporal lobe caused by Listeria monocytogenes 6 months after transplantation which has completely responded to long term ampicillin therapy without surgical intervention. Viral infection or activation of previous virus infection as determined by serological analysis was also common particularly during the height of rejection and inten-

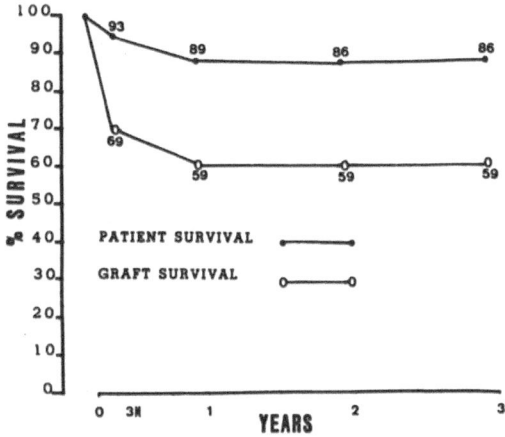

*Fig. 3.* Patient and graft survival in cadaveric donor transplantation in Kuwait.

*Table 5.* Relationship between high risk factors presented in imported cadaveric grafts and subsequent function (N = 30).

| Risk Factors | No. | Immediate diuresis | Functions at 1 month | Loss due to rejection | Functioning at present |
|---|---|---|---|---|---|
| Donor age >50 years | 5 | 4 | 3 | 4 | 1 |
| Multiple vessels | 9 | 6 | 7 | 3 | 6 |
| Surgically damaged | 10 | 9 | 10 | 3 | 7 |
| Medical diseases | 7 | 7 | 7 | 1 | 6 |
| Problem-free grafts | 12 | 11 | 12 | 5 | 7 |
| Donor age <5 years | 4 | 4 | 4 | 1 | 3 |

*Table 6.* The non-infective complications seen after renal transplantation.

| | No. |
|---|---|
| Vascular (renal artery stenosis) | 1 |
| Ureteric necrosis (cadaver) | 2 |
| Lymphocoele | 2 |
| Wound haematoma and/or infection | |
|   L.R.D. (2), Cadaver (2) | 4 |
| Ruptured kidney (cadaver) | 1 |
| Insulin dependent diabetes | 3 |
| Reactivation of D.U. | 3 |
| Gastro intestinal bleeding due to D.U. (cadaver) | 1 |
| Non Hodgkin's lymphoma | 1 |
| Total | 18 |

*Table 7.* The infective complications encountered after renal transplantation.

| | No. |
|---|---|
| *Bacterial* | |
| Bacturia | 60 |
| Re-activation of T.B. | 1* |
| Severe chest infection | 7* |
| Salmonella septicemia | 5* |
| Diabetic foot infection | 2 |
| Wound infection | 3 |
| Listeria cerebral abcess | 1 |
| *Viral* | |
| *Herpes zoster* (3), CMV (4), *Herpes simplex* (19), *Varicella zoster* (1) | 27 |
| *Fungal* | |
| Candida albicans | 10 |
| *Protozoal* | |
| Toxoplasma | 1 |

* In four patients the infection was primary cause of death

sification of immunosuppression. One patient, a physician developed toxoplasmosis which has responded to medical therapy.

## Pediatric transplantation

Nineteen patients in the pediatric age group (5 to 16 years age), 13 males and 6 females, received renal transplantation at our institution. Seventeen of these were given living related donor grafts and 2 received cadaveric grafts. The indications for transplantation were chronic glomerulonephritis in 9, chronic pyelonephritis in 4, congenital medullary cystic disease in 4 and bladder neck obstruction in 2. Two of the patients were HSsAg positive. The patients with congenital disease were 2 pairs of siblings from two different families. One patient had severe renoprival hypertension resulting in pulmonary oedema, hypertensive encephalopathy and cardiac failure which responded only partially to bilateral nephrectomy and daily dialysis. This patient was restored to normal after semi-emergency renal transplantation from his father.

Of the 17 patients who received living donor transplantation 13 came from parents and 4 from siblings. There were 2 HLA identical grafts, 2 without detectable mismatch, 3 with one antigen mismatch and in 12 there were two or more mismatches.

One patient died from interacranial haemorrhage, activation of pulmonary tuberculosis and rejection. Eighteen patients or 95% are alive. Sixteen of the grafts are functioning (84%). The remaining 3 grafts, all living related donors, were lost to rejection at 2 to 4 months including one who had an HLA identical graft from her mother. Actuarial analyses shows patient survival at 1, 2, 3 and 4 years of 95% and graft survival of 89, 84, 84 and 84% for the same period respectively. One of the commonest troubling complications in these children was the development of Cushingoid appearance despite the fact that they received their steroids on alternate days. However, 12 of these children are in full-time ecudation and another 2 have started to work. Appreciable growth has taken place in the younger children but in those older than 12 there has been little change.

**Anti-rejection therapy and maintenance immunosuppression**

In a controlled study involving 66 patients treated for a total of 119 episodes of rejection and followed up for a period of 2 years it was shown that reversal or control of rejection was more effective with antilymphocyte globulin than with high pulse dose steroid therapy, 91% versus 80%. The difference however, was not statistically significant. One and 2 year graft survival in the ALG treated patients was 96% and 83% for the steroid treated group. Again the difference was not statistically significant.

It is a policy of our transplantation unit to reduce steroids as rapidly as possible when the patient is discharged and after the first year they are placed on alternate dose therapy. With this policy many of the complications of corticosteroids are reduced although several patients developed acute rejection and a few of these had to be returned to daily maintenance therapy.

**Other findings**

There were no specific problems in any of the 7 recipients with Hepatitis B associated antigen. Six of these have excellent function at 1 to 4 years although one older patient died of acute myocardial infarction 10 days after transplantation. All 20 recipients who were maintained on pertitoneal dialysis are alive. There was no morbidity related to the peritoneal catheter except in one patient who developed intestinal obstruction after transplantation due to adhesions which were successfully relieved by surgery. All 9 living related donor grafts with 2 to 3 renal arteries are functioning and 7 of 10 cadaveric grafts with 2 to 4 renal arteries are also functioning at 8 to 20 months. None of these grafts were lost to technical or vascular problems.

## Rehabilitation

The rehabilitation of patients after renal transplantation from both living and cadaveric donors has been good. Of the 114 recipients with functioning grafts (97 L.D. & 17 Cadaver), 104 (91%) have returned to employment, to full time education or housework.

## Discussion

The annual incidence of renal failure in the Middle East is estimated to be 70–75 persons per million population. In the part of the Arab World East of the Suez Canal which has a population of 44 million people, about 3000 to 3200 new patients will require renal replacement therapy every year. In Kuwait with a population of 1.5 millions, there are some 125 patients currently on dialysis.

Since transplantation provides a better quality of life and is much less expensive than maintenance dialysis, it is therefore medically preferable and economically desirable that a greater number of patients should be given the opportunity to have renal transplantation. This will require the establishment of a large number of transplant centres in this region of the world in order to cope with the staggering need (Table 8). At present, besides the Transplant Centre in Kuwait, there are only a few smaller units operating in Military Hospitals in some Arab countries: in Saudi Arabia (Dr.Abumelha), in Jordan (Dr.Hananiah) and one each in Egypt and Iraq.

The experience in Kuwait has clearly shown that the establishment of a successful Transplant Programme is not only possible but is extremely worthwhile, since many young patients have been fully rehabilitated and have been spared the inconvenience and the disruption of family life which was the rule when they sought this type of treatment abroad. Also, local governments have been saved vast expense with the establishment of a transplantation service locally. However, it must be seriously borne in mind that in order to establish

Table 8. The estimated incidence of renal failure, the need for renal transplantation programmes in the Arab Middle East.

| | |
|---|---|
| Expected no. of patients requiring renal replacement | = 70/million population per annum |
| Total no. of patients requiring dialysis/transplantation in the arab world east of suez canal (40 million) | = 3000 per annum |
| Total no. of patients requiring dialysis/transplantation in the whole Arab world (154 million) | = 11000 per annum |
| Transplant centres required* | 180 |

* Assuming that each centre will carry out 50–60 transplants per year

successful transplantation service in developing countries of the Middle East, it is of fundamental importance that high quality hospital services and the availability of well trained and well motivated medical and technical man-power be available. It is particularly dangerous and self-defeating to embark on transplantation for reasons of local prestige or to have the procedure carried out by itinerant surgeons who are sporadically invited to some parts of the Middle East and the Gulf region. In our opinion it is imperative that renal transplantation be carried out by transplant surgeons and physicians who are properly trained and committed to the field as is recommended, for example, by the American Society of Transplant Surgeons.

The experience and the results obtained in our living donor series both in terms of patients and graft survival are comparable to those obtained in major North American and European centres (1, 2). The high patient and graft survival rate at 1–5 years was obtained even in the face of poor HLA matching in most of our patients. Our results even in those patients with 2 or more antigen mismatches were as good as those reported by others using Donor Specific Transfusions (3). Although all our patients had received random blood transfusions we did not have a specific policy of transfusing patients before transplantation. We have no particular explanation for this. It is possible that in a society with frequent consanguineous marriages other non-HLA factors are more important (4). More likely however, we believe that in renal transplantation with standard immunosuppression it is the degree of supervision and the quality of care in transplant management that is probably the most important single factor, which determines the final outcome. This is in agreement with the findings of Terasaki and colleagues that the 'good centre effect' may over-ride the disadvantage of poor HLA matching (5). Because of non-availability of cadaveric grafts we resorted to the use of non-related living donors within the family (Husband-wife situation) and the results have been most encouraging. Five of the six recipients who obtained such living grafts are functioning for up to 2 years. Only one graft was rejected in a patient who had already acutely rejected an HLA identical first graft.

The results obtained in our cadaveric recipients are also similar to those obtained by other centres (6, 7) despite the long ischemia times and the fact that many kidneys were 'rejects' from other centres because of serious problems with the kidney or with its donor. We believe that with careful recipient preparation with fluids and mannitol many grafts with long ischemia times can be made to function. Also with meticulous reconstruction and careful handling of the graft it is possible to salvage many suboptimal and damaged kidneys (8). The presence of medical problems in the donor such as diabetes, uncontrolled hypertension, positive urine cultures and donor age greater than 50 or less than 4 years did not seem to mitigate against successful renal transplantation (Table 5). Our longest and best functioning cadaver graft came from a donor 62 years of age (Fig. 4). Two grafts from a 4 year old child with 3 and 4 renal arteries respectively and another from a 6 month old cadaver infant continue to have excellent function in adult recipients (Figs. 5 & 6). Our observation that successful transplantation is possible after preservation in Eurocollin's solution for up to 57 h confirms and extends previous observations by others (9). It implies that preservation and transportation of human cadaveric kidneys should become simpler as well as cheaper, and we now prefer to have all cadaveric kidneys transported to our centre in Eurocollin's solution, providing that the warm ischemia time is very short.

Our experience with pediatric recipient transplantation is also encouraging and it indicates that an excellent patient survival of 95% and good graft survival of 84% for upto 4 years is possible with successful renal transplantation and that most of the children are fully rehabilitated and able to attent full time education. These findings are comparable to those reported recently by the E.D.T.A. (10) and also by the Eurotransplant Foundation (11). Both in our limited experience and in that of others (10, 11) the quality of life after transplantation in children is superior to that on dialysis. Since most of our pediatric recipient group were already over the pubertal age rapid increase in growth could not be observed but 2 children of the series who were under 10 appear to grow normally. This is in agreement with the recent EDTA analysis where growth of children following transplantation was significantly greater than in those on maintenance dialysis at all ages from 4 to 11 years (10). The Cushingnoid effect of steroids in these children is common and troublesome and it is hoped that with the advent of Cyclosporin-A a much more smaller dose of maintenance steroid therapy will be used and this complication will be avoided.

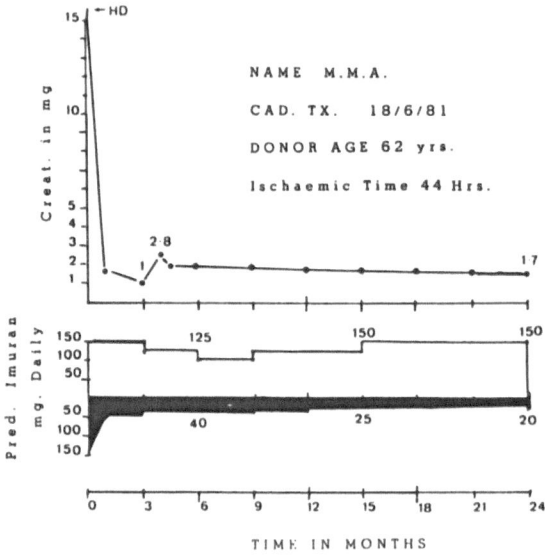

*Fig. 4.* Course of a patient who received a cadaver kidney from an old donor. This kidney had been refused by the Eurotransplant Foundation.

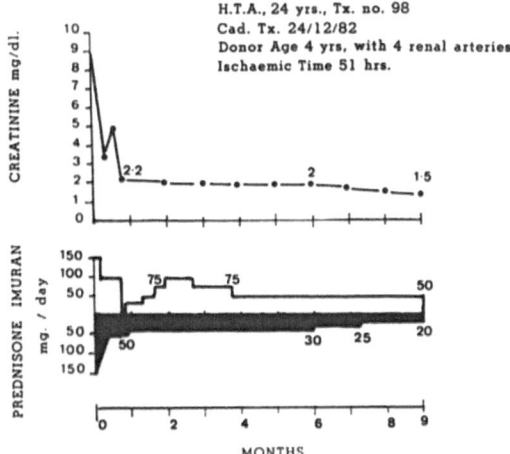

Fig. 5. Course of one of the adult recipients of a cadaveric kidney from a four year old child with 4 renal arteries which was also decapsulated after nephrectomy. The opposite kidney which had 3 renal arteries was also successfully transplanted into another adult recipient. Long aortic cuffs were used in both cases.

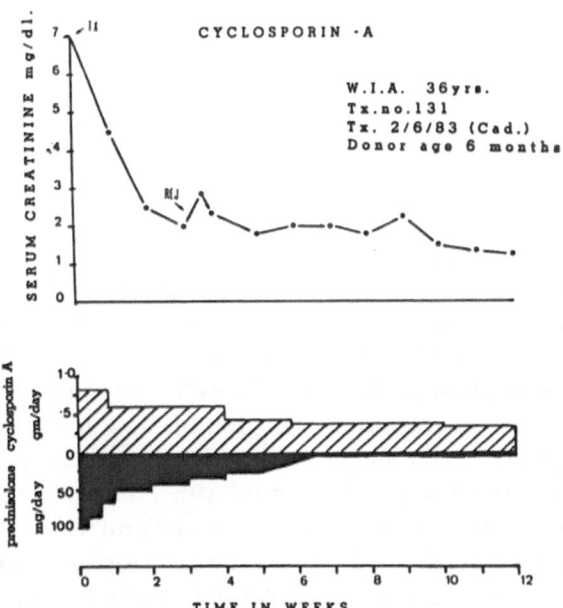

Fig. 6. Course of adult recipient of cadaver kidney from a six month old infant, treated with Cyclosporin-A.

The non infective complications of renal transplantation seen in our experience in Kuwait are relatively small. The early development of lymphoma in one patient (0.7%) is comparable to the general incidence of cancer in transplant recipients (12). The infective complications were common and were largely due to immunosuppression. Viral infections were common in those patients receiving anti-lymphocyte globulin. Bacteriuria was fairly common in our series although we removed the urethral catheter 24–48 h after transplantation. However, bacteriuria had very little effect on renal function in these patients. Our observation in the patient with cerebral Listeria abscess is very interesting since there are very few reports in the literature of his condition being successfully treated by antibiotic therapy alone and without the need for surgical drainage.

The results of our trial with anti-rejection therapy using ALG infusion show a marginal benefit with this form of therapy over standard pulse doses of steroids. Our earlier results with this treatment were much more encouraging, like those reported by Filo (13). However, longer follow-up has shown that the difference between the two methods of treatment is not significant. Of course some of the complications of steroid therapy have been avoided but with increased costs. It is our policy at the present time to use ALG only in steroid resistant rejection or in combination with steroids in early vascular rejections.

The observations that transplantation of kidneys with diabetic nephropathy can function normally and that established diabetic nephrosclerosis regresses after transplantation into non-diabetic recipients will have important implications in regard to the pathogenesis of diabetic nephropathy and in the clinical management of diabetes. It also indicates that kidneys of diabetic donors should no longer be refused (14).

The finding that recipients with hepatitis B associated antigen can be safely transplanted and rehabilitated is important and it is our policy at the present to transplant these patients at the earliest possible moment but taking stringent preventive precautions. The earlier fear that transplantation of patients maintained on peritoneal dialysis might be associated with a greater mortality and morbidity has not materialized. Nineteen of the twenty patients transplanted in this series who had been maintained on peritoneal dialysis had no increased morbidity following transplantation. One patient developed intestinal obstruction from adhesions most probably secondary to peritoneal dialysis but these were successfully released surgically. The transplantation of kidneys with multiple renal arteries does carry a higher risk of vascular problems. However, our experience in this small series of 18 grafts with 2 to 4 vessels, indicates that successful grafting of these kidneys can be achieved providing that extra care and time is taken in such situations. There was no mortality or serious morbidity in any of the 112 living donors in this series. All of them left the hospital within 7 to 10 days and were able to return to their former occupation, with normal renal function, within 1–2 months. Our experience indicates that living related donor transplantation is safe and highly successful and therefore a justifiable procedure.

In view of this, the rapidly increasing demand for renal transplantation and the fact that no more than 30% of our patients have willing related donors we intend to use non-related donors in the future.

The future of renal transplantation in this country and in this region must clearly depend on availability of cadaveric grafts. Unfortunately, until the present time cadaveric organs are not yet available in this part of the world and therefore reliance must continue to be placed on imported cadaveric grafts. This is not an ideal situation since the supply of kidneys from Europe and the United States is insufficient and is usually limited to donors with the less common blood group and in many cases the grafts are less than optimal or have very long ischemia times. Indeed the non-availability of cadaveric grafts is the most important single factor which has hampered the further development of renal transplantation and the introduction of transplantation of other organs such as liver and pancreas in the Middle East. The proper and permanent solution to this problem lies in the provision of the right legal, social and educational environment so that use can be made of hundreds of cadaveric organs from victims of traffic accidents which in Kuwait and in the Middle East have the highest incidences in the World. Due to the efforts of the transplantation team and Kuwait Ministry of Health a law was recently passed by a Kuwaiti Parliament (Law no. 7 1983) making legal the removal of cadaveric kidneys for transplantation providing consent is given by the next of kin or previous permission on a donor card had been made by the decreased during life. It is hoped that with a concentrated and well planned compaign at public education and in the light of this new law it will become possible to use local cadaveric organs for transplantation in the near future.

**Acknowledgement**

We are grateful to the Kuwait Ministry of Health, the Faculty of Medicine of Kuwait University and to many colleagues in various hospitals services for their invaluable help in the development of the Renal Transplantation Programme.

We are thankful for the technical help received from Dr. Ahmed Sayed Mohomad, Dr. E.M. Phillips and Mr. Abdul Redda Abbas and we appreciate the dedicated care given to our patients by Mr. Mahmoud Ashkar, Head Nurse and his Nursing Staff of the Transplantation Department in Kuwait.

# References

1. Howard RJ, Najarian JS: Twenty-four years of Kidney Transplantation. Surgical Rounds 1: 49, 1978.
2. Morris PJ: Results of Renal Transplantation in *Kidney Transplantation*. (Morris PJ ed). Academic Press, 1979, p 377.
3. Salvitierra O, Vincenti F, Amend W, Garovoy MR, Feduska NT: The Enhancement of Graft Survival with Pre-Transplant Blood Transfusion. Heart Transplantation 2: 181, 1983.
4. Abouna GM, Kumar MS, White A, Daddah S, Samhan M, John P, Kusma G, Baissony H: Kidney Transplantation Surgery in Kuwait. Arab Journal of Medicine 1: 5, 1982.
5. Opelz G, Mickey MR, Terasaki P: Calculation of Long-Term graft and patient survival in Human Kidney Transplantation. Transplantation Proceedings 9: 27, 1977.
6. Terasaki PI: Presidental Address: Transplantation Society, 1982. Transplantation Proceedings 15: 14, 1983.
7. Eurotransplant Annual Report (Cohen B ed). Eurotransplant Foundation, Leiden, The Netherlands, 1981.
8. Abouna GM, Kumar AS, White AG, Daddah S, Ommar OF, Samhan M, John P, Soubky AS, Abbas AR, Kremer G: Experience with Imported Human Cadaveric Kidneys having unusual problems and transplanted after 30–60 hours of Preservation. Transplantation Proceedings 16: 61–63, 1984.
9. Squifflet JP, Pirson Y, Gianello P, Van Cangh P, Alexandre GP: Safe Preservation of human renal cadaver transplants by Eurocollin's solution upto 50 hours. Transplantation Proceedings 13: 693, 1981.
10. Donekerwolcke RA, Broyer M, Brunner FP, Brynger H, Jacobs A, Kramer P, Selwood NH, Wing AJ: Combined Report on Regular dialysis and Transplantation of Children in Europe. Proceedings EDTA 19: 60, 1982.
11. D'Amaro J, Cohen B, de Lange P, Persijn GG: Renal Transplantation: Pediatric Recipients. Dialysis and Transplantation 12: 88, 1983.
12. Penn I: Cancer in Transplant Patients. Symposium on Recent Advances in Transplantation, Ankara, Turkey, June 1983 (Abstract).
13. Filo RS, Leapman SB, Smith EJ: American Society of Transplant Surgeons, 9th Annual Meeting, June 1983 (Abstract).
14. Abouna GM, Adnani MS, Kremer GD, Kumar SA, Daddah SK, Kusma G: Reversal of Diabetic Nephropathy in Human Cadaveric Kidneys after Transplantation in non-diabetic Recipients. Lancet 11: 1274–1276, 1983.

# 24. Living related kidney transplantation in Turkey

M. HABERAL, N. BILGIN, N. BUYUKPAMUKCU, U. SAATCI,
M. KARAMEHMETOGLU, Z. ONER, A. BESIM, H. GULAY,
O. DALLAR and Y. SANAC

## Introduction

Since the first successful kidney transplant reported by Murray and his colleagues (1) and due to the development of the highly sophisticated field of immunosuppression, many centres throughout the world including the Middle East are now performing successful organ transplantation (2, 3, 4).

Without doubt kidney and cornea have been the most successful transplants and with the advent of Cyclosporin A improved success has become possible with the transplantation of other organs such as liver, heart, pancreas and bone marrow (5, 6, 7).

Today, because of the ever increasing demand for transplantation it is necessary to obtain more cadaver organs. In countries like Turkey and Kuwait (2) it is largely due to the lack of public education, that cadaver organs are difficult to obtain and the renal transplantation programmes are therefore dependent on living donors. It is clearly essential to meet the growing demand that cadaver organs be utilised.

## Patients and methods

Between November 1975 and September 1982 we transplanted 118 patients with kidneys from living related donors. Of these patients 73.7% were male and 26.3% were females between the ages of 12 and 54 years. The primary kidney diseases in these 118 patients were as follows; undiagnosed end stage kidney disease 33.9%, chronic pyelonephritis 30.5%, chronic glomerulonephritis 28.8%, amyloidosis 4.3% and others 2.5% consisting of one case each of polycystic disease, nephrosclerosis and familial nephronopythises.

The relationship of the kidney donors to the recipients was as follows: Mothers (31.4%), fathers (11.9%), brothers (27.1%), sisters (24.6%) and others 5% (2 sons, 3 uncles, 1 daughter).

Breakdown of the patients into HLA match grade showed that 24.6% were 4 antigen compatible, 27.1% were 3 antigen compatible and 48.3% were 2 antigen compatible.

Prior to transplantation, all patients were on hemodialysis and had open kidney biopsies performed. If the patients hematocrit level was under 25%, whole or packed cell blood was given at least 1 week prior to surgery. Cystouretherograms were performed on all patients. Bilateral pre-transplant or per-transplant nephrectomies were carried out for specific indications of uncontrollable hypertension, pyelonephritis, hemorrhage and ureteric reflux. Three days before transplantation, 1 mg/kg/day prednisone and 3 mg/kg/day azathioprine were started as immunosuppressive agents.

All transplants were performed under general anaesthesia in the supine position with endotracheal intubation. The kidney was always placed extraperitoneally either in the right or the left iliac fossa. Donor nephrectomy was carried out through a standard lateral subcostal extraserous incision, either the left or the right kidney was removed according to the findings of the intravenous pyelogram and arteriogram in the donor. The kidney was removed with an adequate length of ureter and immediately cooled and preserved by perfusion with Perfudex or Ringer's lactate solution at +4°C. If multiple arteries were encountered, they were anastomosed either to individual branches of the hypo-gastric artery and the external iliac artery or to the inferior epigastric artery (Fig. 1).

The ureter was implanted in the bladder in a submucosal tunnel through the open bladder using an anti-reflux technique and everting uretero neo-cystostomy.

A Hemo-Vac system was utilized on all transplants for wound drainage. Six to eight hours after surgery, the patient was on oral feeding, 24 h later was mobile and 72 h later the urethral catheter was removed. Azathioprine dose was adjusted according to the leukocyte count, approximately $2^{1}/_{2}$ to 2 mg/kg/day and prednisone was tapered off to a level of about 20 mg/day at 36 days post-transplant. Acute rejection was treated by methylprednisolone and occasionally by radiotherapy. Prophylactic antibiotics were not used. On average, the patients were discharged after 3 to 4 weeks.

## Results

All patients were followed after transplantation for a period of 4 months to 7 years. Most of the kidney recipients (77.2%) were between the ages of 21–40 years. (Fig. 2). Analysis of the results in relationship to HLA match showed functioning grafts at 1 year is 85.3% in the 4 antigen compatible, 77.3% in 3 antigen compatible and 68.5% in those that had 2 antigens in common. Graft survival when analysed in terms of the relationship between the donor and recipient was 77.5% between siblings, 77.5% from mothers, 60% fathers and other donors 45.5% at one year.

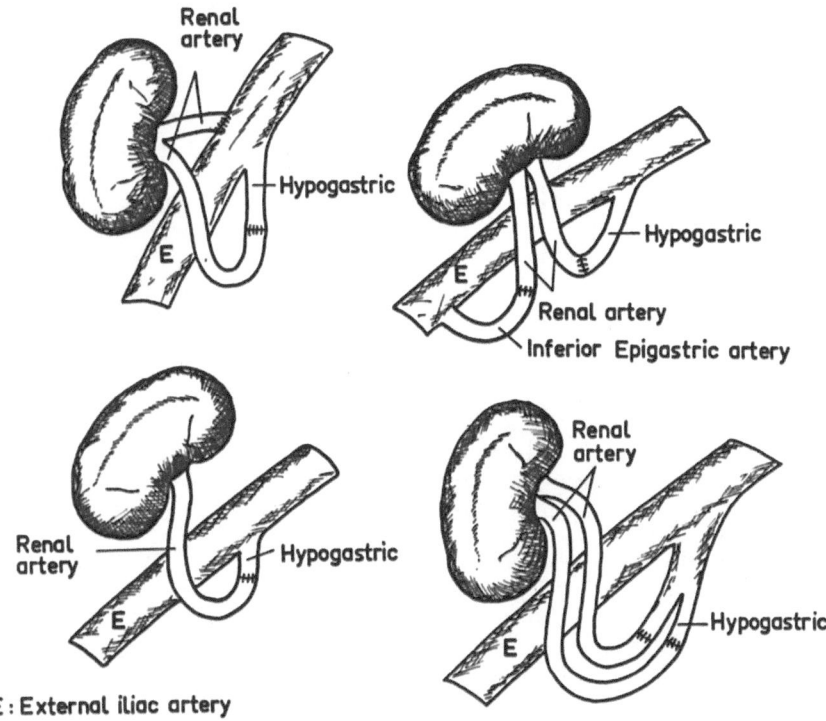

Fig. 1. Methods of vascular anastomoses used in renal transplantation.

Over the 7 year period of the study the patient survival was 73.7% and the graft survival 47.4%. In the first year of our experience the mortality rate was 30% and the graft failure rate 21% and this declined in the second year to 21% and 12% respectively. Since then our mortality rate has fallen to an average of 11.2% per year.

Acute rejection occurred in 38.2% of patients and 8.9% did not recover function after immunosuppressive treatment. The rate of chronic rejection was 37.2% and 39.5% of these required graft nephrectomy. The overall mortality rate in our series was 26.3% and of these 52% died with functioning grafts and 48% whilst on dialysis. The cause of death was infections in 35.8% (fungal 16.3%, bacterial and viruses 16.2%, parasites 3.3%), hepatitis in 17.9% and other causes 46.3%, which included cerebro-vascular accidents 17.2%, sudden death 12.9%, pulmonary embolus 9.8%, pericardial tamponade 3.2% and gastro-intestinal bleeding in 3.2%.

Non-fatal complications were wound infections 16.9%, fungal infection 8.4%, vascular complications 5.9%, lymphocoele formation 4.2%, imuran toxicity 4.2%, urological complications 3.4%, pulmonary abscess 1.7%, gastro-intestinal bleeding 1.7%, diabetes 1.7% aseptic necrosis 0.8% and pancreatitis 0.8%.

212

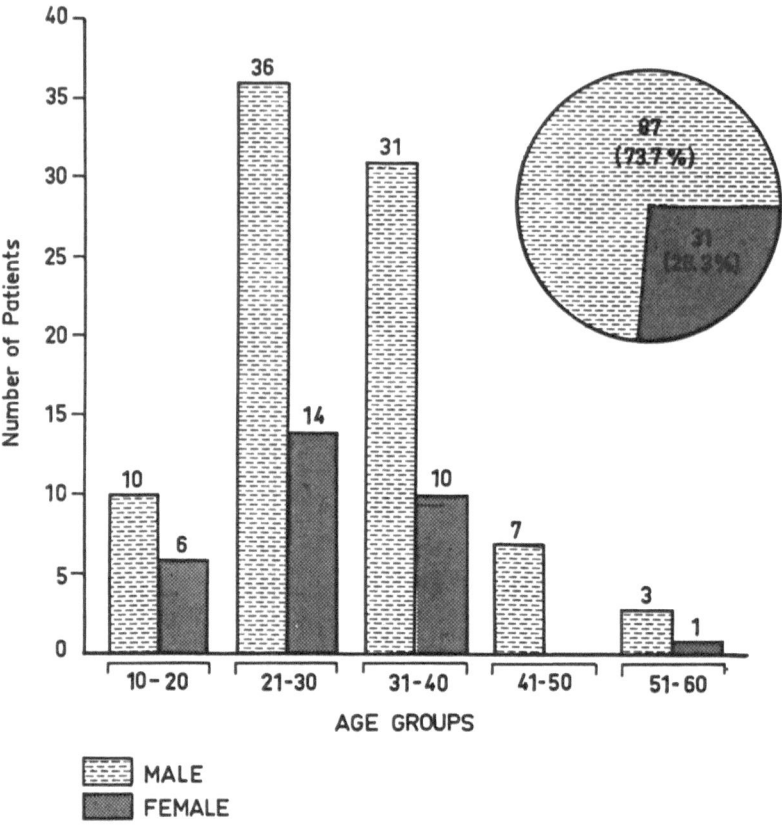

*Fig. 2.* Sex and age distribution of 118 kidney recipients.

## Discussion

Transplantation can be considered as one of the most important medical advances of this century. Like all new ventures in medicine, transplantation is rapidly evolving and the rate of success improving. Since the first kidney transplant and the development of immunosuppressive therapy, over 350 centres are now performing this procedure as part of their daily routine (1, 2, 3, 4). In our centre, kidney transplants are performed from living related donors as well as cadavers on a regular basis.

In the initial 2 years of our programme our mortality and graft failure rate were higher than expected. The reasons for this were that potential recipients were not 'selected' and also we were undergoing a 'learning experience' with personnel being trained. Most of our complications fell in the first 2 years of our experience. In addition when we started transplantation, 21 patients had splenectomy and although the group had a reduced incidence of acute rejection there was a high rate of infection and thrombo-embolic complications (8) leading us to abandon splenectomy. Analysis of our 1 year graft survival shows superior survival in those recipients that received 4 antigen compatible kidneys (85.3%) and this was significantly different from those that received 2 antigen compatible (68.3%).

Out of our series of 118 patients who received living donor kidneys 56(47.4%) are currently alive with functioning grafts and are rehabilitated.

In Turkey as well as in other countries (2) the demand for transplantation is such that use must be made of cadaver organs. Intensive education of the public and also of the medical profession should be carried out in order to make them aware of the benefits of organ transplantation to both patient and society. Only when this is achieved will optimal utilisation of cadaver organs be possible.

## References

1. Murray JE, Tilney NL, Wilson RE: Renal Transplantation; a 25 year Experience. Ann Surg 184: 565, 1976.
2. Abouna GM, Kumar A, White AG, Dadah S, Samhan M, John P, Kusma G, Baissony H: Kidney Transplantation Surgery in Kuwait, The Results in the first 72 Recipients. Arab Journal of Medicine 1(8): 5–11, 1983.
3. Howard RJ, Pfaff WW et al: 500 Renal Transplants at the University of Florida, 1966–1982. J Fl MA 69: 849, 1982.
4. Williams GM: Status of Renal Transplantation Today. Surg Clin North Amer 58: 273–284, 1978.
5. Calne RY, Rolles K, White DJG, Thiru S, Evans DB, Henderson R, Hamilton DL, Boone N, McMaster P, Gibby O, Williams R: Cyclosporin 'A' in Clinical Organ Grafting. Transplant Proc 8: 349–358, 1981.
6. Oyer PE, Stinson EB, Jamieson SW, Hunt SA, Billingham M, Scott W, Bieber CP, Reitz BA, Shumway NE: Cyclosporin A in Cardiac Allografting: A preliminary experience. Transplant Proc 1247–1257, 1983.
7. Kennedy MS, Deeg HJ, Storb R, Thomas ED: Cyclosporin in Marrow Transplantation: Concentration – Dependent Toxicity and Immunosuppression in Vivo. Transplant Proc 15: 471–473, 1983.
8. Engin A, Haberal M, Bilgin N: The Effect of Splenectomy on the sensitivity to infection in related renal Haemotransplants. Microbial Bull 13: 211, 1979.

# 25. Clinical pancreas and islet transplantation: registry statistics and an overview

DAVID E.R. SUTHERLAND

## Introduction

Interest in the application of clinical pancreas transplantation has increased dramatically recently, as evidenced by the fact that nearly as many pancreas transplants have been performed in the last two years (1981–1982) as in the preceding 14 years following the first pancreas transplantation in 1966 (14). The potential of pancreas and islet transplantation as treatments for Type I diabetes approximates that of kidney transplantation for treatment of end stage renal disease.

The evidence that the complications of diabetes are secondary to disordered metabolism is overwhelming (3). New methods of exogenous insulin delivery have been developed in attempts to maintain nearly constant euglycemia, but these techniques also have risks (33), specifically hypoglycemia (34), which, as immunosuppressive techniques become safer and more effective, may equal or exceed those of pancreas transplantation. Internal insulin pumps, implanted in some Type II diabetics (4), deliver insulin at a constant rate (although some can be induced to give an intermittent bolus), but until they can be coupled to a glucose sensor with automatic changes in delivery rate (and thus mimic a beta cell), they will not be suitable for most Type I diabetics.

Pancreas or islet transplantation is the most physiological approach to treatment of diabetes. Their application is currently limited by technical and immunological problems, but, at least for pancreas transplantation, these can be overcome and several patients currently have functioning grafts.

The American College of Surgeons/National Institutes of Health (ACS/NIH) kept an Organ Transplant Registry until June 30, 1977 (10). The ACS/NIH Registry did not tabulate cases of islet transplantation, but recorded information on 57 pancreas transplants in 55 patients from December 17, 1966 until the Registry closed. Three pancreas transplants (one primary, two secondary) performed in 1976, missed by the ACS/NIH Registry, were reported to the new International Human and Pancreas Transplant Registry (24). The new Registry, formed under the auspices of the Scientific Studies Committee of the American Society of Transplant Surgeons and located in Minneapolis, has tabulated all known cases of clinical islet transplantation since 1970 and all known cases of pancreas transplantation since July 1, 1977 (24). In addition, the records of the old ACS/NIH Registry have been incorporated into the total Registry data. The information in the Registry on pancreas and islet transplant cases performed through December 31, 1982, and followed to February, 1983, are summarized in the following sections.

**Pancreas transplant registry**

*Number of pancreas transplants and overall results*

Between December 17, 1966, and December 31, 1982, 264 pancreas transplants performed in 34 institutions were reported to the Registries. Sixteen patients received second transplants and one received a third transplant after primary grafts failed, so the transplants were performed in 247 patients. The 57 transplants in the ACS/NIH Registry and 3 of the transplants in the new Registry were placed in 56 patients before June 30, 1977. The other 204 transplants were performed in 193 patients, but 2 of these patients (1 Lyon and 1 Stockholm) had had previous transplants recorded by the ACS/NIH Registry, so the total number of new patients recorded by the new Registry after July 1, 1977, is 191.

The six institutions with the largest, as well as the most recent experiences, Minnesota (18, 27, 28), Lyon (7), Stockholm (11, 12), Zurich (2), and Cambridge (5, 9) and Detroit (32) have published the details on all except their latest cases of pancreas transplantation. Some of the other institutions have also published reports on their pancreas transplants, most of which are referenced in recent comprehensive review articles (26,29).

Currently (June, 1983), 34 patients have functioning grafts and are insulin independent, 21 for more than one year (Table 1). Nine other grafts functioned for more than a year before the recipients either died with functioning grafts (one Minnesota and one New York patient in the ACS/NIH Registry and one Lyon patient in the new Registry), or the grafts failed and the patients resumed exogenous insulin (two Cambridge, two Lyon, one Birmingham and one Minnesota patient in the new Registry). The other 219 grafts ceased to function at less than one year because of technical complications, rejection, or death of the recipient. All of the grafts currently functioning were transplanted since 1977.

Not only is the success rate of pancreas transplantation improving, but the procedure is definitely becoming safer. Of the 56 patients who received transplants before July 1, 1977, 29 (52%) either had a transplant related death or died soon after transplantation, and no more than 14 of the patients (25%) are still alive. In contrast, of the 193 patients who received transplants between July 1, 1977 and December 31, 1982, only 35 (18%) died with transplant or preoperative related problems or within the first 3 months of diabetic complications, and 134

*Table 1.* Pancreas transplant (1 PD, 8 whole, 191 segmental) association with kidney transplants from July 1, 1977 to December 31, 1982.[a]

| Association | No. of cases | Grafts currently functioning[b] | | |
|---|---|---|---|---|
| | | No. | % | Duration (months) |
| Pancreas before kidney | 2 | 0 | 0 | – |
| Pancreas alone | 51 | 7 | 14 | 3–26 |
| Pancreas after kidney | 54 | 9 | 17 | 3–55 |
| Pancreas plus kidney | 93[c] | 22 | 24 | 3–42 |
| Total | 200 | 38 | 19 | 3–55 |

[a] Leeds case not included because technique and outcome not known
[b] Insulin-independent as of February, 1983
[c] Two patients had previous kidney transplants

(69%) of the patients are currently alive.

It is also clear that pancreas transplantation can restore carbohydrate metabolism to normal, or nearly normal, in some but not all patients. There is some variability in the response and, in at least one recipient, diabetes seemed to recur in the transplanted pancreas without evidence of rejection (27). It is hoped that such an occurrence is rare. Example of metabolic profiles and glucose tolerance tests after successful transplants of pancreas allografts in three patients from the Minnesota series are depicted in Figure 1.

## *Results of pancreas transplants according to association with kidney transplants*

Most recipients of pancreas transplants have had diabetic nephropathy or other far advanced complications of diabetes, and transplantation was carried out at a time when the risks of immunosuppression and surgery were high. Kidney transplants were performed either before, simultaneous with or after most of the pancreas transplants (Table 1).

Of 193 patients reported to the Registry since July 1, 1977, 49 were said not to have end stage diabetic nephropathy, but proteinuria and other clinical manifestations of nephropathy were present in some members of this group.

Most doubly grafted patients have had both organs transplanted simultaneously. Even though the pancreas transplant success rate has been approximately the same with either a synchronous procedure or with the dysynchronous procedure of pancreas transplantation after a successful kidney transplant, the patient survival rate and the kidney graft survival rate has been much higher in those who have had a pancreas transplant subsequent to, rather than simultaneous with, a kidney transplant (23). It thus appears that restoration of renal

218

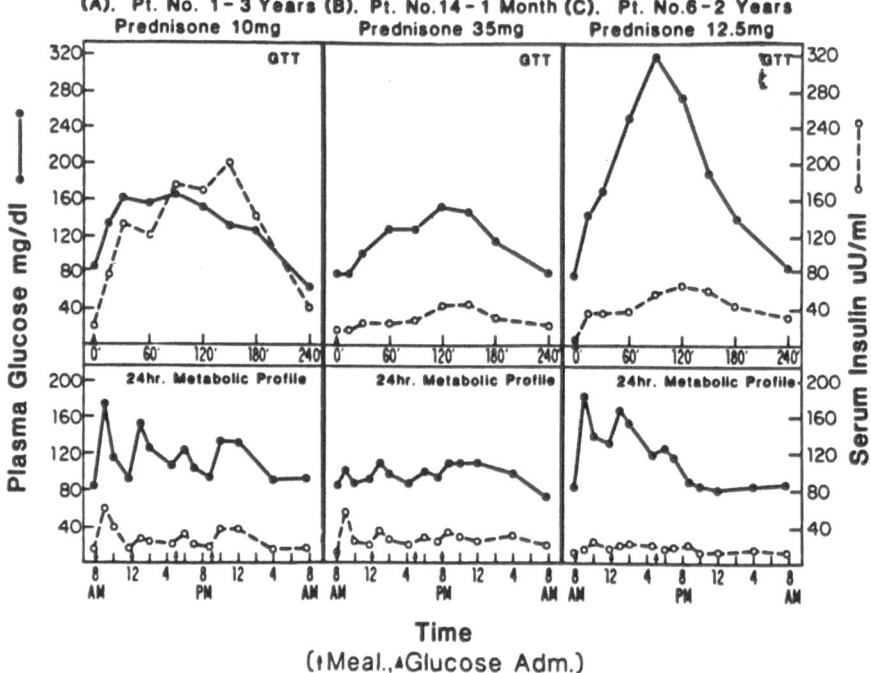

Fig. 1. Results of glucose tolerance tests and 24 hour metabolic profile in the absence of exogenous insulin in three recipients of segmental pancreas transplant in the Minnesota series, illustrating the variability in response of individual patients.

function is of more immediate importance than total endocrine replacement therapy in an uremic diabetic (31).

## Results in pancreas transplants according to technique

The most important technical issue in pancreas transplantation is the provision for handling the exocrine secretions. In the ACS Registry nearly half (27 cases) of the transplants were pancreaticoduodenal (PD); only one in the New Registry (London) was by this technique. A variety of methods have been used in recent years (Table 2). Eight of the transplants performed between July 1, 1977 and December 31, 1982 were whole pancreas without the duodenum; the others were segmental (hemi-pancreas) grafts. The three open duct grafts currently functioning are long term (>3 years), as are 11 of the grafts injected with synthetic polymers and 4 grafts anastomosed to recipient bowel (>1 year). The other functioning grafts have a shorter follow-up. Suppression of exocrine function by injection into the duct is currently the most popular technique. The complication rate has been relatively low, but some injected grafts may have failed because fibrosis was induced by the injected agent and involved the islets (7, 27). It is not

*Table 2.* Techniques used for 8 whole and 191 segmental pancreas transplants from July 1, 1977 to December 31, 1982[a]

| Method | No. of cases | Grafts currently functioning[b] | | |
|---|---|---|---|---|
| | | No. | % | Duration (months) |
| Ducto-cysto-or-ureterostomy | 5 | 1 | 20% | 6 |
| Duct-ligation | 9 | 0 | 0% | – |
| Open Duct Intraperitoneal | 16 | 3 | 19% | 39–55 |
| Pancreatico-enterostomy | 41 | 10 | 24% | 4–18 |
| Duct-Injection c̄ Polymers | 128[c] | 24 | 19% | 3–42 |
| Total | 199 | 38 | 19% | 3–55 |

[a] Leeds case not included because technique and outcome not known

[b] Insulin independent as of February, 1983

[c] Neoprene in 35 (6 Fxn), Prolamine in 36 (8 Fxn), Silicone in 28 (5 Fxn), Polyisoprene in 20 (5 Fxn), Cyanoacrylate in 9 (0 Fxn)

clear at this time which technique is best, and the physiological approach of pancreatico-enterostomy has been used in recent cases at Minnesota (27), Stockholm (11) and Cambridge (5).

### Results of pancreas transplantation according to immunosuppression

Cyclosporine with or without other agents (usually prednisone) is known to have been used in 76 recipients of pancreas allografts, of whom 18 (24%) currently have functioning grafts. Azathioprine and prednisone (with or without anti-lymphocyte globulin preparations) is known to have been used for immunosuppression in 124 recipients of pancreas allografts since July 1, 1977, of whom 16 (13%) currently have functioning grafts. Technical as well as immunological failures are included in the calculations.

### Results of pancreas transplantation according to preservation

Many of the clinical pancreas transplants have been performed by immediate transfer of the organ from the donor to the recipient, but when preservation has been employed the simple cold storage technique has been used almost exclusively (22). The immediate function rates have been approximately the same for all storage times up to 24 h.

**Islet transplant registry**

There is information on 76 islet allotransplant procedures in 71 diabetic patients, but only 3 islet allotransplants have been reported to the Registry since 1980. A variety of tissue sources, methods of preparation, sites of implantation, and immunosuppressants have been used, but almost all attempts have failed (26). Four patients were reported to be insulin independent for sustained periods after islet transplantation, but insufficient details are available in these cases for critical analysis. The best documented case is that of Largiader *et al.* (17) in Zurich. A 32 year old diabetic simultaneously received a kidney transplant and an intrasplenic injection of collagenase dispersed tissue prepared from the pancreas of a 4 year old cadaver donor. This patient, an insulin dependent diabetic for 22 years, was withdrawn from exogenous insulin therapy at 9 months after transplantation. She remained insulin independent for 10 additional months, and then rejected the kidney. Simultaneous with return to hemodialysis, she became hyperglycemic, and had to resume exogenous insulin. She died 1 month later, 20 months after transplantation (15). No C-peptide measurements were done. According to a report forwarded to the Registry by Largiader no islets were identified in the spleen at autopsy. Even if islets did engraft, their absence at autopsy would be expected if rejection occurred one months before death.

Almost all of the reports on islet transplantation submitted to the Registry have omitted specific information on preservation. Thus, it is impossible to speculate on the role that preservation may have had on the unsatisfactory results of clinical islet transplantation. Almost all of the attempts to date have been made using relatively unsophisticated techniques, and the recent innovations in experimental islet allotransplantation (6, 25) have not yet been applied clinically.

**Comments**

There has been an obvious resurgence of interest in pancreas transplantation in recent years, emphasized by the fact that more than one-quarter of the pancreas transplants performed since 1966 were done in 1982. The success rate is still relatively low, but long term graft function has been sustained in several patients. The mortality and morbidity is also much lower than in previous years.

Most pancreas transplants have been performed in patients with far advanced secondary complications. Ideally, pancreas transplants should be performed early, but only a few non-uremic, non-kidney transplant patients have received pancreas transplants; the largest series includes 19 patients at Minnesota and 6 at Stockholm.

The new immunosuppressive drug, Cyclosporine, has been associated with an improvement in the results of pancreas transplantation. The results, however, are still not nearly as good as those reported for kidney transplantation (5). It is also likely that some technically successful pancreas grafts ceased to function for reasons other than rejection. for example, at least two of the Cambridge patients have had other organ grafts (One liver and one kidney), transplanted from the same donor as the pancreas, continue to function after the pancreas failed at more than one year after transplantation (5). Although Cyclosporine may be a more effective immunosuppression with a better therapeutic ratio than the standard immunosuppression used in earlier years, it is still a generalized immunosuppressant, and its use by itself will not greatly expand the patient population than can be considered for pancreas transplantation.

Clinical attempts at islet allotransplantation have been largely unsuccessful. The procedure is a safe and simple procedure for the recipient, but the manipulations that lead to a relatively high success rate in experimental animal models (25) have not been possible in the clinical situation (26). Islet transplantation is not simpler for the transplant team. Procurement of a sufficient quantity of viable islet tissue from pancreases is a major problem (16). More effective techniques are needed for preparation of islets. Improvements are needed in immunosuppression, and techniques that can alter graft immunogenicity need to be made practical (8). If the new methods currently being investigated in animals are effective for isolation and reduction of immunogenicity of human islets, a rationale basis for future attempts at clinical islet transplantation will be established (6).

Pancreas transplantation can be applied to selected diabetic patients at this time. The limiting factor is the need for generalized immunosuppression. Thus, pancreas transplantation is currently restricted to patients whose secondary complications of diabetes are, or predictably will be, more serious than the potential side effects of anti-rejection therapy. Such patients include those who have had or who require a kidney transplant and in whom immunosuppressive therapy is obligatory.

When abrogation of a specific immune response in humans is possible, and the risks of transplantation are minimal, the limiting factor will be the availability of donor pancreases as a source of islets for free grafting or as intact organs for transplantation as immediately vascularized grafts. This problem would appear to be solvable. Approximately 5000 kidney transplants are done per year in the United States (13) . The incidence of new cases of Type I diabetes in the U.S. is approximately 10,000/year, of which less than half develop serious complications (35). According to Bart *et al.* (1) only a small proportion of potential donors are currently used, but there is no inherent reason why donor procurement should be any more difficult for pancreas transplantation than for kidney transplantation. New methods, such as measurement of joint stiffness, may be able to identify patients whose diabetes cannot be adequately controlled by exogenous insulin and who are at high risk to develop secondary complications (21). It may also be possible to identify those diabetics who are most likely to have hyperglycemic reactions on insulin pump or other intensified insulin therapy regimens, such as those with impaired epinephrine responses (34). Patients with these characteristics may be those who are most likely to benefit from a pancreas or islet transplant, and a sufficient number of pancreases should be available for this select group.

Reliable preservation will be needed for either pancreas or islet transplantation to be logistically feasible on a scale as large as envisioned in the preceding paragraph. For pancreas transplantation, preservation times of 24 to 72 h should be sufficient to ensure that all donor organs are used (9). However, the longer the preservation capabilities, the more extensive can sharing be between institutions. Institutions not performing pancreas transplants could ship pancreases to those that do, or if HLA matching is deemed important, pancreases could be exchanged between various institutions transplanting this organ to diabetic recipients in order to achieve the best match. The effect of HLA matching on the results of kidney transplantation is controversial (20). Preliminary evidence indicates that matching for HLA DR exerts a greater effect on graft survival than matching for HLA A and B loci. Since a very high proportion of Type I diabetics are DR 3 or 4 or both, even if complete sharing between institutions was possible, at current cadaver donor procurement rates, not more than 25% of recipients could be matched for both DR antigens. Thus, if matching is to be used, the current donor procurement rate must also be increased by at least 4 fold. If HLA matching turns out not to be important (certainly a strong possibility as more effective means to prevent rejection are developed), a sufficient number of donors are currently available to supply pancreases for the number of diabetics who could theoretically benefit from the procedure.

The current kidney transplant rate in the U.S.A. is similar to the current incidence of complication prone Type I diabetes. If preservation is improved to the point that it is as reliable for the pancreas as the kidney, pancreas transplantation could be carried out on a semi-emergent basis, as is kidney transplantation when a cadaver donor becomes available. Related donors could be used for hemi-pancreas transplantation to some diabetics (30) as is the current practice at Minnesota for both kidney (31) and pancreas (27) transplantation.

In conclusion, clinical pancreas transplantation is a procedure being applied with increasing effectiveness for the treatment of diabetes. Islet transplantation remains a laboratory exercise. Three rationales for pursuit of the clinical islet transplantation exist. First, if islet yield can be improved, the potential exists for one donor to treat more than one recipient. Second, islet transplantation is a smaller operation for the recipient (although it certainly increases the maneuvers necessary on the part of the transplanter). Third, isolated islets can potentially by manipulated *in vitro* to reduce immunogenicity. Until the techniques necessary to achieve the first and third rationales can be adapted for the human situation, pancreas transplantation is the only option for total endocrine replacement therapy in diabetes. Pancreas transplantation potentially could be applied on as large a scale as kidney transplantation. Ultimately early pancreas transplantation could prevent the development of diabetic nephropathy and replace kidney transplantation in the management of complication prone diabetic patients.

## Acknowledgements

Janet Sanders, Lori Anderson-Tepley, and Nancy Hanson prepared the manuscript and Mary Brozic prepared the figure. The reports from the transplant teams of the various institutions cited were, of course, essential for compiling the Registry data, and their contributions are gratefully acknowledged.

## References

1. Bart KJ, Macon EJ, Whittier FC, Baldwin PJ, Blaunt JH: Cadaveric kidneys for transplantation. A paradox of shortage in the face of plenty. Transplantation 31: 374–382, 1981.
2. Baumgartner D, Largiader F, Uhlschmid G, Binswanger U: Rejection of simultaneous pancreas and kidney transplants. Transpl Proc 15(1): 1330–1331, 1983.
3. Brownlee MC, Cahill GF: Diabetic control and vascular complications. Atherosclerotic Reviews, Vol 4 (Paoletti R, Gatto AM eds). Raven Press, New York, pp 29–70, 1979.
4. Buchwald H, Rupp WM, Rhode JD, Barbosa J, Dorman FD, Blackshear PJ, Varco RL, Steffes MW, Mauer SM: Implantable insulin pump: insulin infusion in animals and man. Trans Am Soc Art Int Organs 28: 687–690, 1982.
5. Calne RY, White DJG: The use of cyclosporine in clinical organ grafting. Ann Surg 196: 330–337, 1982.
6. Clark WH (ed): Proceedings of a Workshop on Preventing Rejection of Transplanted Pancreas or Islets. Diabetes 31 (Suppl 4): 1–111, 1982.
7. Dubernard JM, Traeger J, Possa G et al: Clinical experience with 31 pancreatic transplants in man. Transpl Proc 15 (1): 1318–1321, 1983.
8. Faustman D, Hauptfeld V, Lacy P, Davie J: Prolongation of murine islet allograft survival by pretreatment of islets with antibody directed to Ia determinants. Proc Natl Acad Sci USA 78: 8, 5156–5159, 1981.
9. Florack G, Sutherland DER, Heil J, Zweber B, Najarian JS: Long term preservation of segmental pancreas autografts. Surgery 92: 260–269, 1982.
10. Gerrish EW: Final Newsletter, American college of Surgeons/National Institutes of Health Organ Transplant Registry, June 30, 1977.
11. Groth CG, Lundgren G, Klintman G et al: Successful outcome of segmental pancreas transplantation with Roux-en-Y jejunal diversion after modification in technique. Lancet 2: 522–524, 1982.
12. Groth Cg, Lundgren G, Ostman J, Gunnarsson R: Experience with nine segmental pancreatic transplantations in pre-uremic diabetic patients in Stockholm. Trans Proc 12 (No 4, Suppl 2): 68–71, 1980.
13. Health Care Financing Administration (HCFA) Office of Special Programs. End-Stage Renal Disease Program Medical Information System, Facility Survey Tables, Department of Health and Human Services, USA, HCFA. January 1-December 31, 1981.
14. Kelly WD, Lillehei RC, Merkel FK, Idezuki Y, Goetz FC: Allotransplantation of the pancreas and duodenum along with the kidney in diabetic nephropathy. Surgery 61: 827–837, 1967.
15. Kolb E, Largiader F: Transplantation of pancreatic microfragments in patients with juvenile diabetes. In: Islet Isolation, Culture and Cryopreservation (Eds. Federlin K, Bretzel eds). RG

Georg Thieme Verlag, Stuttgart-New York, pp 188–194, 1981.

16. Lacy PE, Lacy ET, Finke EH, Yasunami Y: An improved method for the isolation of islets from the beef pancreas. Diabetes 31 (Suppl 2): 109–111, 1982.

17. Largiader F, Kolb E, Binswanger U: A long term functioning human pancreatic islet allotransplant. Transplantation 39: 76–77, 1980.

18. Lillehei RC, Simmons RL, Najarian JS, Weil R III, Uchida H, Ruiz JO, Kjellstrand CM, Goetz FC: Pancreaticoduodenal allotransplantation. Experimental and clinical experience. Ann Surg 172: 405–436, 1970.

19. McMaster P, Gibby OM, Calne RY et al: Pancreatic transplantation. J Roy Soc Med 75: 47–51, 1982.

20. Opelz G, Terasaki PI: International study of histocompatibility in renal transplantation. Transplantation 3: 87–95, 1982.

21. Rosenbloom AL, Silverstein JH, Lezotte DC, Richardson K, McCallum RN: Limited joint mobility in childhood diabetes mellitus indicates increased risk for microvascular disease. N Eng J Med 305: 191–194, 1981.

22. Sutherland DER: Current status of clinical pancreas and islet transplantation with comments on need for and complications of cyrogenic and other preservation techniques. Cryobiology (1983, in press).

23. Sutherland DER: Current status of pancreas transplantation: Registry statistics and an overview. Transpl Proc 15(1) (1983, in press).

24. Sutherland DER: International human pancreas and islet transplant registry. Transpl Proc 12 (No 4, Suppl 2): 229–236, 1980.

25. Sutherland DER: Pancreas and islet transplantation. I. Experimental Studies. Diabetologia 20: 161–185, 1981.

26. Sutherland DER: Pancreas and islet transplantation. II. Clinical trials. Diabetologia 20: 435–450, 1981.

27. Sutherland DER, Goetz FC, Elick BA, Najarian JS: Experience with 49 segmental pancreas transplants in 45 diabetic patients. Transplantation 34: 330–338, 1982.

28. Sutherland DER, Goetz FC, Elick BA, Najarian JS: Pancreas transplantation for diabetes: Clinical experience and metabolic studies in 54 recent cases at the University of Minnesota. Transpl Proc 15(1): 1322–1326, 1983.

29. Sutherland DER, Goetz FC, Najarian JS: Pancreas Organ Transplantation. Clin Endocrin & Metabol 11: 549–578, 1982.

30. Sutherland DER, Goetz FC, Najarian JS: Living related donor segmental pancreatectomy for transplantation. Transpl Proc 12 (No 4, Suppl 2): 19–25, 1980.

31. Sutherland DER, Morrow CE, Fryd DS, Ferguson RM, Simmons RL, Najarian JS: Improved patient and renal allograft survival in uremic diabetic patients. Transplantation 34: 319–325, 1982.

32. Toledo-Pereyra LH, Mittal VK: Segmental pancreas transplantation. Arch Surgery 171: 505–508, 1982.

33. Ungar RH: Meticulous control of diabetes: Benefits, risks and precautions. Diabetes 31: 479–483, 1982.

34. White N, Skor DA, Cryer PE, Levandoski PA, Bier DM, Santiago JV: Identification or Type I diabetic patients at increased risk for hypoglycemia during intensive therapy. N Engl J Med 308: 485–491, 1983.

35. West KM: Epidemiology of diabetes and its vascular lesions. Elsevier, New York, 1978.

# 26. Pancreas transplantation in Lyon 1976–1983

J.M. DUBERNARD, J. TRAEGER, G. KAMEL, E. BOSI,
A. GELET, S. EL-YAFI, F. CANTON, M.C. MALIK, H. CODAS
and J.L. TOURAINE

## Introduction

The first pancreatic transplant at the Herriot Hospital of Lyon was performed in October 1976. Between then, and May 1983, 39 pancreatic allografts were performed in 37 insulin-dependent diabetic patients.

Thirty-eight of the 39 pancreatic transplants were segmental and 1 was total. In all the cases the handling of the exocrine secretion was obtained by Neoprene injection into the pancreatic duct system. In 11 cases pancreas was transplanted alone, in 2 cases it preceded and in one case it followed a kidney transplant, while in 25 instances kidney and pancreas were transplanted simultaneously. Organs were always removed from cadavers, and in the double simultaneous pancreatico-renal transplants the two organs were provided by the same donor. Currently (1 June 1983) 10 patients have a pancreatic graft functioning and are insulin independent. The clinical experience of these 39 pancreas transplants is reviewed and summarized herein.

## Patients

The 37 patients were all insulin-dependent diabetic patients aged 34, 9 ±8, 6 years with a duration of diabetes of 20, 4 ± 6, 1 years (Mean ± S.D.).

All of the patients were affected by severe degenerative diabetic complications, seven of them being completely blind at the time of transplantation.

Diabetic nephropathy was present at a preuremic degree in 6 recipients of single pancreatic transplants; all the others were affected by end-stage renal failure and they were maintained on hemo and peritoneal dialysis. Donors were heart-beating cadavers selected for ABO compatibility and negative cross-match. HLA and DR typing were routinely performed but not considered for matching donors and recipients.

**Surgical technique**

The segmental transplant technique with neoprene-injection experimented first in dogs has been developed in humans (1). The segment including the body and the tail of the pancreas is removed from the donor, with a patch of the celiac or aortic arteries and a patch of the portal vein. The suppression of the pancreatic exocrine secretion is obtained by injecting into the Wirsung duct a variable amount of neoprene, a liquid synthetic rubber. Due to the different pH, a flocculation occurs at the contact between neoprene and pancreatic juice leading to the obstruction of the ductal system and consequently to an extended fibrosis of the exocrine parenchyma. The pancreas is then placed in the iliac fossa. The graft vein and artery are end-to-side anastomosed to the external iliac vein and to the common or external or internal iliac artery, respectively.

Starting from case 7, an additional procedure of omentoplasty was performed in order to provide a mechanism of reabsorption of the residual pancreatic exocrine secretion: the omentum is attracted through a short peritoneal incision and wrapped around the graft, which is then placed totally or partially extraperitoneal. When a simultaneous pancreatico-renal transplant is performed, the kidney is placed extraperitoneally on the opposite iliac fossa.

*Immunosuppression*

Different protocols of immunosuppressive treatment have been employed during our experience in pancreas transplantation.

*Protocol A*. Upto May 1981 all the recipients of pancreatic transplants (21 cases) were treated beginning the day of transplantation with azathioprine (2,5 mg/kg/day), prednisone (1 mg/kg/day and antilymphocyte globulin (ALG) (8 mg/kg/day of purified equine IgG); ALG was discontinued after 4 to 12 weeks of treatment, while azathioprine and corticoids were progressively decreased to a maintainance dose of 1 and 0, 5 mg/kg/day respectively. Doses of prednisone were eventually increased in case of rejection, and reduced after normalisation of renal function.

*Protocol B*. In June 1981 Cyclosporin A (CyA) became available for clinical use at our institution. Since then 7 pancreatic transplant patients were allocated in a protocol of therapy including CyA (14 to 18 mg/kg/day) from the day of transplantation in association with ALG at the same doses and timing of protocol A. In 3 cases CyA was initially given by i.v. route and switched to oral administration 4–5 days after.

*Protocol C*. Because of the difficulties occurring in handling the CyA dosage in the immediate post-operative period and in distinguishing between rejection and drug-nephrotoxicity, we presently prefer to employ an initial course with conventional treatment (protocol A), and to switch to CyA after stabilization of renal function. Ten patients were allocated in this protocol of combined immunosuppression. Of them 7 recent cases have not yet been switched to CyA. Except two cases, all the recipients had received, randomly, blood transfusions. A continuous lymph drainage was attempted by means of a thoracic duct fistula in 9 patients, resulting in a removal of more than $20 \times 10^9$ lymphocytes in 6 of them. The drainage was stopped after a period of 2–3 weeks, and the pancreas transplants performed within the next three months.

## Results

*Patient and graft survival.* The rate of survival of the 37 patients undergoing primary pancreatic transplantation was 75% at 6 months, 65% at 1 year and 49% at 2 years. The overall survival rate of the pancreatic transplants was 49% at 3 months, 36% at 6 months, 21% at 1 year and 13% at 2 years (Fig. 1). Different rates of transplant survival were obtained according to the different techniques and immunosuppressive treatments employed.

*Single pancreatic transplant series.* Of the 13 single pancreatic transplants, only two survived more than three months, allowing the patients to receive a kidney allograft at a second time (Fig. 2).

The causes of failure were early vascular thrombosis in four cases, vascular thrombosis or rejection in two cases, rejection in four cases, and a death from cardiac failure with the pancreas functioning in one case. Of the two patients who received a renal graft after pancreas, one returned to insulin therapy 9 months after pancreatic transplantation because of chronic rejection, the other died of meningitis 11 months after pancreatic transplantation with both pancreas and kidney functioning. The only pancreas transplanted after kidney was a second graft after pancreatic failure of a primary simultaneous double transplant, with the kidney still functioning: the patient remained insulin-independent for four

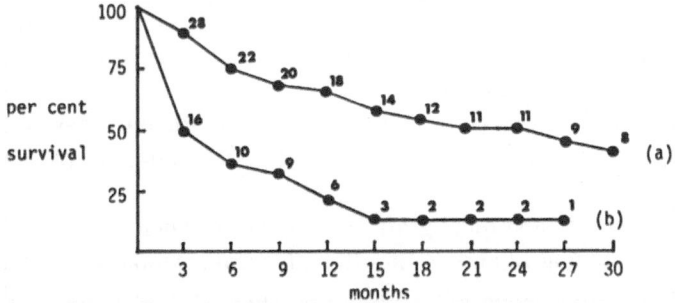

*Fig. 1.* Patient (a, n = 37) and pancreatic graft survival (b, n = 39) after pancreas transplantation.

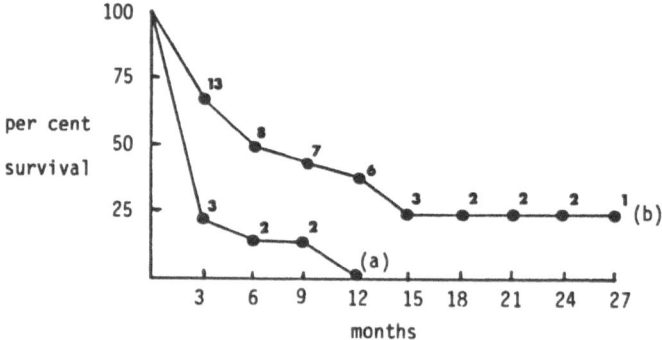

*Fig. 2.* Pancreatic graft survival after: (a) single pancreatic transplant or dysynchromous pancreas and kidney transplant (n = 14); (b) simultaneous pancreatic and renal transplant (n = 25).

months, until resumption of insulin therapy was necessary because of the recurrence of hyperglycemia, most likely due to rejection.

In this series, only two patients received CyA as part of immunosuppressive treatment.

*Simultaneous kidney plus pancreas transplant series.* Better results were obtained in the 25 simultaneous pancreatic and renal transplants. The success rate of the pancreatic grafts was 67, 50, 38 and 24% survival at three, six, twelve and twenty-four months respectively (Fig. 2).

Seven of the 25 transplants performed failed within 3 months of transplantation: in two cases the pancreatic function was compromised by a partial or total venous thrombosis which occurred in the immediate post-operative period. In two patients pancreatic failure occurred during the third month after transplantation, presumably from rejection. Three patients died with the pancreatic graft functioning: one of mesenteric infarction, one of disseminated intravascular coagulation consequent to irreversible kidney rejection and one of a lymphoproliferative syndrome.

Fourteen pancreatic transplants survived more than three months: in 4 of them rejection occurred and insulin therapy was resumed 5, 11, 12 and 14 months after transplantation; four patients died with functioning pancreatic grafts, one of myocardial infarction at 3 months and 2 weeks, one of lymphoproliferative syndrome at 5 months, one of carebral vascular accident at 7 months and one of chronic hepatitis at 29 months.

Ten patients have currently (1 June 1983) functioning renal and pancreatic transplants and are insulin independent 1, 1, 2, 2, 2, 5, 6, 14, 18 and 26 months after transplantation.

Two patients retained renal graft function after pancreatic failure. These are currently functioning 12 and 34 months after transplantation. The use of CyA from the day of transplantation (protocol B) did not greatly improve the pancreatic graft survival at 3 months (71 vs 62 and 69 percent of protocols A and C, respectively).

However, at long-term the treatment with CyA seemed to be beneficial for the pancreatic graft, attaining 30% survival at 2 years (protocols B and C) in comparison with 12% with the conventional therapy.

*Control of diabetes.* The successful cases of pancreatic transplantation led to the correction of the clinical signs of diabetes (hyperglycemia, glycosuria, ketosis, etc.) and restored insulin-independence within a few days from transplantation.

In many cases insulin therapy had to be temporarily resumed in concomitance with acute steroid treatment for rejection episodes, but it was discontinued as the steroid doses were reduced.

All the successful transplants rapidly achieved a substantial normoglycemia which was maintained for the duration of pancreatic function, irrespective of the type of immunosuppressive treatment, although provocative tests revealed individual variations in patterns of endocrine secretions from the grafts.

The glycosilated haemoglobin values (Hb Alc) were usually in the normal non-diabetic range from the first months after transplantation.

## Discussion

After the early unsatisfactory attempts, the re-evaluation of pancreas transplantation as an approach in the management of endstage insulin-dependent diabetes mellitus, was made possible by the availability of new techniques of grafting which made the surgical procedure safer and simpler than previously (1, 4).

At present, the success rate of pancreas transplantation, although still below that of kidney and liver, has improved and this procedure could be advised for a larger number of patients. Until now the usual technique has been that of segmental pancreatic graft with duct occlusion by injection of polymers (5). Although the more physiological technique of pancreatico-enteric anastomosis has recently been reconsidered with preliminary encouraging results (6), we prefer to continue with the polymer (i.e. neoprene) technique: indeed this procedure, which was developed in our laboratory, has been validated by experimental studies and by many long-term transplant survivals in our as, in other, clinical series.

Two reasons indicate pancreas transplantation in those diabetic patients who also need a kidney transplant. Firstly patients who require a kidney transplant have to be immunosuppressed and therefore the pancreatic transplant does not increase the related risks. Secondly, the success rate of pancreatic grafts has increased when associated with kidney transplantation: in our series of 13 single pancreatic transplants, only 2 survived more than three months, while all the long-term pancreatic transplants belonged to the pancreaticorenal series. One explanation could be that the chronic renal failure and haemodialysis treatment prior to transplantation induce an immunodeficiency which can contribute to reduce the host responsiveness. Furthermore, for reasons still unclear, the kidney has the tendency to be rejected before the pancreas, and the monitoring of plasma creatinine can be useful also in preventing pancreatic rejection by an adequate treatment of renal rejection. This peculiar timing of rejection for kidney and pancreas has recently been confirmed by experimental studies (7). In our experience the causes of pancreatic failure were due to technical, vascular and immunological reasons or to the death of the patients.

The introduction of CyA improved the pancreatic graft survival at 2 years, but did not succeed in reducing the rate of the early failures. Because of our still limited experience and of the uncertainty about the causes of many graft failures, a correct estimation of the capability of CyA in preventing pancreatic rejection is not yet possible.

However, a further motivation for the use of CyA in pancreatic transplantation rises from the necessity of abolishing, or at least reducing the diabetogenic effect of the steroid treatment: indeed the patients treated by CyA alone exhibited a better degree of glucose tolerance after OGTT than those receiving steroids (3).

In conclusion, the success rate of pancreas transplantation is improving and the validity of this therapeutic approach is sustained by some long-term transplant survivals. A clarification of the immunological events occuring after this heterotopic graft as well as a further improvement of the transplant techniques are needed in order to make this procedure applicable to a larger number of patients. At present, the association of kidney and pancreas transplants seems to offer more chances of success than the transplantation of the pancreas alone. The metabolic control obtained after successful pancreatic transplants is a promising tool for the prevention of degenerative diabetic complications and possibly the improvement of immunosuppressive therapy will permit grafting earlier in the course of the disease.

## References

1. Dubernard JM, Traeger J, Neyra P, Touraine JL, Tranchant D, Blanc-Brunat N: A new method of preparation of segmental pancreatic grafts for transplantation. Trials in dogs an in man. Surgery 84: 633–639, 1978.
2. Pozza G, Traeger J, Dubernard JM, Secchi A, Pontiroli AE, Bosi E, Malik MC, Tuiton A, Blanc N: Endocrine responses of type 1 (insulin-dependent) diabetic patients following successful pancreas transplantation. Diabetologia 24: 244–248, 1983.
3. Traeger J, Dubernard JM, Pozza G, Bosi E, Secchi A, Pontiroli AE, Touraine JL, Betuel H, El-Yafi S, Da-Ponte F, Cantarovich D, Diab N, Cardozo C, Martin X, Kamel G, Gelet A: Influence of immusuppressive therapy on the endocrine function of segmental pancreatic allografts. Transplant Proc 15: 1326–1329, 1983.
4. Sutherland DER: pancreas and islets transplantation. II. Clinical trials. Diabetologia 20: 435–450, 1981.
5. Sutherland DER: Current status of pancreas transplantation: Registry statistics and an overview. Transplant Proc 15: 1303–1307, 1983.

6. Groth Cg, Collste H, Lundgren G, Wilczek H, Klintmalm G, Ringden O, Gunnarsson R, Ostman J: Successful outcome of segmental human pancreatic transplantation with enteric exocrine diversion after modifications in technique. Lancet II: 522–524, 1982.
7. Severyn W, Olson L, Miller J, Kyriakides G, Rabinovitch A, Flaa C, Mintz D: Studies on the survival of simultaneous canine renal and segmental pancreatic allografts. Transplantation 33: 606–616, 1982.

## 27. Pancreas transplantation at the University of Minnesota: experience with 68 recent cases

DAVID E.R. SUTHERLAND, FREDERICK C. GOETZ, PATRICIA L. CHINN, BARBARA A. ELICK, RICHARD L. SIMMONS and JOHN S. NAJARIAN

### Introduction

Efforts to transplant immediately vascularized pancreas grafts or free grafts of dispersed pancreatic islet tissue have been made almost continuously at the University of Minnesota since 1966. The work of Lillihei and colleagues with 14 pancreas transplants performed before 1974 have been reported previously (5, 6), as have 18 of our 20 attempts at islet transplantation since that time (8, 13).

An entirely new series of pancreas transplants was begun in July of 1978, and to the present (March, 1983) includes 68 pancreas transplants in 62 diabetic patients. This experience is summarized herein.

### Materials and methods

Of the 62 pancreas transplant recipients (26 male, 36 female), 44 had had functioning renal allografts placed 6 months to 9 years previously for treatment of end-stage diabetic nephropathy, while 23 patients had not had a kidney transplant. Two of the latter had a kidney transplant subsequent to the pancreas transplant. Of the 67 pancreas grafts, 39 were procured from cadaver donors, and 28 from living related donors. All of the related and 24 of the cadaveric grafts were of the standard (hemi-pancreas) segmental type, 5 were extended segmental grafts, and 10 were whole pancreas grafts. With the latter two techniques the hepatic-pancreatico-duodenal and splenic arteries both remain intact from their origin on the celiac axis, and the tail, body and part of the head and uncinate process (extended segmental), or the entire gland (whole pancreas without the duodenum), are transplanted, as previously described (9).

All of the grafts were placed intraperitoneally and the donor pancreas vessels were anastomosed to the iliac vessels of the recipients. Five different techniques have been used for duct drainage (Table 1). Silicone rubber injections or pancreatico-jejunostomys have been used exclusively during the past year.

The details of our immunosuppressive protocols have been described (8). Briefly, 20 recipients of pancreas allografts were treated with azathioprine,

*Table 1.* Outcome after pancreas transplantation in Minnesota cases according to technique, donor source and immunosuppression.

| Technique | No. of txs (rel/cad) | CsA/Aza | Technical failures | Late loss of function | Grafts currently functioning– | |
|---|---|---|---|---|---|---|
| | | | | | No. | Duration (months) |
| Duct ligated | 2 (0/2) | 0/2 | 2(100%) | 0(0%) | 0(0%) | – |
| Prolamine inj. | 4 (1/3) | 2/1 | 0(0%) | 4(100%) | 0(0%) | – |
| Duct open | 15 (5/10) | 1/14 | 8(53%) | 4(27%) | 3(20%) | 40, 45, 56 |
| Pancreatico-jej. | 19 (19/0) | 11/5 | 6(32%) | 3(16%) | 9(47%) | 1, 1, 1, 4, 7, 8, 14, 17, 19 |
| Silicone inj. | 28 (3/25) | 23/5 | 2(8%) | 18(64%) | 6(21%) | 1, 4, 6, 13, 26, 27 |
| Total | 68 (28/40) | 37/27 | 18(26%) | 28(41%) | 18(26%) | 1–56 |

* As of March, 1983, (12/28) (43%) related and 6/40 (15%) cadaver grafts were functioning. Of technically successful allografts, 7/14 (50%) treated with Azathioprine (Aza) are functioning (all 3 open duct cadaver grafts, and the 4 and 27 month Silicone-injected and the 1 and 17 month pancreatico-jejunostomy related grafts); and 10/34 on Cyclosporin (CsA) are functioning (4 Silicone-injected cadaver grafts and 6 Pancreatico-jejunostomy related grafts). One of the latter is currently on Aza. Four recipients of grafts (1 Prolamine-injected, 3 Pancreaticojejunostomys) from identical twins (1 functioning) were not immunosuppressed. Three patients with technically successful transplants (2 silicone injected, 1 pancreatico-jejunostomy) died with functioning grafts.

prednisone and anti-lymphocyte globulin (ALG); 7 with azathioprine and prednisone only; 9 with cyclosporine (CsA) for maintenance immunosuppression after an initial course of conventional immunosuppression; and 28 with CsA and prednisone beginning immediately after transplantation (Table 1). four of the latter were switched from cyclosporine to azathioprine between 3 and 6 months after transplantation; one had no change in graft function and remains insulin independent at >1 year after transplantation, while the other three had decline of graft function and had to resume exogenous insulin between 2 and 6 months after conversion. Thirteen pancreas grafts in conventionally and two in CsA immunosuppressed patients failed for technical reasons.

## Results

Fifty-two of the 62 patients are currently (March, 1983) alive and 19 have functioning primary pancreas allografts and are insulin independent, 9 for >1 year, the longest for 4.7 years after transplantation (Table 1). Seventeen pancreas grafts failed for technical reasons, the details of which have previously been published (8, 9, 11). Five recipients of unsuccessful grafts died between one and 3 months after transplantation. Three patients died with functioning grafts between 1 and 6 weeks after transplantation, while 28 grafts functioned between 1 and 12 months before hyperglycemia recurred and resumption of exogenous insulin was necessary in the recipients. All but two of the latter are alive and well between 2 and 53 months after loss of graft function. The two exceptions died from myocardial infects at 21 and 51 months posttransplant.

Of the 28 technically successful grafts that eventually ceased to function, 15 (4 open duct, 2 prolamine, 8 silicone, 1 panc-jej) were not biopsied or removed at the time, and so the cause of loss of function is uncertain. Of the 13 grafts that were biopsied, one was from an identical twin (prolamine injected), and fibrosis was almost certainly the cause of loss of function two months after transplantation (12). Ten other allografts injected with either prolamine or silicone rubber also showed fibrosis. But elements of rejection were present as well. One recipient of a related graft (pancreaticojejunostomy) had hyperglycemia occur at 8 months, two months after conversion from Cyclosporine to Azathioprine. Biopsy of the graft showed mononuclear cell infiltration consistent with rejection. the patient was treated with ALG and prednisone and currently has C-peptide levels above baseline, but requires insulin for postprandial hyperglycemia. One related graft (pancreatico-jejunostomy) was biopsied at 6 months after transplantation, 4 months after resumption of exogenous insulin was necessary; it was normal in every regard except for the absence of beta cells in otherwise intact islets, in distinct contrast to the presence of beta cells in the islets at the time of transplantation; rejection seems an unlikely explanation and this case may illustrate a type of patient in whom the original disease recurrs in the grafted organ (9).

Recurrence of hyperglycemia was presumptively diagnosed as rejection and was treated in 14 recipients of 8 cadaver and 6 related grafts with an increase in prednisone dose or with ALG administration. Five recipients (two cadaver and three related grafts) reverted to euglycemia and insulin independence after antirejection treatment; the treatment had no effect in the patient who, on biopsy, had a normal pancreas graft except for the absence of beta ccells (9).

Of the patients with functioning grafts who are insulin independent, some, but not all, have normal or nearly normal glucose tolerance tests (15). The results of a recent glucose tolerance test and metabolic profile in the patient who is currently the longer survivor with a functioning pancreas graft (4.5 years) is illustrated in Figure 1. The particular patient received an open duct segmental pancreas graft from a cadaver donor 6 years after a kidney had been transplanted from her mother. A biopsy of her renal allograft before the pancreas transplant showed an increase in glomerular mesangium matrix, and linear staining for albumin on tubular and glomerular membranes; biopsies of the kidney at 2 and 4 years after the pancreas transplant showed regression of these changes on light microscopy (observations by S.M. Mauer).

The related donors of 28 segmental grafts, along with 2 previous related donors of hemi-pancreases (11) for islet grafts (13) are alive and well. Two (7%) required re-operation, one for a splenectomy and one to religate the pancreatic duct at the line of transection. The spleens remained viable in 27 (97%) of the donors, as determined by technetium scans. Minor changes in glucose tolerance results

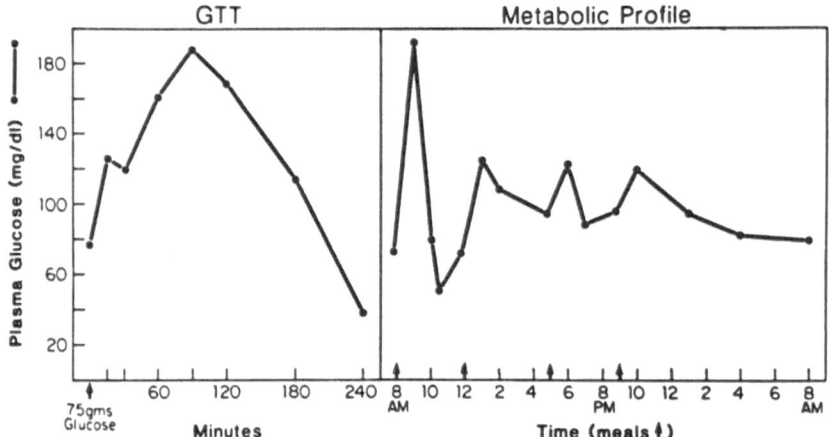

Fig. 1. Oral glucose tolerance test and metablic profile in a patient 4 years after transplantation of an open-duct segmental pancreas graft.

occurred after hemi-pancreatectomy in some donors, but were judged to be physiologically significant only in one obese donor (2).

## Discussion

Our current protocol for pancreas transplantation is derived from lessons learned during 96 endocrine replacement therapy attempts in 83 patients at the University of Minnesota since 1966 (12 pancreaticoduodenal, 20 islet, 9 whole and 55 segmental pancreas transplants. Many of the current features of our program are also similar to those of other groups who are applying pancreas transplantation to the treatment of diabetes, including the use of cyclosporine for recipient immunosuppression (7) and either duct injection (3) for suppression of exocrine function or pancreatico-enterostomy for physiological drainage of graft exocrine secretions (4).

Our approach to the uremic diabetic in recent years has differed from that of most other groups. We are not performing synchronous kidney and pancreas grafts. The results of kidney transplant alone in uremic diabetics are now excellent (14); it has not been shown that simultaneous pancreas transplants improves the renal allograft survival rate, and thus we prefer to delay pancreas transplantation until after the renal graft is well established. However, since complications of diabetes continue to progress after kidney transplantation, and since these patients already require immunosuppression, pancreas transplantation is a logical therapy and, until recently, recipients of previous renal allografts made up the largest proportion of our pancreas transplant population.

Ideally, pancreas transplantation should be done early in the course of the disease. Because generalized immunosuppression is required, such an approach can not be taken unless the recipients clearly have, or are developing, diabetic complications which are more serious than the potential side effects of the anti-rejection therapy. We have performed pancreas transplantation in 21 non-uremic patients. During 1982, 13 of our 24 pancreas transplant recipients had progressive retinopathy, neuropathy or early nephropathy as indications for pancreas transplantation. Out of 19 patients with currently functioning grafts (12 related, 7 cadaver), 8 (7 related, 1 cadaver) had not had previous kidney grafts.

We are still not sure which technique of pancreas transplantation is best. Pancreatico-jejunostomy is the most physiological, but because of the risk of bacterial contamination at the time of operation we have used this approach only in recipients of related grafts who receive less immunosuppression. Currently, we use duct injection with silicone rubber (16) for recipients of cadaveric grafts; in an attempt to preserve the maximal amount of endocrine tissue, should fibrosis occur as a result of duct injection, we have transplanted the whole pancreas in 10 recent cases.

Most of our efforts have focused on simply achieving an acceptable pancreas graft functional survival rate with a low morbidity and mortality in the recipients. However, it is also important to study the pancreas transplant recipients for the effect on secondary complications, and the increased success rate of pancreas transplantation should allow many fundamental questions related to diabetes to be answered (1). Preliminary observation on the kidney in our patient followed for the longest time (>4 years) after pancreas transplantation, suggests that not only prevention, but actually a reversal of early lesions is possible. With the use of both related and cadaver donor, we see no reason why pancreas transplantation could not eventually have the same impact on the treatment of diabetes as kidney transplantation has on the treatment of end-stage renal disease.

In summary, of 81 pancreas transplants in 76 patients at the University of Minnesota, 67 of them were performed in 62 patients since 1978. Currently (March, 1983), 19 patients have functioning grafts, 9 for more than one year. Pancreas transplantation can be performed with some expectation that long term function will be sustained. Concurrent advances in immunosuppression (cyclosporine), technique (duct injection or pancreatico-enterostomy) and patient selection have been associated with an increase in the success rate of pancreas transplantation.

**Acknowledgements**

Supported by NIH Grants AM 19269 and RR-400.

238

## References

1. Barker CF, Naji A, Perloff LJ, Dafoe DC, Bartlett S: Invited commentary: An overview of pancreas transplantation – biologic acpects. Surgery 92: 113–137, 1982.
2. Chinn P, Sutherland DER, Goetz FC, Elick BA, Najarian JS: Metabolic effects of hemi-pancreatectomy in living related graft donors. Transplant Proc (in press).
3. Dubernard JM, Traeger J, Neyra P, Touraine JL, Traudiant D, Blanc-Brunat N: A new method of preparation of segmental pancreatic grafts for transplantation: Trials in dogs and in man. Surgery 84: 633–639, 1978.
4. Groth CG, Collste H, Lundgren G, Gunnarsson R, Colste H, Wilczek H, Ringden O, Ostman J: Successful outcome of segmental pancreatic deversion after modifications in technique. Lancet 2: 522–524, 1982.
5. Lillehei RC, Ruiz JO, Acquino C, Goetz FC: Transplantation of the pancreas. Acta Endocrinol 83 (Suppl 205): 303–320, 1976.
6. Lillehei RC, Simmons RL, Najarian JS, Weil R, III, Uchida H, Ruiz JO, Kjellstrand CM, Goetz FC: Pancreaticoduodenal allotransplantation. Experimental and clinical experience. Ann Surg 172: 405–436, 1970.
7. McMaster P, Gibby OM, Calne RY, Evans DB, Thirn S, Rolles K, Bevan R, Smith J: Pancreatic transplantation. J Roy Soc Med 75: 47–51, 1982.
8. Najarian JS, Sutherland DER, Matas AJ, Steffes MW, Goetz FC: Human islet transplantation: A preliminary experience. Transplant Proc 9: 233–236, 1977.
9. Sutherland DER, Goetz FC, Elick BA, Najarian JS: Experience with 49 segmental pancreas transplants in 45 diabetic patients. Transplantation 34: 330–338, 1982.
10. Sutherland DER, Goetz FC, Najarian JS: Intraperitoneal transplantation of immediately vas-cularized segmental pancreatic grafts without duct ligation: A clinical trial. Transplantation 28: 485–491, 1979.
11. Sutherland DER, Goetz FC, Najarian JS: Living related donor segmental pancreatectomy for transplantation. Transpl Proc 12(Suppl 2): 19–25, 1980.
12. Sutherland DER, Goetz FC, Rynasiewicz JJ, Baumgartner D, White DC, Elick BA, Najarian JS: Segmental pancreas transplantation from living related and cadaver donors: A clinical experience. Surgery 90: 159–169, 1981.
13. Sutherland DER, Matas AJ, Goetz FC, Najarian JS: Transplantation of dispersed pancreatic islet tissue in humans: Autografts and allografts. Diabetes 29 (Suppl 1): 34–44, 1980.
14. Sutherland DER, Morrow CE, Fryd DS, Ferguson RM, Simmons RL, Najarian JS: Improved patient and primary renal allograft survival in uremic diabetic recipients. Transplantation 34: 319–325, 1982.
15. Sutherland DER, Najarian JS, Greenberg BZ, Senske BJ, Anderson CE, Francis RC, Goetz FC: Hormonal and metabolic effects of an endocrine graft: Vascularized segmental transplantation on the pancreas in insulin-dependent patients. Ann Int Med 95: 537–541, 1981.
16. White DC, Sutherland DER, Najarian JS: Endocrine function and histology of the canine pancreas after exocrine ablation by ductal injection of silicone rubber adhesive: A preliminary report. J Surg Res 31: 371–374, 1981.

# 28. Cardiac transplantation

STUART W. JAMIESON, PHILIP E. OYER, EDWARD B. STINSON
and NORMAN E. SHUMWAY

## Introduction

The first serious attempts at experimental cardiac transplantation were carried
out by Alexis Carrel, at the University of Chicago, shortly after the turn of the
century (1). He achieved the beating of transplanted puppy hearts in the necks of
adult mongrel dogs for a number of hours. Though these hearts did not support
the circulation, this was a remarkable achievement at the time considering the
lack of heparin and the very crude nature of the surgical techniques and materials
used.

It was not until Mann and his colleagues renewed this work in the Mayo clinic in
the mid 1930's (2), that awareness of rejection occurred. They noted that some of
the transplanted hearts would beat for a number of days and then failed for what
was termed 'biological manipulation'. Since there was no immunosuppression at
this time of course, work in cardiac transplantation once more essentially ceased.
It was Shumway's group in San Francisco that seriously addressed the potential
clinical problems in cardiac transplantation, beginning with work in dogs in the
late 1950's (3). By 1961 they had achieved survival for one year after orthotopic
transplantation in dogs. The next decade was spent in solving the many problems
involved with the diagnosis and treatment of rejection, and perfecting the technical aspects of cardiac transplantation. The operative technique and methods of
cardiac transplantation. The operative technique and methods of cardiac preservation were worked out, and working methods for the diagnosis and treatment of
graft rejection were established. The effects of anatomic denervation on cardiac
performance were studied.

The first human cardiac transplant was carried out by James Hardy in Mis-
sissippi in 1964 (4). The donor was a chimpanzee whose heart was not big enough
to sustain the circulation, and the recipient died after a period of hours. The first
human to human cardiac transplant was carried out in 1967 in Capetown (5), and
the following month the clinical program was initiated at Stanford. In the calen-
dar year of 1968, 101 cardiac transplants were performed by 64 teams in 22
countries of the world. This unprecedented display of enthusiasm for an untried
clinical prcedure, especially in centers that had little or no previous experience in

the experimental aspects of the work, resulted in a predictably poor survival rate, and the cessation of heart transplantation in almost every center. The program at Stanford, founded on a decade of thorough experimental activity, continued, and in the decade between 1970 and 1980 performed over half the total cardiac transplants in the world.

Continued laboratory research at this center after the inception of the clinical program allowed several major improvements. Numbered amongst these were the introduction of rabbit antithymocyte globulin (6), the endomyocardial biopsy technique for the diagnosis of rejection (7), methods for monitoring the immunological status of the patient (8), and long-distance transport of the donor heart (9). More recently, protocols for the use of the new immunosuppressive agent cyclosporine have been determined (10) and clinical heart and lung transplantation has been successfully transferred from the laboratory to the clinical arena (11).

As a result of the now demonstrated efficacy of cardiac transplantation as a therapeutic procedure, other centers throughout the world are once more commencing clinical programs.

**Donor procurement**

The recognition of brain death as absolute was pivotal to the development of successful cardiac transplantation. Removal of the heart after anoxic arrest is not compatible with effective cardiac transplantation, and the definition of irreversible coma by the AD Hoc Committee of the Harvard medical school in 1968 (12) was an important advance. Guidelines established in this report furnished the basis for the legal pronouncement of death on the basis of total and irreversible cerebral injury, regardless of continued artificial support of the circulation respiration.

The donor must have a negative history of heart defects, together with an electrocardiogram interpreted to be within normal limits. It should be noted that electrocardiograms of people that are neurologically dead often have abnormalities in the ST segments, and commonly atrial premature contractions. These may be ignored provided no other abnormalities are found. Hypothermia, diabetes insipidus, pulmonary insufficiency, or arterial hypertension secondary to autonomic nervous system dysfunction may all contribute to cardiovascular instability in donors. This generally responds to fluid administration.

The shortage of donors has required most active centers to resort to distant heart procurement. Two thirds of all donor hearts at Stanford are removed from distant sites (up to 500 miles away). After arrest with hypothermic cardioplegic solution inserted into the aortic root, the heart is excised and stored in cold saline (4°C). The longest ischemic time at Stanford has been 3.5 h, and we have been unable to detect a difference between the function of hearts from on site and distant donors, either by immediate cardiac function or by light and electron microscopic examination of ventricular biopsies at the time of surgery.

The causes of brain death in donors in the Stanford program are shown in Table 1.

## The recipient

Stringent selection criteria are used for potential recipients. At the present time patients must be less than 55 years of age, have a stable psycho-social outlook, be medically compliant and have an absence of any active infection. Similarly, any disease process that would independently limit survival, such as malignancy, or predispose to infection or other complications, such as insulin dependent diabetes, is also a contraindication. Needless to say, life expectancy must be judged in terms of months, and all other therapeutic measures, both surgical and medical, must have been exhausted. The average life expectancy of those patients selected to the program who die before a donor is made available is two months, and none of these patients have lived more than nine months. The recipient pool, then, represents patients truly in the end-stages of their disease.

The evaluation of potential recipients includes a full history and physical examination, a full biochemical and hematological investigation, and hemodynamic and angiographic studies. Occasionally cardiac biopsy may be indicated. The pulmonary vascular resistance must be less than six Wood units (the normal donor right ventricle cannot acutely accommodate high resistance), and only mild or moderate renal or hepatic dysfunction secondary to cardiac failure should be present. This is especially true since the introduction of cyclosporine as an immunosuppressant agent, it being both hepato- and renal toxic.

The presenting diagnoses of the recipients is shown in Table 2. About half the

Table 1. Stanford cardiac transplantation: donors etiology of brain death.

|  | On site | Distant |
| --- | --- | --- |
| Cranial trauma |  |  |
| Vehicular | 89 | 59 |
| GSW | 22 | 18 |
| Other | 25 | 9 |
| CVA | 37 | 11 |
| Anoxic brain death | 9 | 4 |
| Other | 2 | 2 |
|  | 184 | 101 |

Age: mean 25; range (12–51)
Sex: men 224; women 61

*Table 2.* Stanford cardiac transplantation: recipient diagnosis.

|  | No. of patient |
| --- | --- |
| Coronary artery disease | 127 |
| Cardiomyopathy | 113 |
| Valve disease with CM | 16 |
| Congenital heart disease | 4 |
| Cardiac tumor | 1 |
| Coronary artery emboli | 1 |
| Post traumatic aneurysm | 1 |
| Total | 263 |

patients have end-stage coronary artery disease, the other half suffer from end-stage idiopathic cardiomyopathy. Fewer patients are currently being transplanted for end-stage coronary artery diseasy, this probably being a result of the ability to perform coronary artery surgery safely on a higher proportion of these patients.

**The operation**

The technical aspects of the operation have been fully described elsewhere (11) but the basic technique consists of cannulation for cardiopulmonary bypass high in the ascending aorta, with low caval cannulation. The recipient heart is excised, leaving the atria (with the exception of the appendages) *in situ*. The donor heart is then sewn in place after opening out the donor left and right atria. Continuous running prolene sutures are used, and anastomosis commences with the left atrium, then the atrial septum, followed by the right atrium. The aortic anastomosis is then performed, and finally the pulmonary anastomosis. After removal of all air from the heart the aortic crossclamp is removed.

Immediate postoperative care is similar to that of routine cardiac surgery save that immunosuppression is instituted and the patient is initially nursed in isolation. Since the denervated donor heart is rate-dependent for its cardiac output an infusion of isoproteranol is commenced, together with dopamine at a dose of 3 mg/kg/min to augment renal perfusion. This is helpful in recipients who are at present treated with cyclosporine as the primary immunosuppressive agent.

**Results**

Between january 1968 and May 1983, 287 cardiac tranplants were performed in 263 patients at Stanford. All of these were orthotopic cardiac transplants save one, a heterotopic transplant which was performed in a patient who was dying and in whom the only heart available was judged to be too small to maintain the circulation alone, and was therefore placed in the heterotopic position. We do not favor heterotopic transplantation since the patient who receives such a transplant is exposed to the same risks of immuno-suppression as one receiving an orthotopic transplant, and in addition retains in the native heart a potential source of systemic emboli, and a substrate for the development of endocarditis. Another possible indication for heterotopic transplantation may be the presence of severe pulmonary hypertension, though in the latter case heart and lung transplantation may be a preferred alternative.

A total of 140 patients have survived one year or more after transplantation and 106 are currently alive, the longest now nearly 14 years after transplantation. The current survival rate for transplanted patients is shown in Figure 1, which also demonstrates the survival rate for those patients who were accepted for transplantation but who died before a suitable donor could be found. The survival during the first six years of clinical experience at Stanford is also shown together with the survival from 1974 to 1980, after the introduction of immunological monitoring, the use of the endomyocardial bioptome, and rabbit antithymocyte globulin.

The one year survival of patients operated on during 1968, the first year of the program and Stanford, was 22%. The survival rate at one year has steadily increased, to a level of 83% for the sixteenth program year. This improvement in survival can be directly attributed to the advances in post-operative management that were developed and tested in the laboratory before clinical use.

**Out-patient care**

Patients are discharged four to eight weeks after operation. They are evaluated at twice-weekly intervals initially, and then weekly. In the outpatient clinic elec-

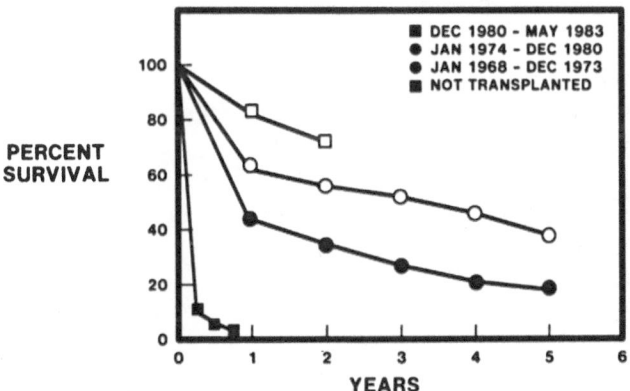

*Fig. 1.* Stanford cardiac transplantation.

244

trocardiograms, chest X-rays, and full blood screens are performed. In the absence of complications, patients return to their home towns after two to four months, and are then under the care of their own cardiologists. Close communication is maintained with Stanford, and the patients return yearly for admission to hospital, at which time cardiac catheterization, coronary arteriography, left ventriculography and endomyocardial biopsy are performed.

Immunosuppression is always required. With 'conventional' therapy, the usual maintenance regimen includes prednisone at a dose of approximately 0.25 mg/kg/day, and azathioprine at 1.5 to 2.0 mg/kg/day. Cyclosporine patients are maintained according to periodic measurement of drug levels, and generally tolerate a much lower dose of prednisone. Long-term survivors continue to sustain the risks of graft rejection and the infectious complications of immunosuppression, as well as the development of accelerated graft coronary atherosclerosis, probably as a result of repetitive endothelial injury with circulating antibody. When patients are noted to have severe coronary atherosclerosis on yearly arteriograms retransplantation is advised and this has been carried out in fifteen patients. An additional fifteen patients died from accelerated coronary atherosclerosis that remained undiagnosed.

Other causes of death in the series are shown in Table 3.

## Conclusion

Cardiac transplantation has now been shown to provide a therapeutic option when other forms of therapy have been exhausted for patients with end-stage heart disease. However, the limitations of the immunosuppressive regimens

*Table 3.* Stanford cardic transplantation: primary cause of death – 157 patients.

|  | No. of patients |
| --- | --- |
| Infection | 85 |
| Acute rejection | 26 |
| Graft arteriosclerosis |  |
| A. Proliferative | 6 |
| B. Atherosclerotic | 9 |
| Malignancy | 11 |
| Pulmonary hypertension | 7 |
| CVA | 3 |
| Sudden death | 4 |
| Pulmonary embolus | 2 |
| Cerebral edema | 1 |
| Myopathy | 1 |
| Suicide | 1 |
| Acute graft falure | 1 |

currently available mean that only highly selected patients can be offered transplantation. The use of cardiac transplantation in a larger group of patients will depend on other immunosuppressive measures that control the immune response more specifically. This would simplify the postoperative management of such patients and reduce the cost of transplantation. Cyclosporine offers substantial advantages over conventional therapy, but retains significant side-effects. Further research is likely to identify more refined immunosuppressive regimens.

## References

1. Carrel A: The Surgery of Blood Vessels. Bull Johns Hopkins Hosp 18: 18, 1907.
2. Mann FC, Priestley JT, Markowitz J, Yater WM: Transplantation of the Intact Mammalian Heart. Arch Surg 26: 219–224, 1933.
3. Lower RR, Shumway NE: Studies in Orthotopic Homotransplantation of the Canine Heart. Surgical forum 11: 18–19, 1960.
4. Hardy JD, Chavez CM, Kurrus FD, Neely WA, Eraslan S, Turner D, Fabian L, Labecke D. Heart Transplantation in Man. JAMA 188: 1132, 1964.
5. Barnard CM: The operation. A human cardiac transplant: an interim report of a successful operation at Groote Schuur Hospital, Capetown. S Afr Med J 41: 1271–1274, 1967.
6. Bieber CP, Griepp RB, Oyer PE, Wong J, Stinson EB: Use of Rabbit Antithymocyte Globulin in Cardiac Transplantation: Relationship of Serum Clearance Rates to Clinical Outcome. Transplantation 22: 478, 1976.
7. Caves PK, Stinson EB, Billingham ME, Shumway NE: Percutaneous Transvenous Endomyocardial Biopsy in Human Heart Recipients. Ann Thorac Surgery 16: 325, 1973.
8. Bieber CP, Griepp RB, Oyer PE, David LA, Stinson EB: Relationship of Rabbit ATG Serum Clearance Rates to Circulatory T-cell Levels, Rejection Onset, and Survival in Cardiac Transplantation. Transplant Proc 9: 1031, 1977.
9. Watson DC, Reitz BA, Baumgartner WA, Raney AA, Oyer PE, Stinson EB, Shumway NE: Distant Heart Procurement for Transplantation. Surgery 86: 56, 1979.
10. Oyer PE, Stinson EB, Jamieson SW, Hunt SA, Billingham M, Scott W, Bieber CP, Reitz BA, Shumway NE: Cyclosporin A in Cardiac Allografting: A Preliminary Experience. Transplantation Proc 15: 1247–1252, 1983.
11. Jamieson SW, Baldwin J, Reitz BA, Stinson EB, Oyer PE, Hunt SA, Billingham ME, Theodore J, Modry D, Bieber CP, Shumway NE: Combined Heart and Lung Transplantation. Lancet 1: 1130–1132, 1983.
12. A definition of Irreversible Coma. Report of the Harvard Medical School to Examine the Definition of Brain Death. JAMA 205: 85, 1968.

# 29. Heart-lung transplantation

STUART W. JAMIESON, EDWARD B. STINSON,
PHILIP E. OYER, JAMES THEODORE, SHARON HUNT
and NORMAN E. SHUMWAY

## Introduction

The Russian surgeon Demikhov was responsible for the first serious experimental work in combined heart and lung transplantation (1). In 1946 he achieved survival of a dog for two hours after heart-lung transplantation. His efforts were hampered by the lack of cardiopulmonary bypass, and Webb and Howard, using cardiopulmonary bypass (2) then achieved survival for 22 h. Lower and associates in 1961 (3) achieved six day survival with these techniques, but it was noted that disturbance of the respiratory pattern, presumably as a result of denervation, was the primary impairment to long-term survival. The longest reported survival after cardiopulmonary transplantation in dogs was accomplished by Grinnan and associates in 1970 (4), with one 10 day survivor from 25 transplants.

Nakae (5) then showed that normal respiratory control was not possible after pulmonary denervation in the dog, which presumably is highly dependent on the Hering-Breuer reflex for respiratory control. Primates were noted to have normal respiratory patterns following denervation.

Clinical experience with heart-lung transplantation began when Cooley and associates performed a heart-lung transplant in a two month old infant in 1968 (6). The child died fourteen hours after operation. A second human heart-lung transplant was performed by Lillehei in 1970 (7). The recipient was a 43 year-old man with advanced emphysema and pulmonary hypertension, and although he initially did well, he died eight days after surgery from progressive respiratory failure. A third patient underwent this operation in Cape Town in 1971 (8). This patient was a 49 year old man with chronic obstructive lung disease who then lived for 23 days.

Clinical efforts in heart-lung transplantation at Stanford were postponed until cardiac transplantation was thoroughly established, and available immunosuppressive techniques were modified in such a way as to provide better healing of the tracheal anastomosis. The advent of cyclosoporine (9) indicated that further investigation of heart and lung transplantation might be promising, and this drug was applied to experimental models of cardiac transplantation in the rat (10) and monkey (11), and to heart and lung transplantation in monkeys (12). It was then introduced into the clinical cardiac transplantation program in December 1980. After the initial experience in isolated cardiac transplantation had confirmed the efficacy of this agent (13) and longterm survival after heart and lung transplantation had been achieved in several monkeys, it was judged appropriate to proceed with a clinical trial of cardiopulmonary transplantation.

**Recipient selection**

Although many patients might be potential recipients for heart and lung transplantation, our operations have thus far been restricted to those with pulmonary hypertension, either primary or secondary to congenital heart disease (Eisenmenger's syndrome). These patients are good candidates for the operation, since there is almost always significant cardiac involvement even in the primary form of this disease, and the patients are relatively young. Many patients with Eisenmenger's syndrome have had one or more palliative operations which, in the presence of coagulation abnormalities due to hepatic dysfunction and the development of large collateral vessels, can make surgery hazardous.

Other categories of patients, such as those with end-stage chronic obstructive lung disease, interstitial fibrosis, and cystic fibrosis may also be candidates for heart-lung transplantation. However, the fact that the tracheo-bronchial tree is rarely sterile, the possibility of other organ involvement, and uncertainty about recurrence of disease make these groups less than optimal candidates.

Of the fourteen candidates to have received transplantation at Stanford, four had primary pulmonary hypertension, the remaining had Eisenmenger's syndrome. There were four women and ten men, ranging in age from 22 to 45 years. Five patients had primary pulmonary hypertension, and the remainder had congenital heart disease with secondary pulmonary vascular changes. Three patients in the latter category had received palliative or reconstructive procedures prior to heart-lung transplantation. Cardiac catheterization had demonstrated high, fixed pulmonary vascular resistance in all patients.

**Donor selection**

It has been more difficult to identify suitable donors for heart-lung transplantation than for heart transplantation alone. Pulmonary infection occurs early in patients who have suffered brain death, and neurogenic pulmonary edema or thoracic trauma will eliminate other donors. Less than 20% of potential heart donors have lungs that are suitable for heart-lung transplantation.

A further requirement that is not applicable to cardiac transplantation is a close size match, since the donor lungs have to fit within the fixed capacity of the recipient's thoracic cage. To compress the donor lungs within the recipient would lead to significant atelectasis and shunting, though a relative mismatch in the opposite direction; the transplantation of small donor lungs into a large thoracic cavity is unlikely to be as detrimental.

Additional requirements for donors are to have satisfactory gas exchange, with an arterial $PO_2$ of more than 100 on forced inspiratory oxygen (F102) of 40%, a good lung compliance with peak inspiratory pressures of less than 30 mm mercury with normal tidal volumes, and an absence of obviously infected pulmonary secretions. The chest X-ray should be clear. The length of time that the patients have been ventilated is not as critical as the care that they have received during this time, and we have used donors that have been ventilated for five days, whereas others have been unsuitable as a result of pneumonic changes within 12 h.

### The operation

An essential aspect of the operation is to maintain the integrity of the phrenic, vagus, and recurrent laryngeal nerves. In addition, in cyanotic patients, the bronchial arteries are large and tortuous, and must be adequately secured. We have found that visualization is better if the heart and lungs are removed separately.

The vagus nerves run immediately behind the hilum of the lung on each side, and lie anterior to the oesophagus. The recurrent laryngeal nerve winds about the ductus ligament, immediately posterior to the bifurcation of the pulmonary artery, and the phrenic nerves pass anterior to the hilum on each side, closer to the right hilum than the left.

There are generally several large bronchial vessels on either side that run posterior to the trachea and both bronchi, arising from the aorta. These vessels become large in patients with Eisenmenger's syndrome, and may give rise to major bleeding if not adequately identified and secured. Control of bleeding from these vessels is difficult after implantation of the donor heart and lungs.

After institution of cardiopulmonary bypass the heart is removed, leaving a posterior cuff of right atrium in place for subsequent reimplantation. The left lung is then excised, followed by the right lung.

Implantation of the donor organs commences with the tracheal anastomosis, followed by the atrial anastomosis, and lastly anastomosis of the aorta. All anastomoses are performed with continuous polyropylene sutures.

### Postoperative management

Recipients are given cyclosporine orally (18 mg/kg) as soon as a donor is found to be satisfactory, and oral cyclosporine is continued post-operatively after extuba-

250

tion. Immunosuppression is augmented with azathioprine 1.5 mg/kg/day orally in order to avoid using steroids, which might impair tracheal healing. Rabbit anti-thymocyte globulin (RATG) is given on the day of operation, and for two or three days thereafter, until the measured level of circulating T-lymphocytes (rosette tests) falls to below 5%. After 14 days, azathioprine is replaced with oral pred-nisone at 0.2–0.3 mg/kg daily. Oral steroids are commenced at fourteen days, at low levels (0.2–0.3 mg/kg), and maintenance immunosuppressive therapy after two weeks is with cyclosporine and prednisone. Azathioprine is discontinued.

Serial transvernous endomyocardial biopsies are performed on a weekly basis. Early rejection episodes are treated with one gram of methylprednisolone daily for three days, but one month after transplantation rejection episodes may be treated merely with augmented oral prednisone.

Our experience thus for indicates that significant pulmonary rejection does not occur without detection of rejection on the cardiac biopsy. The frequency and severity of rejection episodes is not greater than with cardiac transplantation alone, and the frequency of rejection episodes, as with cardiac rejection, is highest within the first 60 days after transplantation. Rejection episodes requiring one or more courses of augmented immunosuppression have occurred in five of the ten long-term survivors. Satisfactory resolution of rejection occurred in each case.

Healing of air-way anastomoses has been a major concern in lung transplanta-tion, but thus far there has been no tracheal necrosis, rupture, or late stenosis in our patients, or amongst the primate survivors of heart-lung transplantation in the laboratory. Late arteriograms performed in animals, and coronary arterio-grams in patients between ten and twelve months after operation have shown the development of collaterals to the area of the suture-line from the donor coronary circulation, and from the recipient bronchial arteries. In this regard heart-lung transplantation is likely to be superior to lung transplantation alone, where there is no immediate bronchial supply to the airway anastomosis in the latter proce-dure.

**Results**

Four patients died within one month of operation. One patient died during operation as a result of failure of the donor lungs to provide adequate gas exchange. Another patient died on the fourth post-operative day as a result of severe haemorrhage sustained intraoperatively; this patient with transposition of the great vessels had undergone three previous cardiac procedures, and pre-sented with greatly distorted cardiac anatomy. One patient died sixteen days after operation having never been extubated: she suffered early and severe acute respiratory distress with renal and hepatic failure. The remaining patient died 24 days after surgery, with multi-system failure beginning with renal failure.

*Table 1.*

| Patient | diag. (death) | Rejection | Infection | Discharge-days |
|---------|---------------|-----------|-----------|----------------|
| 1. MG f45 | PPH | 2 | Herpes (cutaneous) | 85 |
| 2. CW m30 | E | 0 | CMV (systemic) | 46 |
| 3. KW f29 | E | X | X | (4) |
| 4. BD m40 | E | 0 | 0 | 46 |
| 5. DM f37 | PPH | 2 | 0 | 64 |
| 6. NL f29 | PPH | X | X | (23) |
| 7. JMD m22 | E | X | X | (0) |
| 8. RG m40 | E | 0 | Bacteroides (blood and lung) CMV (systemic) | 40 |
| 9. PMG m22 | E | 2 | Enterococcus (lung) | 38 |
| 10. FLF m28 | E | 2 | 0 | 39 |
| 11. DV m38 | E | 0 | 0 | 38 |
| 12. FF m33 | E | 0 | CMV (systemic) | 46 |
| 13. SS m | E | 1 | Serratia (pulmonary) CMV (systemic reactivation) | 60 |
| 14. ST f | PPH | X | Candida (systemic) | (16) |

E: Eisenmenger's syndrome; PPH: Primary pulmonary hypertension; Rejection: Acute rejection episodes in hospital requiring IV methylprednisolone; CMV: Cytomegalovirus; X: Not considered at risk for rejection or infection

The remaining patients have done well. They have maintained a normal functional capacity, and exercise freely and without limitation. Four of these patients have now survived more than 12 months after operation, and the first patient is alive and well two and a half years after operation. Catheterization studies between 8 and 12 months in 4 patients have demonstrated normal pulmonary vascular resistance and cardiac function. Respiratory function tests in all survivors have been normal. A summary of the patients is shown in Table 1.

## Discussion

Primary pulmonary hypertension resistant to medical therapy is progressive and fatal. In Eisenmenger's syndrome cardiac transplantation alone is not possible since the normal donor right ventricle cannot increase its work-load acutely to accommodate an inordinately elevated pulmonary vascular resistance. Heart and lung transplantation constitutes the only realistic therapeutic option for these patients with end-stage disease.

We believe that combined heart and bilateral lung transplantation is likely to prove a more successful approach than unilateral lung transplantation for patients with end-stage pulmonary disease. Advantages of the combined operation are that all diseased pulmonary tissue is removed, thus preventing both recurrent infection and ventilation/perfusion imbalance caused by the remaining lung. A tracheal anastomosis, since it receives a better blood supply, is more likely to heal than a bronchial anastomosis; this is further aided in the combined operation since coronary – bronchial anastomosis in the 'en-bloc' graft are preserved. An additional advantage is provided by the ability to sequentially biopsy the heart since both clinical and laboratory experience to date have shown a close correlation between cardiac and pulmonary rejection. clinical experience with heart-lung transplantation has thus far have been encouraging.

## References

1. Demikhov VP: Some Essential Points of the Techniques in Transplantation of the Heart, Lungs and Other Organs. In: *Experimental Transplantation of Vital Organs,* Moscow, 1960, Medgiz State Press for Medical Literature in Moscow, Chapter II. Translated from Russian by Basil Haigh, Consultants Bureau, New York, 1962, pp 29–48.
2. Webb WR, Howard HS: Cardiopulmonary Transplantation. Surg Forum 8: 313, 1957.
3. Lower RR, Stofer RC, Hurley EJ, Shumway NE: Complete Homograft Replacement of the Heart and Both Lungs. Surgery 50: 842–845, 1961.
4. Grinnan GLB, Graham WH, Childs JW, Lower RR: Cardiopulmonary Homotransplantation. J. Thorac Cardiovasc Surg 60: 609–615, 1970.
5. Nakae S, Webb WR, Theodorides T, Gregg WL: Respiratory Function Following Cardiopulmonary Denervation in Dog, Cat and Monkey. Surg. Gynecol Obstet 125: 1285, 1967.
6. Cooley DA, Bloodwell RD, Hallman GL, Nora JJ, Harrison GM, Leachman RD: Organ Transplantation for Advanced Cardiopulmonary Disease. Ann Thorac Surg 8: 30–42, 1969.
7. Lillihei CW: In: Discussion of Wildevuur CRH, Benfield JR. A review of 23 Human Lung Transplantations by 20 Surgeons. Ann Thorac Surg 9: 489–515, 1970.
8. Barnard CN, Cooper DKC: Clinical Transplantation of the Heart: A Review of 13 years' Personal Experience. J R Soc Med 74: 670–674, 1981.
9. Borel JF, Feurer C, Gubler HU, Stahelin H: Biological Effects of Cyclosporin A: A New Antilymphocytic Agent. Agents Actions 6: 648, 1976.
10. Jamieson SW, Burton NA, Bieber CP, Reitz BA, Oyer PE, Stinson EB, Shumway NE: Cardiac Allograft Survival in Rats Treated with Cyclosporin-A. Surgical Forum 30: 289–291, 1979.
11. Jamieson SW, Burton NA, Oyer PE, Reitz BA, Stinson EB, Shumway NE: Cardiac Allograft Survival in Primates Treated with Cyclosporing-A. Lancet 1: 545, 1979.
12. Reitz BA, Burton NA, Jamieson SW, Pennock JL, Stinson EB, Shumway NE: Heart and Lung Transplantation: Auto and Allotransplantation in Primates with Extended Survival. J Thorac Cardiovasc Surg 80: 360–371, 1980.
13. Oyer PE, Stinson EB, Jamieson SW, Hunt SA, Billingham M, Scott W, Bieber CP, Reitz BA, Shumway NE: Cyclosporin A in Cardiac Allografting: A Preliminary Experience. Transplantation Proc 15: 1247–1252, 1983.

# 30. Immunosuppressive therapy for cardiac transplantation

STUART W. JAMIESON, PHILIP E. OYER, EDWARD B. STINSON
and NORMAN E. SHUMWAY

## Introduction

The immunosuppression of cardiac transplantation recipients is required indefinitely. Acute rejection episodes occur in most patients, and must be identified early and treated effectively. Acute rejection is seen most frequently during the first three postoperative months with both 'conventional therapy' and patients treated with cyclosporine. With standard immunosuppression, 90% of patients experience at least one rejection episode during this interval; with cyclosporine the incidence of this is somewhat less. The frequency of acute rejection declines substantially after 12 months (one episode per 748 patient days, compared to 1 per 35 patient days during the first three months) (1).

Immunosupression at Stanford between 1968 and 1980 consisted of steroids, azathioprine, and antihuman thymocyte globulin derived from rabbits (RATG). This regimen is still used at many centers, but at Stanford a new drug, cyclosporine, has been the primary agent of immunosuppression since December 1980. This will be discussed further, but since cyclosporine is not yet generally available, conventional therapy will be described first.

## Conventional immunosuppression

Conventional immunosuppression consists of azathioprine (2 mg/kg IV) administered immediately prior to surgery. Rabbit anti-human thymocyte globulin (RATG) is injected into the thigh muscles in divided doses (2.5 mg of IgG/kg IM). Immediately following surgery, 500 mg methylprednisolone is administered IV, followed by 125 mg for three doses, or until oral intake resumes. Oral administration of azathioprine is begun on the first postoperative day, and maintained at the maximum level tolerated without leukopenia or thrombocytopenia (usually one to two mg/kg). RATG is given daily for the first three days, and then every other day as determined by individual kinetics of the rabbit globulin, and the degree to which the depression of thymic derived lymphocytes (as measured by the e-Rosette tests) is obtained. The aim of RATG therapy is to reduce the rosette count to less than 5% (normally over 60%), and to keep it low for the first three weeks.

After the initial course of intravenous steroids, prednisone is started at a dose of 1.5mg/kg/day. The daily dose is then tapered until a maintenance level of one mg/kg is reached, by about two months postoperatively. Further gradual reduction of the daily dose is then continued in order to achieve a level of approximately 0.25 mg/kg/day by the end of the first year after transplantation. The rate of decrease of prednisone, and the established maintenance dose of this drug is determined by the degree to which an individual rejects the graft.

Immunological surveillance for rejection is carried out by monitoring the daily rosette count, the daily sum of the QRS voltages on the EKG, and measuring the serum level of circulating rabbit globulin twice weekly. A rise in the rosette count means an increase of circulating T-cells, and, this, especially if it is associated with a clearance of circulating rabbit globulin, is generally a sign of impending rejection. A cardiac biopsy should be performed. The EKG voltage falls with established rejection, and such a fall should also prompt a biopsy. Two disadvantages with the EKG measurement are that false positive results are possible, due to fluid overload or changes in the lung, and, for the voltage to drop, rejection must have already occurred. Great reliance is therefore placed on the rosette test, to try and predict rejection before it becomes established. However, this test is only valuable for the first few weeks after transplantation, after which the rosette count rises regardless of rejection.

The diagnosis of graft rejection is, in the final analysis, made by percutaneous transvenous endomyocardial biopsy. Using local anesthesia the biopsy forceps are passed through a cardiac catheterization sheath into the right internal jugular vein (2). The bioptome is then advanced into the region of the apex of the right ventricle using fluoroscopy, and three or four biopsy specimens are obtained. This procedure is extremely safe, and over 5,000 such biopsies have been performed at this center with no mortality or serious morbidity. The procedure may also be performed on an outpatient basis. Graft biopsy is performed routinely at intervals of 5 to 7 days, and also upon suspicion of graft rejection. The ability to repetitively and safely biopsy the transplanted heart provides a unique advantage for cardiac transplantation that is not available in the management of recipients of other types of solid organ grafts. It should also be pointed out that it is this technique that has made heart-lung transplantation relatively safe, by virtue of the ability to detect lymphocytic infiltration of the transplanted tissue mass.

Early acute cardiac rejection is marked histologically by infiltration of the graft with mononuclear cells, initially in a perivascular distribution, and then diffusely throughout the interstitium. Congestion of small vessels and interstitial edema also occur. More advanced rejection is marked by myocyte necrosis and hemorrhage. Unfortunately, the histological features of rejection are somewhat different with 'conventional therapy' and with cyclosporine. With the latter drug, a degree of lymphocytic infiltration is almost invariable, though the lymphocytes are smaller and not always pyroninophilic. Edema is rarely seen, even with moderately severe rejection. This latter feature may explain the lack of decrease of EKG voltage accompanying rejection in cyclosporine-treated patients.

When rejection is diagnosed the dose of oral prednisone is increased to 1.5 mg/kg/day once again, and in addition one gram intravenous pulses of methylprednisolone are given for three days. If the rosette count has risen, rabbit antithymocyte globulin is given for a further three days. Assessment of the histological response to treatment by serial graft biopsy is vital, both to assess the response of rejection to therapy, and to minimize the total corticosteroid dose.

## Cyclosporine

Cyclosporine is a fungal metabolite manufactured by Sandoz Ltd., and has been used as the principle immunosuppressive agent at Stanford since December 1980. It is thought to have an effect somewhat similar to that of azathioprine, and has therefore been administered in combination with prednisone. An initial course (three to four single doses) of rabbit antithymocyte globulin was also used in the first 27 patients, but since then RATG has only been used for resistant rejection.

Cyclosporine is given orally at 18 mg/kg/day commencing immediately prior to surgery. It is continued postoperatively, and given twice daily, down the nasogastric tube while the patient remains intubated. We do not use intravenous preparations of this drug. Cyclosporine levels are performed twice weekly, and the cyclosporine dosage is thereafter modulated according to these levels.

A major disadvantage of cyclosporine therapy is that monitoring for rejection, which was previously based on serial EKG voltage drop, and immunological monitoring by measurement of serum rabbit globulin and rosette counts, appears to be no longer relevant. The diagnosis of rejection in cyclosporine patients pivots upon the histological examination of allograft tissue. Regular biopsies are thus an important feature of the management of patients on cyclosporine, even once patients are discharged from hospital.

Though cyclosporine therapy carries this major disadvantage, the rejection process appears to progress more slowly than with conventional treatment, and possibly is also more easily treatable than in patients receiving azathioprine. Furthermore, hemodynamic compromise has not yet been observed with severe rejection in patients receiving cyclosporine.

## Complications of immunosuppression

Most of the strict selection criteria established for tranplantation candidates are required because the toxicity of generalized immunosuppression causes considerable side-effects. Infection is the commonest complication, and indeed, the majority of deaths after cardiac transplantation have been the result of infection.

Since suboptimal cardiac function is rarely tolerated, the general level of immunosuppression required after cardiac transplantation is higher than that for other organ transplants. This of course renders the recipient highly susceptible to opportunistic organisms, most particularly during the early postoperative months when immunosuppression is highest.

The primary cause of death of recipients transplanted in the sixteen-year period between 1968 – 1983 is shown in Table 1. The causative agents of infection are shown in Table 2. Most of the infections encountered in the transplant series were bacterial, though viral, fungal, protozoan, and nocardial infections are also encountered.

The most common site of infection is the lung, and lung infections have included pneumonias, empyemas, and cavitating pulmonary infections caused by Aspergillus, nocardia, and various aerobic and anaerobic organisms. Other common sites of infection are shown in Table 3.

*Table 1.* Stanford cardiac transplantation: primary cause of death – 157 patients.

| | |
|---|---|
| Infection | 85 |
| Acute rejection | 26 |
| Graft arteriosclerosis | |
|     A. Proliferative | 6 |
|     B. Atherosclerotic | 9 |
| Malignancy | 11 |
| Pulmonary hypertension | 7 |
| CVA | 3 |
| Sudden death | 4 |
| Pulmonary embolus | 2 |
| Cerebral edema | 1 |
| Myopathy | 1 |
| Suicide | 1 |
| Acute graft failure | 1 |

*Table 2.* Stanford cardiac transplantation: total infections.

| | No. of infections | No. of patients |
|---|---|---|
| 1. Bacterial | 402 | 172 |
| 2. Viral | 167 | 129 |
| 3. Fungal | 97 | 87 |
| 4. Protozoan | 42 | 38 |
| 5. Nocardia | 28 | 28 |
| Total | 736 | |

*Table 3.* Stanford cardiac transplantation: infectious episodes.

| | No. of episodes | No. of patients |
|---|---|---|
| Pulmonary infection | 306 | 160 |
| Empyema | 11 | 11 |
| Septicemia | 78 | 63 |
| Urinary tract infection | 43 | 30 |
| Disseminated fungal | 14 | 14 |
| Central nervous system | 24 | 24 |
| Hepatitis | 15 | 14 |
| Miscellaneous | 220 | 147 |
| Retinitis | 8 | 7 |
| Osteomyelitis | 1 | 1 |

The incidence of infection is somewhat lower in cyclosporine treated patients. However, the incidence of viral infection is about the same as that previously seen in azathioprine treated patients. Infectious complications in cyclosporine treated patients are more easily treatable than was the case previously.

It is essential to maintain a high level of vigilance for infectious complications, and aggressive diagnosis, with specific and effective therapy, is essential for survival. Daily chest X-rays must be obtained. When a pulmonary infection is suspected, transtracheal aspiration is carried out as a primary diagnostic step. Bronchial aspiration of the lung is performed if the radiological findings suggest a fungal or protozoan infection. A successful outcome can be expected in the majority of cases if specific therapy is started early. Seventy per cent of long-term surviving patients in the Stanford series have sustained potentialy lethal infections. Fungal infections are associated the highest mortality (50%), but those can successfully be treated with amphotericin B, sometimes in conjunction with 5-fluorocytosine, if the diagnosis is accomplished before the organism becomes disseminated.

All immunosuppressed patients are subject to a higher risk of *'de novo'* malignancy. There have been 15 lymphomas diagnosed in the Stanford series. The original cardiac disease was coronary artery disease in six of these. Interestingly, only two patients with coronary artery disease as a presenting diagnosis developed lymphoma during the thirteen years that 'conventional therapy' was used for immunosuppression, whereas during this same time period eight patients with an original diagnosis of cardiomyopathy developed this complication. In the two years since cyclosporine therapy has been instituted there have been five cases of lymphoma, four in patients with coronary artery disease, one in a patient with end-stage valvular disease, and none in patients with cardiomyopathy (Table 4).

It is interesting that there have been no cases of lymphoma in patients with

*Table 4.* Presenting diagnosis of patients developing lymphoma.

| Presenting diagnosis | Conventional therapy | Cyclosporine therapy |
|---|---|---|
| Coronary artery diasease | 2 (1.9% of 104) | 4 (25% of 16) |
| Cardiomyopathy | 8 (8.7% of 92) | 0 (0% of 22) |
| Valve disease | 0 (0% of 11) | 1 (50% of 2) |
| Total | 10 | 5 |

cardiomyopathy since cyclosporine therapy has been instituted, though the incidence of lymphoma in this group of patients was previously high. This perhaps suggests a different etiological mechanism for this disease process. Whether this trend in the distribution of patients developing lymphoma will continue remains to be seen. The high incidence of lymphoma in the patients treated with cyclosporine, corticosteroids and RATG has prompted the omission of RATG therapy as routine, and this drug is now only used in the treatment of resistant rejection. Recent evidence suggests the possibility that these tumors are Epstein Barr virus (ABV) associated, and the development, or reactivation of, EBV disease appears to be enhanced by RATG therapy, and further aggravated by the ability of cyclosporine to inhibit T cell cytotoxic responses to EBV-infected autologous B cells.

Side-effects of cyclosporine therapy also include renal dysfunction, hepatic dysfunction, hypertension, hirsutism and mild tremors. Renal dysfunction following cyclosporine administration has been observed in most patients, and in some instances has required the termination of the drug, particularly when concomitant administration of other renal toxic agents, including aminoglycoside antibiotics and amphotericin B, has been necessary. Dialysis may be required for temporary support during renal dysfunction. We have not yet encountered irreversible cessation of renal function.

With cyclosporine therapy, since RATG is no longer used routinely, the predictive value of the rosette tests, and the levels of circulating antithymocyte globulin are lost. In addition, possibly because even in severe rejection histological edema is no longer seen, the total EKG votage no longer drops in the presence of rejection. All non-invasive parameters of monitoring for rejection have therefore been lost, and this is a serious restriction in the use of cyclosporine therapy, since the diagnosis of rejection is only by invasive monitoring by frequent endomyocardial biopsy. Though this is easily accomplished while the patient is in hospital, it presents distinct tactical problems upon discharge.

With cyclosporine treated patients, the diagnosis of rejection results in treatment with three grams of methylprednisolone as given for rejection during 'conventional immunosuppression', but the oral prednisone dose is not augmented. In addition, RATG is no longer given except for advanced and resistant rejection.

# References

1. Jamieson SW, Bieber CP, Oyer PE: Immunosupression in Clinical Cardiac Transplantation. In: *Immunosuppressive Therapy*. (Salaman JR ed) MTP Press, pp 177–199, 1981.
2. Caves PK, Stinson EB, Billingham ME, Shumway NE: Percutaneous Transvenous Endomyocardial Biopsy in Human Heart Recipients. Ann Thorac Surgery 16: 325, 1973.

# 31. Current status of liver transplantation

THOMAS E. STARZL, SHUNZABURO IWATSUKI and
BYERS W. SHAW

## Introduction

I would like to cover the experience which we have had with liver transplantation
and to try to indicate where I think developments in this field will be going. There
has been some interesting administrative movement in the United States which
may have relevance to the objectives of workers in Europe and the Middle East.

Liver transplantation has been considered to be an experimental undertaking
and for that reason (and the consequent inability to fund these efforts) it has been
difficult for centers other than the ones where I have worked to get started.
However, the perception has grown in the last two or three years as results have
improved with the introduction of cyclosporine that the procedure really is not
experimental. There is in process in the United States an administrative chain of
events known as a Consensus Development which came to completion in June
1983 and which will almost certainly lead to a government decision that liver
transplantation is in fact therapeutic.

When that time comes, we believe that a network of centers capable of
providing liver transplantation will spring up in the United States almost over-
night. We think that the number of centers will be 20 or 30. There are already
several active groups and there are, in training, several other teams. The steps in
making liver transplantation a widespread service are following somewhat the
same format as the development of renal transplantation about 20 years ago in
our country.

## The dimensions of the problem

Data about the need for hepatic transplantation is being accumulated. It has
become obvious that the numbers of potential candidates are far higher than
anyone had realized. Until recently no one had taken a good look at this question,
perhaps because it was perceived to be a non-issue, but my estimate is that at an
equilibrium level the number of liver transplantations in the United States will be
in the 5,000 per year range. Many of you know that this is about the number of

renal transplantations in the United States per year. In our country, liver disease is the fourth most common cause of death.

Although a significant proportion of these deaths are alcohol related, a surprising percentage are free of the alcohol taint. Moreover, there is no reason to arbitrarily exclude patients with alcoholic cirrhosis from treatment. A number of years ago it was estimated that there might be as many as 5,000 potential candidates for liver transplantation in the British Isles and 20,000 in the United States (1). Although these figures are probably too high, it is clear that liver transplantation will be a common form of transplantation with numbers that may be competitive with the kidney. Realization of the objective of making liver transplantation a common service will depend upon the progress which I will describe in the following sections.

## Hepatic rejection and its prevention

Rejection of liver grafts is not different in principle than that which is seen with other transplanted organs. In untreated dogs after 4 or 5 days, the typical findings include massive infiltration of mononuclear cells which are heavily concentrated around the portal tracts and central veins. Parenchymal necrosis and interstitial edema are other classical findings (1, 2).

Almost two decades ago, the feasibility of hepatic transplantation in patients with end stage liver disease was established with the chronic survival of many dogs whose livers were replaced with grafts from non-related mongrel donors under treatment with azathioprine (1, 2). More than a dozen of the animals had therapy discontinued after about 4 months. Rejection did not supervene (1) and one of these dogs lived from more than a decade. The observation that therapy could often be stopped in these dogs as well as later work in Paris, Bristol, Cambridge, and Denver with pigs suggested that the liver could be at the 'easy' end of the scale in terms of controlling rejection. That advantage, if it does exist, can be easily overstated because rejection occurs frequently after human liver transplantation in spite of all efforts to prevent this process.

The first extended survivals after human liver transplantation were obtained in the summer of 1967 (1). In January 1970 a child was treated who became the human counterpart of the canine experiment in that her survival first equalled and then superceded that of the famous dog. She is now $14^{1}/_{2}$ years post transplantation. I should say in passing that George Abouna was a member of the team that took care of this little girl. Her treatment was with azathioprine, prednisone, and ALG.

## Indications for liver transplantation

The indications for liver transplantation in 237 consecutive cases are shown in Table 1. The heterogenous nature of the diseases that can be treated is obvious. Chronic aggressive hepatitis, or more accurately non-alcoholic cirrhosis, was a leading indication, cutting across all age barriers. Biliary atresia was very common in pediatric patients.

With all the indications in Table 1, we have tried to formulate some idea about the technical difficulties that the surgeons can anticipate at the time of transplantation, the average degree of metabolic abnormalities that can be expected from the original hepatic disease, the difficulties (if any) in deciding the propriety of candidacy, and finally the question of recurrence of the disease which had destroyed the native liver.

In Table 2 is a brief declaration of these issues in patients with biliary atresia. With this disorder, the decision about candidacy is a very easy one. Willis Potts, the great pediatric surgeon in Chicago, once wrote that biliary atresia had provided the blackest chapter in the history of pediatric surgery. His remarks were apt, since at that time nothing could be done for these children who required

*Table 1.* Influence of disease upon one year and subsequent survival in 237 patients.[a]

|  | Conventional therapy | | | Cyclosporine-steroids | | |
|---|---|---|---|---|---|---|
|  | No. | 1 Year | Now[b] | No. | 1 Year | Now[c] |
| Biliary atresia | 51 | 14 (27%) | 7 (14%) | 11 | 6 (54.5%) | 6 (54.5%) |
| Non alcoholic cirrhosis | 46 | 16 (34.8%) | 10 (21.7%) | 16 | 9 (56.3%) | 8 (50%) |
| Primary liver malignancy | 18 | 5 (27.8%) | 1 (5.6%) | 9 | 6 (66.7%) | 4 (44.4%) |
| Alpha-1-antitrypsin deficiency | 11 | 6 (54.5%) | 5 (45.5%) | 6 | 3 (50%) | 3 (50%) |
| Other inborn errors[d] | 4 | 2 (50%) | 1 (25%) | 4 | 4 (100%) | 4 (100%) |
| Alcoholic cirrhosis | 15 | 4 (26.7%) | 3 (20%) | 0 | – | – |
| Primary biliary cirrhosis | 6 | 1 (16.7%) | 1 (16.7%) | 6 | 5 (83.3%) | 5 (83.3%) |
| Sclerosing cholangitis | 7 | 2 (28.6%) | 0 (0%) | 3 | 2 (66.7%) | 1 (33.3%) |
| Secondary biliary cirrhosis | 4 | 3 (75%) | 2 (50%) | 5 | 1 (20%) | 1 (20%) |
| Budd-chiari syndrome | 1 | 1 (100%) | 1 (100%) | 3 | 3 (100%) | 1 (33.3%) |
| Miscellaneous[e] | 7 | 2 (28.6%) | 1 (14.3%) | 4 | 3 (75%) | 3 (75%) |

[a] The same case material was analyzed in detail elsewhere (2) but with shorter followups. The followups have been brought up to date to June 15, 1983.

[b] Followups 3½ to 13½ years.

[c] Followups 1 to 3 ¼ years.

[d] Wilson's disease (3 examples), Tyrosinemia (2 examples), Glycogen storage disease (2 examples), Sea blue histiocyte syndrome (1 example).

[e] Neonatal hepatitis (3 examples), Congenital hepatic fibrosis (2 examples), Byler's disease (2 examples), Adenomatosis, Hemachromatosis, Protoporphyria, Acute hepatitis B (1 example each).

*Table 2.* Factors of candidacy from experience with 237 consecutive patients. Biliary atresia, 62 of the 237 cases.

| Decision of candidacy | Easy |
|---|---|
| Previous surgery | 100% |
| Metabolic abnormalities | Moderate |
| Technical difficulties | Moderate[a] |
| Disease recurrence | None |

[a] Unless there are anomalies.

a major social, economic and medical input, but from whom nothing could be expected. The victims of biliary atresia became pariahs as they entered the downhill slope of their life with the development of numerous secondary complications. The breakdown of parent-offspring relationships in which the children became objects of despair and sometimes even hatred has been documented by social scientists. Thus the decision to operate on a child with biliary atresia is an easy one.

All patients with biliary atresia have had previous surgery, and this is an adverse factor, but not such a serious one as in adults. The most important technical problems with children with biliary atresia have come from associated anomalies, such as hypoplasia of the portal vein. The metabolic abnormalities at the time of transplantation have ranged from minor to very severe, but usually they have not been unreasonable. In the past many of these children have died from the complications of biliary atresia while still possessing good synthetic functions of their liver.

The same questions shown in Table 2 can be asked about all the major diseases for which transplantation might be indicated. Prospective recipients with non-alcoholic cirrhosis have been murderously difficult from a technical point of view and especially so when previous operations have been carried out within the abdomen. The degree of metabolic decay has been unusually severe in such patients. Finally patients with chronic active hepatitis who are B virus carriers have had a marked tendency to recapitulate in their graft the same disease as destroyed their native liver. It now appears that the recurrence rate will be in the 80% range. Clearly, the full exploitation of liver replacement in such recipients will depend upon better ways of preventing a recurrence of the hepatitis. The use of hyperimmune specific globulin, or the use of interferon are two possibilities.

The inborn errors of metabolism (Table 1) have provided for surgical scientists and for biochemists a unique opportunity. It was discovered almost two decades ago that a new liver provided new protein phenotypes for the recipient and that these donor specific phenotypes were retained for the life time of the graft. This principle of donor specificity of the liver homograft implies that hepatic based inborn errors of metabolism are curable by liver transplantation, and this implication has been proved on a number of occasions. The inborn errors shown in Table

1 (footnote) have all been metabolically 'cured' with the possible exception of the sea-blue histiocyte syndrome. With congenital tyrosinemia and the glycogen storage diseases, there is a known and highly specific enzyme deficit in the livers; it has been shown that these enzymes when brought to the recipient with the new liver are thereafter present as long as the liver is viable. In other diseases such as Wilson's disease and alpha-1-antitrypsin deficiency in which the exact enzyme deficit (if any) is not known, these disorders are also cured in spite of this ignorance about the basic pathogenesis.

Some of the most difficult decisions about candidacy have been in patients with hepatic malignancies (1, 3). The reason is that the incidence of recurrence in patients whose livers were replaced because primary tumors could not be removed with subtotal resection have exhibited a very high incidence of recurrence, more than 80% in our initial experience. In recent years, the incidence of recurrence has been lower (3) but this may only have reflected a better case selection. Many of the recipients with hepatic malignancies treated in the last several years have had the so called fibrolamellar hepatomas which are late to metastasize, or the hepatomas which occur as incidental findings in livers destroyed by other diseases such as tyrosinemia, alpha-1-antitrypsin deficiency, and the seablue histiocyte syndrome. The role of liver replacement in the treatment of patients with otherwise nonresectable hepatic tumors has yet to be fully defined, but it is certain that the minority of patients would qualify.

A number of diagnoses which are not well represented in Table 1 are certain to be more common in candidates for liver transplantation in the future. The most important of these diseases will be primary biliary cirrhosis and sclerosing cholangitis. The technical ease with which liver replacement can be carried out in primary biliary cirrhosis is remarkable. Patients with this disorder have normal or sometimes larger than normal livers, with relatively modest portal hypertension, and with a disease evolution that is slow enough so that therapies can be carried out early before terminal deterioration of health. The diagnosis of sclerosing cholangitis has a less favorable set of circumstances on average since so many patients with this disease have either had total colectomy for the underlying disease of ulcerative colitis or else efforts at biliary tract reconstruction.

## Technical aspects of transplantation

The preservation methods which can be used today are limited, but good enough to permit the harvesting of organs in various parts of the United States with transfer of the hepatic grafts for thousands of miles. In Europe, similar networks have been set up leading to English, German and Dutch centers.

The techniques of the actual transplantation have been so well described that there is little point in discussing these here (1, 3). A recent development which is going to play a major role in permitting transplantation to be used on a broad scale has been the use of veno-venous pump driven nonheparin bypasses. With such bypasses, the blood from the occluded vena caval system as well as from the portal vein can be shunted around the upper abdomen during the period of obligatory venous obstruction and channeled into the axillary vein or some other vein of the upper half of the body. The physiologic stress imposed in the past during the so called anhepatic phase has been largely eliminated by this method which has been used for the last 20 or 25 adults. It is probable that the perfection of these nonheparin bypasses has been the most important technical development in almost 2 decades.

In the early days of liver transplantation complications of biliary tract reconstruction were both frequent and lethal. These have been virtually eliminated in recent years. In our center the preferred form of biliary reconstruction is with duct to duct anastomosis over a T-tube. Obviously, this option does not exist for many patients (and by definition never with biliary atresia) but a very satisfactory alternative procedure is choledocojejunostomy using a Roux limb.

**Survival**

*With conventional immunosuppression (1963–1979).* From 1963 to the end of 1979 170 consecutive patients were treated, and average case load of less than a dozen a year. Fifty-six (32.9%) of the recipients lived for at least one year and 32 (18.8%) are still alive with followups of $3^1/_2$ to $13^1/_2$ years. Six of the residual group are more than 10 years postoperative and 26 are more than 5 years. Only one patient who lived for as long as 5 years has subsequently died.

The predominant mortality was in the first 3 postoperative months and was due mainly to technical surgical accidents, acceptance of some recipients with hopelessly advanced disease, the use of damaged liver grafts, the inability to control rejection, and a variety of infections. The majority of the deaths subsequent to this time were due to chronic rejection.

*With cyclosporine-steroid therapy (1980–1981).* Fourteen patients were treated in 1980 and 26 in 1981; followups of 18 to 38 months are available for those still living. The one year survival was 28/40 (70%). Three of the one year survivors died in the 13, 16, and 20th months of recurrent cholangiocarcinoma, recurring Budd-Chiari syndrome and chronic rejection (with an unsuccessful attempt at retransplantation) respectively.

*The breakout year of 1982.* In 1982, 2 important events occurred which demonstrated that liver transplantation could be exploited in many centers. For one thing, a large number of transplantations were carried out, 80 in all, an unprecedented number since the highest total in any previous year was only 30. In addition, fellows and residents began to do the operations, and contributed almost half of the cases. During 1982, half of the recipients have survived with followups of 5 to 15 months. The losses still occurred perioperatively.

The trials with the non-heparin bypass during the actual transplantation were begun late in our experience and the results in 1983 will have to be assessed before a final decision about the influence of this achievement will be forthcoming.

In the meanwhile the movement of liver transplantation from an experimental to a service undertaking can be illustrated by studying the first 67 consecutive cases in what have been known as the cyclosporine era. The comparison of the results using this drug with those in all previous experience is shown in Table 1. Results have been about twice as good as in the past.

*Prospect for the future.* The revitalization of interest in hepatic transplantation has dated from the better immunosuppression that became available $3^1/_2$ years ago. Since that time the number of successful liver replacements has sharply increased.

Forty-two patients have been followed for at least a year after liver transplantation under cyclosporine-steroid therapy. The mystique surrounding liver transplantation has largely been dispelled during this time. Since 1980 other units in the United States and in other countries have been able to mount new and effective programs. Thus liver transplantation has been developed to the point of a service operation, the exploitation of which depends on the establishment of multiple regional centers. The increased use of this procedure will permit the delivery of optimal health care to victims of end stage liver disease.

### Acknowledgements

Supported by research grants from the Veterans Administration; by project grant AM-29961 from the National Institutes of Health and by grant RR-00084 from the General Clinical Research Centers Program of the Divisions of Research Resources, National Institutes of Health.

### References

1. Starzl TE (with the assistance of Putnam, CW): *Experience in hepatic transplantation.* Philadelphia, WB Saunders CO, 1969.
2. Starzl TE, Marchioro TL, Porter KA, Taylor PD Faris TD, Herrmann TJ, Hlad CJ, Waddell WR: Factors determining short- and long- term survival after orthotopic liver homotransplantation in the dog. *Surgery* 58: 131–155, 1965.
3. Starzl TE, Iwatsuki S, Van Thiel DH, Gartner JC, Zitelli BJ, Malatack JJ, Schade RR, Shaw BW Jr, Hakala TR, Rosenthal JT, Porter KA: Evolution of liver transplantation. *Hepatology* 2: 614–636, 1982.

# 32. Current status of bone marrow transplantation

E. DONNALL THOMAS

## Introduction

Based on studies in murine systems, bone marrow transplantation was undertaken in human patients in the late 1950s. Most of these early attempts failed except for occasional transplants between identical twins. In the late 1950s and early 1960s, marrow transplants were carried out in the canine model which defined the problems and some of the solutions of marrow grafting in an outbred species. Particularly important was the finding that marrow grafts between DLA-matched canine littermates resulted in a high proportion of long-term survivors. Advances in human histocompatibility typing and improved supportive care of the patients without a functioning marrow (isolation techniques, antibiotics, platelet and granulocyte transfusions) made it feasible to return to studies of human marrow grafting by the end of the 1960s.

## Histocompatibility typing

The technical success of kidney transplantation and the problems of graft rejection provided the major impetus to the development of knowledge about human tissue typing. Human leukocyte antigens (HLA) were found to the governed by the major histocompatibility complex, and during the 1960s rapid strides were made in the understanding of the HLA region of chromosome 6. Because it comprises a series of major loci, this region has been referred to as a supergene. Three of these loci are thought to be of major importance in determining the success or failure of a graft. They are HLA-A and HLA-B, detected serologically, and HLA-D/DR, detected by serologic typing of B cells or by reactivity in the mixed leukocyte culture. Other loci in the HLA region, not yet defined, may also play a role in graft rejection and/or graft-versus-host disease. Each of the three main loci are characterized by a large number of alleles which make it difficult to find phenotypically matched unrelated donors. However, within a family there are only four HLA haplotypes, and therefore typing within a family is relatively easy. Marrow grafts have generally employed one of three types of donors: (1) an identical twin – donor and twin are matched not only for HLA but for all other genetic loci; (2) an HLA-matched sibling – donor and recipient are matched for HLA but may or may not be matched for other histocompatibility loci known as 'minor' transplantation antigen systems. In humans incompatibility for these minor antigen systems, for which typing techniques are not available, may result in a severe graft-versus-host reaction and/or life-threatening graft-versus-host disease; and (3) donor and recipient are partially matched family members or phenotypically matched unrelated individuals. It is apparent that some disparity of HLA antigens can be tolerated (described below), but the limits of tolerable disparity have not yet been defined.

**Preparation of the recipient**

Except for transplants between identical twins or in recipients with severe combined immunologic deficiency, the marrow graft recipient is immunologically competent and immunosuppression must be given so that a graft will be accepted. For nonmalignant diseases the usual preparative regimen has consisted of large doses of cyclophosphamide. For malignant diseases this regimen has usually included cyclophosphamide and total body irradiation. Such preparation of the recipient involves destruction of most or all of the patient's own normal marrow. Since 2–4 weeks is usually required before a marrow transplant begins to function, there is always a period of profound marrow aplasia which implies intensive supportive care of the recipient with transfusions of blood products, with isolation techniques, and with broad-spectrum antibiotics.

**Clinical data on marrow transplantation for nonmalignant diseases**

Table 1 lists the nonmalignant diseases for which marrow transplantation has been carried out. Marrow grafts involve not only the transplantation of erythroid and myeloid cells but also transplantation of donor lymphoid and monocyte-macrophage cell systems. In patients with severe combined immunologic deficiency disorders, the principal objective is to transplant the donor lymphoid system. Result of these studies have been described elsewhere.

In the nonmalignant disease, the Seattle Marrow Transplant Team has placed its emphasis on marrow transplantation for severe aplastic anemia. Initially these studies were undertaken in patients after failure of supportive care, including steroids, androgens, and multiple blood transfusions. These patients were prepared with cyclophosphamide (50 mg/kg on each of 4 days) followed by marrow infusion from HLA-identical siblings. Methotrexate was given in the first 100 days in an effort to suppress the graft-versus-host reaction. In the early series of patients, long-term survival and cure was achieved in only 45% of the cases.

*Table 1.* Bone marrow transplant for nonmalignant disorders.

---

Aplastic anemia
Immunodeficiency syndromes
Thalassemia
Genetic disorders of hematopoiesis
Inborn errors of metabolism

---

Approximately 30% of the failures were due to graft rejection. Studies in the canine system had indicated that transfusion of blood products could sensitize the recipient and set the stage for subsequent graft rejection. Presumably, graft rejection is mediated by some host lymphoid cells which are not destroyed by the preparative regimen and with subsequently mount an immunologic attack against the donor cells.

Two approaches have considerably reduced the likelihood of graft rejection. The first is to carry out the marrow transplant for severe aplastic anemia before transfusions are given. Long-term survival and cure in these patients is now approximately 80%.

The second approach is to give additional donor buffy coat cells. A pint of blood is obtained from the donor and centrifuged, and the white blood cell buffy coat at the interface between the plasma and the red blood cell layer is separated. The plasma and red blood cells are then returned to the donor. Four such units of buffy coat cells are obtained each day for 5 days. The supplementation of the marrow graft by these buffy coat cells has resulted in a significant lowering of the incidence of graft rejection, but the mechanism involved is not well understood. Long-term survival and cure of patients with severe aplastic anemia who have had blood transfusions before coming to marrow graft is now approximately 70% in patients given supplemental buffy coat cells.

The remaining problems are principally those of graft-versus-host disease and opportunistic infections which will be described below.

## Clinical data on marrow transplantation for malignant diseases

Most effective agents for cancer therapy also destroy the normal bone marrow. Thus, marrow toxicity is a common limiting factor in the application of these agents. Bone marrow transplantation, whether autologous, syngeneic or allogeneic, avoids the lethal consequences of marrow damage and makes it possible to give 'superlethal' chemoradiotherapy in an effort to kill a greater fraction of malignant cells.

Marrow transplantation has now been utilized in therapy of a variety of malignant diseases as shown in Table 2.

Clinical data are most extensive for patients with leukemia. Initially, marrow

*Table 2.* Bone marrow transplant for malignant disease.

---

Acute lymphoblastic leukemia
Acute nonlymphoblastic leukemia
Chronic granulocytic leukemia, chronic phase
Chronic granulocyte leukemia, blast crisis
Hairy cell leukemia
Lymphoma
Hodgkin's disease
Myeloma
Myelofibrosis
Selected solid tumors

---

transplants were carried out for patients with end-stage acute leukemia who had failed combination chemotherapy. In Seattle, patients were prepared with cyclophosphamide, 60 mg/kg on each of 2 days, followed by 1000 rad total body irradiation delivered from dual opposing cobalt-60 sources at dose rates of 5–6 rad/min. Fifty-four patients with acute nonlymphoblastic leukemia (ANL) and 46 patients with acute lymphoblastic leukemia (ALL) were treated on this regimen and given marrow grafts from HLA-identical siblings. There were many deaths from advanced illness, opportunistic infections, graft-versus-host disease (GVHD), and recurrences of leukemia. However, 12 of these patients are living in unmaintained remission 7–11 years later and are apparently cured of their disease. Other marrow transplant teams report long-term disease-free survival of 5–15% for patients transplanted in relapse.

Many patients with ALL may be cured by combination chemotherapy, but once relapse has occurred the prognosis is grim. The Seattle Marrow Transplant Team therefore undertook marrow transplantation for patients with ALL who had relapsed at least once and had been put back into remission with chemotherapy. It was thought that the possibility of long-term survival and cure would be improved by carrying out the transplant with the patient in good clinical condition and with a minimal body burden of leukemic cells. The actuarial survival, with all patients followed more than 5 years, was 27%. The major problem was recurrence of leukemia with an overall incidence of approximately 60% from the actuarial analysis. Nevertheless, the apparent cure of approximately one-fourth of these patients represents a significant advance in comparison to the results of chemotherapy. In a prospective study carried out at the Children's Orthopedic Hospital in Seattle, patients with ALL in second remission were treated with chemotherapy in the absence of marrow donors and with marrow transplantation if matched siblings were available. With a follow-up of 3–6 years, all 21 patients treated with chemotherapy have relapsed and only one is alive while 8 of 24 marrow transplant recipients continue in unmaintained remission.

Patients with ANL who achieve complete remissions on chemotherapy have a poor prognosis with a median first remission duration of approximately 8–18 months. Therefore, marrow grafting was undertaken in these patients in first remission. The initial series of 22 patients were prepared with cyclophosphamide and 920 rad total body irradiation. Now, with all patients followed for more than 5 years, 12 of the 22 patients are living in unmaintained remission.

A prospective, randomized study of fractionated irradiation was carried out in an effort to improve these results. In theory, fractionated irradiation might be effective in killing leukemic cells while reducing damage to normal tissues. Patients with ANL in first remission were given cyclophosphamide. Twenty-seven patients were randomized to receive 1000 rad in a single exposure while 26 patients were randomized to receive 200 rad on each of 6 days. They were then given marrow transplants from HLA-identical siblings followed by a regimen of methotrexate given in the first 100 days in an effort to prevent GVHD. With a minimum follow-up of 2.5 years, approximately 50% of the patients are living in unmaintained remission. Survival was somewhat better ($p = 0.05$) for patients given the fractionated regimen.

Several marrow transplant teams have reported the long-term survival and apparent cure of slightly more than one-half of the patients transplanted for ANL in first remission using total body irradiation and chemotherapy.

To compare the results of chemotherapy to the results of marrow transplantation, a prospective study has been carried out in the Pacific Northwest. Patients between the ages of 18 and 50 with ANL were treated with daunorubicin (70 mg/ $m^2$ on days 1, 2 and 3) and cytosine arabinoside (100 mg/m$^2$ intravenously every 12 h on days 1–9) along with 6-thioguanine and prednisone on days 1–9 and vincristine on days 1 and 8. The complete remission rate for 111 patients so treated was 81%. Patients who did not have HLA-identical sibling donors were continued on chemotherapy including consolidation and intensification at 6 and 12 months. Patients with HLA-identical siblings were offered marrow transplants. Prognostic parameters, including age, were equivalent in the two groups. At present the follow-up time ranges from 1 to 6 years. A Kaplan-Meier analysis of overall survival indicates a 5-year survival of 20% for the 45 patients treated with chemotherapy and 50% for the 32 patients who received marrow transplants ($p<0.01$). Two patients who had matched siblings relapsed before the transplant could be carried out. Both were subsequently transplanted and one is a long-term survivor. Eleven patients with matched siblings declined transplants and were treated with chemotherapy. Ten of these patients have died of leukemia and one continued in remission.

For the past $2\frac{1}{2}$ years the Seattle Marrow Transplant Team has been carrying out a study of the new immunosuppressive agent cyclosporine. Patients with ANL in first remission have been prepared with cyclophosphamide and 200 rad on each of 6 days. They were then randomized to receive methotraxate (42 patients) or cyclosporine (36 patients) following the transplant. The difference in survival is not statistically significant. Also, the probability of relapse and the probability of developing GVHD are not different. The methotrexate regimen is somewhat more marrow-suppressive, and methotrexate may potentiate the mucositis following chemotherapy and irradiation. Cyclosporine does not have these undesirable properties, and the patients given cyclosporine have an earlier functioning marrow graft and less mucositis. Cyclosporine is nephrotoxic, however. This study has recently been terminated, but patients must be followed for approximately 2 more years before a final evaluation can be made.

Based on the experience gained and the improved survival observed in patients transplanted for acute leukemia, marrow transplant teams are now exploring marrow grafting for patients with chronic granulocytic leukemia (CGL). CGL is a clonal disease with, in most cases, the Philadelphia chromosome as a cytogenetic marker. CGL has not been cured by any chemotherapeutic regimen. The disease is easy to control in the chronic phase, but when acceleration occurs, which appears to be a random event, the prognosis is grim. The remissions induced by chemotherapy in some patients are almost always of short duration. Initial efforts to transplant patients with CGL in blast crisis were disappointing. More recently, there has been some improvement. The survival resembles that for patients with acute leukemia transplanted in relapse with about one-fourth of the patients becoming long-term survivors free of the Philadelphia chromosome.

By analogy with results obtained for patients with acute leukemia transplanted in remission, it seemed reasonable to think that results might be improved by undertaking marrow transplantation for patients with CGL in chronic phase. To assess the antileukemic effects of the preparative regimen without the problems associated with allogeneic grafts, these studies were initially undertaken in patients who had identical twins to serve as donors. Eight of the first 12 patients are living in remission without the Philadelphia chromosome 3–7 years following the syngeneic graft. Encouraged by these results, we undertook marrow grafting for patients with CGL in chronic phase using HLA-identical siblings as donors. Our results and the results of four other marrow transplant teams are similar with long-term survival on the order of 60–70%. The continued absence of the Philadelphia chromosome in almost all these patients suggests that they may be cured, but a much longer follow-up will be necessary before final evaluation.

In theory marrow transplantation should be effective for any malignant disorder that shows a steep dose-response curve to therapy in which marrow toxicity is the dose-limiting factor. However, marrow grafting has not been studied extensively in the other malignant diseases listed in Table 2. Using the standard regimen of cyclophosphamide and total body irradiation, the Seattle team carried out syngeneic transplants in eight patients with end-stage non-Hodgkin's lymphoma. Five of these patients are alive, four in continued complete remission 2–12 years after grafting. Seven patients with advanced multiple myeloma have been given syngeneic marrow transplants in Seattle. Two died early, two responded but progressed again at 6 and 17 months, and three are in remission after 7, 10 and 41 months. One patient with hairy cell leukemia appears to have been cured with a follow-up of more than 5 years. Some patients with carefully selected solid tumors may benefit from intensive chemoradiotherapy and marrow grafting. For example, in Seattle one patient with extensive small cell lung cancer refractory to chemotherapy was prepared with cyclophosphamide and total body irradiation and given a marrow graft from an HLA-identical sibling. A complete remission ensued until the patient died of an intracranial recurrence 10 months later. This and other anecdotal experiences indicate the need for further study, keeping in mind the experience with acute leukemia which showed that the best results are achieved by undertaking marrow grafting before the patient is in the terminal stages of the disease.

**Autologous marrow transplantation**

With the improving results of syngeneic and allogeneic marrow transplantation, there has been a resurgence of interest in the transplantation of the patient's own marrow. However, there are a number of major problems in the use and evaluation of autologous marrow transplants. These problems are not related to preserving viable marrow, although there is room for technical improvement. It is now well established in both animals and humans that fresh or cryopreserved autologous marrow can be effective in bringing about hematopoietic reconstitution. The major problems are as follows:

1) Is the autologous marrow necessary to rescue the patient following the preparative regimen? With 'supralethal' total body irradiation, an exogenous source of marrow is clearly necessary for hematopoietic recovery. With most other regimens, this is not at all clear. With autologous marrow there is, of course, no blood genetic marker to provide proof of engraftment. Further, with improved supportive care techniques, patients can be kept alive and in good condition long enough for autogenous marrow regeneration to occur following intensive treatment regimens. Finally, there are the ethical problems of designing a study in humans where controls not given autologous marrow might have a fatal outcome.

2) Is marrow toxicity the limiting toxicity? An autologous marrow transplant will protect a patient against the lethal consequences of marrow toxicity consequent to high-dose regimens but will not protect against other toxicities. Many of our best chemotherapeutic agents are known to have major toxic effects on other organs in a narrow dose range above that of marrow toxicity.

3) Is there a significant therapeutic effect with the preparative regimen employed? In some otherwise incurable diseases in carefully selected patients and with a few preparative regimens, it has been shown that curability is an obtainable goal when syngeneic or allogeneic marrow is utilized (see above). Comparable studies of similar patients must be carried out in evaluating the role of autologous marrow. With a variety of tumors and a variety of unproven regimens, it is

virtually impossible to assess any role for autologous marrow transplantation. Certainly, the conduct of these studies in end-stage patients is not likely to prove informative.

4) Are tumor cells present in the marrow? This question and the corollary of how to remove or destroy the contaminating tumor cells occupies a good deal of interest at the present time. Tumor cells might be killed by chemotherapy of the marrow in vitro but at the risk of damage to normal stem cells. In one study in a mouse model it has been possible to show that an immunotoxin can specifically kill tumor cells in a marrow inoculum. Efforts are being made to kill leukemic cells *in vitro* with the use of monoclonal antibodies. One should keep in mind the above three questions which must be answered before the question of removing tumor cells from the marrow inoculum becomes relevant.

5) When should the marrow be stored and when should aggressive treatment be carried out? Some tumors which show a steep dose-response curve to chemotherapeutic regimens, and are therefore attractive targets for the use of autologous marrow, respond well to current conventional regimens. Examples are Hodgkin's disease, non-Hodgkin's lymphomas, testicular tumors, and ovarian tumors. The storage of marrow soon after diagnosis cannot be justified, as yet, because many of these patients will be cured on conventional regimens. Further, it is difficult to justify very aggressive and potentially lethal therapy until the disease has progressed despite conventional therapy, by which time it may well be too late to achieve a significant benefit from the aggressive therapy.

In summary, although there is much enthusiasm for the simple concept of using the patient's marrow and thereby avoiding the problems of an allogeneic graft, there are major problems to be considered before autologous marrow transplantation will have any real role in the treatment of malignant disease.

**Transplants from partially matched donors or unrelated donors**

A major limitation to the wider application of marrow grafting is the fact that a majority of patients will not have HLA-identical siblings. In Seattle we have undertaken a study of the use of partially matched donors. By a search of the extended family, a donor may sometimes be identified who has one HLA haplotype genotypically identical with the patient and the other haplotype phenotypically compatible for at least one of the three major loci. Eighty patients with acute leukemia have now been transplanted using this type of donor. Most have been in relapse or in second remission, and the survival curve is not demonstrably different from that of comparable patients given marrow transplants from HLA-identical siblings.

Another approach designed to extend the availability of compatible donors involves the use of unrelated individuals who are phenotypically HLA-identical with the patient. One such transplant was successfully carried out in Seattle. The recipient did not have GVHD and did well until relapse of leukemia 17 months after the transplant. With computerization of HLA-A, -B and -DR typing, it is now technically feasible to have a large panel of volunteer unrelated donors. Data concerning the use of such donors should now accumulate rapidly.

**Recurrent leukemia**

As indicated above, the recurrence of leukemia following marrow grafting has been a major problem, particularly in patients with ALL. We have studied patients with acute leukemia given marrow grafts from donors of opposite sex who subsequently relapsed. Of 54 patients studied, 48 were found to have relapsed in host-type cells, in 3 the results were equivocal, and in 3 the relapse was in donor-type cells. Thus, the vast majority of relapses are apparently the result of regrowth of the original leukemic clone which was not eradicated by chemoradiotherapy nor by the graft-versus-leukemia effect.

Since the majority of recurrent leukemias are of the original host type, current efforts are directed toward improving methods of eradicating the leukemic clone. At Sloan-Kettering in New York, Dinsmore et al are studying a regimen of hyperfractionated total body irradiation (1320 rad) with cyclophosphamide given after the irradiation. The preliminary results are encouraging in that the occurrence of leukemic relapse seems to be distinctly less than that previously observed. In Minnesota the transplant team is giving additional chemotherapy after the marrow graft in an effort to prevent recurrence. In Seattle we have been carrying out a randomized study of patients with ALL given marrow grafts from HLA-identical siblings who then receive or do not receive interferon during the first 80 days after the transplant in the expectation that the antileukemic effect of interferon might be most evident when the body burden of leukemic cells is minimal. In Cleveland a preparative regimen of high-dose cytosine arabinoside is being evaluated. The results of all these studies are awaited with great anticipation.

In two of our patients, both with ALL, the relapse was in donor-type cells with the morphologic appearance of the original leukemia. Several recurrences in donor-type cells have now been described. The Seattle Team has reported a 5-year-old male with ALL given a marrow graft from a sister. The patient died of an immunoblastic sarcoma 55 days after grafting. The tumor was shown to be of female type and monoclonal. The tumor DNA hybridized with cloned probes showed multiple copies of Epstein-Barr virus genome. Cytomegalovirus genome could not be detected. DNA from the tumor of one of the original Seattle patients with recurrence in donor-type cells failed to show the presence of either Epstein-Barr virus or cytomegalovirus. Fortunately, the development of second tumors in marrow-grafted patients has been a rare event but can be expected to occur as it has in immunosuppressed patients following other organ grafting.

## Immunological recovery after grafting

Regardless of whether the marrow transplant is syngeneic or allogeneic, marrow graft recipients all show evidence of a slow recovery of immune defense mechanisms. Depending upon the parameter being measured, recovery may take weeks or months. For example, the absolute lymphocyte count usually reaches normal levels in 2 or 3 months, but the absolute number of T helper cells and recovery of skin test reactivity often require as long as 1 year. In general, patients who develop GVHD take much longer to recover because of either the GVHD or its treatment. Efforts to accelerate immunological recovery as, for example, with the use of thymic implants or thymic hormones, have been unsuccessful.

## Tolerance

The nature of the tolerance displayed by the chimeric animal or patient, healthy despite the presence of foreign lymphoid cells, continues to be a puzzle. Some studies favor the clonal deletion hypothesis while other studies suggest a role for suppressor cells. For up to 1 year after grafting, we have observed a reversal of the OKT4/OKT8 ratio in healthy chimeras, indicating an imbalance in the helper cell-suppressor cell functions. However, the significance of this inverse ratio is not clear because it is also seen following syngeneic and autologous marrow grafting. Tsoi et al. (1) in studies of human chimeras, have observed that healthy chimeras display specific suppressor cell populations, presumably preventing a reaction of the graft against the host, while chimeras with GVHD show nonspecific suppressor cells that suppress the chimeric lymphocyte responses to antigens other than those of the host.

## Graft-versus-host disease

GVHD is considered to be an illness brought about by the reaction of donor lymphoid cells against the tissues of the host. Target organs are the skin, the liver, and the gut. Even when donor and recipient are HLA-identical siblings and despite the use of methotrexate or cyclosporine postgrafting, GVHD can be a severe illness. In the grading system commonly used, grade 0 refers to those patients with no evidence of GVHD, and grade I refers to those with only a transient skin rash. In most analyses these two grades have been compared to grades II–IV which represent progressive severity of GVHD with multiple-organ involvement. One of the problems in evaluating the prophylaxis of GVHD is the wide variability of its occurrence. This variability indicates the need for carefully controlled trials with an adequate number of patients before firm conclusions can be reached regarding regimens used to prevent GVHD. Based on studies in rodents and in dogs, the Seattle team has routinely administered methotrexate during the first 100 days after grafting to prevent GVHD and/or reduce its severity. We were unsuccessful in an attempt to prevent GVHD with the use of horse antithymocyte globulin. The role of cyclosporine in preventing GVHD is now under investigation (see above). Santos et al. (2) have attempted to prevent GVHD by the administration of cyclophosphamide. In a randomized trial, Ramsay et al. (3) showed that a regimen of methotrexate, antithymocyte globulin and prednisone was superior to methotrexate alone in preventing acute GVHD in young patients.

Treatment of established GVHD with high-dose steroids, antithymocyte globulin, or cyclosporine is unsatisfactory because some patients respond to treatment but many do not. Chronic GVHD, a scleroderma-like illness involving the skin and sometimes the liver or gut, may occur more than 100 days after grafting, either as a continuation of acute GVHD or de novo. Early diagnosis and treatment with azathioprine and steroids has considerably improved the prognosis of patients with chronic GVHD. Both forms of GVHD are associated with an increased mortality from nonleukemic causes because of GHVD or because GVHD and/or its treatment increases the likelihood of opportunistic infections.

**Treatment of donor marrow**

Based on many studies in animals, it is thought that human GVHD is the consequence of donor T cells contained in the marrow inoculum which recognize major or minor transplantation antigens on recipient cells and mount an immunologic attack against the tissues of the host. In rodents it has been shown that the graft-versus-host reaction can be avoided by removing donor T cells from the marrow inoculum. Attempts are now being made to remove T cells from marrow of human donors. One method involves removal of T cells by sedimentation after lectin agglutination and rosetting with sheep red blood cells. An initial report from the Sloan-Kettering team shows a striking reduction in the expected incidence of GVHD in infants with severe combined immunodeficiency given haplotype-incompatible donor marrow after removal of T cells. Such transplants into immunocompetent recipients may be more difficult since the removal process involves the loss of many cells from the donor marrow inoculum.

Monoclonal antibodies directed at T cells or T cell subsets are being explored as a means of removing donor T cells from the inoculum. Initial reports suggesting a beneficial effect by *in vitro* treatment of the donor marrow with antibody OKT3 without complement have not been confirmed. In Seattle, HLA-identical donor marrow was treated *in vitro* with a cocktail of eight anti-T cell monoclonal antibodies without complement. Three of nine patients developed moderately severe acute GVHD, and we concluded that the use of these antibodies without complement is not likely to be effective. Several teams are now studying the use of anti-T cell monoclonal antibodies with complement or combined with a toxic agent (immunotoxins) for *in vitro* treatment of donor marrow. The results of these studies will require careful evaluation, not only for the effect on GVHD but also for the effect on the graft-versus-leukemia reaction.

## Opportunistic infections

During the first 2–3 weeks after grafting, marrow graft recipients are profoundly granulocytopenic and are subject to bacterial infections. Ultra-isolation techniques and prophylactic granulocyte transfusions have been shown to be effective in reducing the incidence of bacterial infections. With these techniques and a modern arsenal of antibacterial agents, only a few marrow graft recipients are lost to these infections in the first month after grafting. At greatest risk are those transplanted in relapse who often have established infections at the time of transplant. During the first 3 months after grafting, regardless of the granulocyte level, patients are at risk for development of almost any kind of opportunistic infection including bacterial, fungal, viral and parasitic infections. The physician must be particularly alert for these problems, especially in patients with GVHD, so that early diagnosis and treatment can be carried out.

## Interstitial pneumonia

Interstitial pneumonia is the primary cause of death among patients given marrow grafts for leukemia during the first 3 months after grafting. Approximately one-half of the Seattle marrow graft recipients developed some form of nonbacterial pneumonia during the period 1971–1976. The incidence has now decreased to approximately 30% of the patients. A recent evaluation of the entire Seattle experience shows the following frequencies of nonbacterial pneumonia: idiopathic, 0.10; cytomegalovirus, 0.16; *Pneumocystic carinii,* 0.04; other viral agents, 0.03; clinical diagnosis without biopsy, 0.05; incidence of all types of nonbacterial pneumonia, 0.36. The incidence of these pneumonias is greater in patients with GVHD and also increases slightly with the age of the patient. The 'idiopathic' pneumonias are those in which extensive study, including an open-lung biopsy, fails to identify an etiologic agent. These pneumonias probably represent, at least in part, pulmonary toxicity of chemoradiotherapy. Their incidence has decreased slightly with the use of fractionated irradiation. The incidence of cytomegalovirus pneumonia is much greater in patients who have antibodies to cytomegalovirus at the time of admission for transplantation and in those patients without such antibodies who are given granulocyte transfusions from donors having cytomegalovirus antibodies. Mortality from cytomegalovirus pneumonia is approximately 80% regardless of treatment which has included adenine arabinoside, interferon, acyclovir, and combinations of these agents.

The incidence of cytomegalovirus pneumonia can be decreased by the administration of immune globulin, as shown in two recent studies. Efforts are now underway to reduce the incidence of cytomegalovirus pneumonia in patients who do not have cytomegalovirus antibodies at the time of transplantation by administration of blood products obtained only from donors who do not have cytomegalovirus antibodies and who are therefore presumed not to be infected with the virus.

Studies in recipients of identical-twin marrow have shown a decreased incidence of interstitial pneumonia as compared to allogeneic graft recipients. The incidence of idiopathic interstitial pneumonia is approximately the same, which is consistent with the hypothesis that these pneumonias are due to the effects of chemoradiotherapy on the lung. The incidence of cytomegalovirus pneumonia is much less in the syngeneic recipients. The difference in the incidence of cytomegalovirus pneumonia between the two groups does not appear to be related to a difference in exposure to cytomegalovirus since the rates of seroconversion are similar in twins and nontwins. In animal studies the presence of an allogeneic reaction may be associated with suppression of specific antibody production and activation of virus, thereby enhancing dissemination of cytomegalovirus. The low incidence of this complication in identical twins suggests that it may also be low following autologous transplantation and also suggests that better methods to prevent GVHD after allogeneic transplantation may also result in a lower incidence of pneumonia.

**Veno-occlusive disease**

Following an allogeneic marrow transplant, hepatic disorders are frequent and perplexing problems with the differential diagnosis including GVHD, viral hepatitis, fungal and bacterial infections, parenteral nutrition, drug reactions, and leukemic infiltrates. Veno-occlusive disease, an obliteration of small enterohepatic central venules, has emerged as an additional problem. In the Seattle experience approximately 15% of marrow graft recipients were found to have veno-occlusive disease which was life-treatening or lethal in onehalf. Predictive factors were abnormal liver function tests before transplant and the use of more vigorous chemotherapy regimens. The increasing use of vigorous chemotherapy regimens in the treatment of patients with acute leukemia may lead to a greater incidence of veno-occlusive disease of and when these patients come to marrow transplantation.

**Graft versus leukemia**

Although we usually think of the graft-versus-host reaction as being harmful to the patient, there are some advantages. Studies in murine systems have shown that a graft-versus-host reaction can also injure malignant cells, the so-called graft-versus-leukemia effect. Initial studies in humans were difficult to evaluate because of the problems of increased mortality from nonleukemic causes in patients with GVHD. More recently, with improvements in the management of patients with GVHD, a graft-versus-leukemia effect has become apparent in those patients with a high incidence of recurrent leukemia such as patients with ALL transplanted in second or subsequent remission. In these patients survival is actually better for those patients with GVHD because of the reduced likelihood of relapse of leukemia following transplantation. These observations do not necessarily indicate the existence of leukemia-associated antigens but are compatible with the interpretation that leukemic cells were eradicated because they were perceived to be of host origin. Furthermore, the antileukemic effect may be due to the treatment of GVHD or to other unknown mechanisms. The clinical observations indicate that we must learn to moderate rather than prevent GVHD.

## Marrow transplantation versus chemotherapy for the treatment of leukemia

The increasing success rate in the treatment of leukemia with marrow grafting and particularly the increased likelihood of cure has raised some controversy as to which form of treatment is better. Such a controversy need not exist. In the first place, the best results for a patient given marrow grafts have been in those patients who achieved a remission on combination chemotherapy. Further, the improving results of marrow transplantation must be considered in relation to the improving results of chemotherapy. For children and young adults marrow transplantation, whether carried out in remission or in relapse, is clearly superior to combination chemotherapy alone in all categories except the children with good-risk ALL. However, the results of marrow grafting in patients ages 30–50 have not yet been demonstrated to be superior to combination chemotherapy. Patients older than age 50 are currently not accepted by most marrow transplant centers and must usually be treated by combination chemotherapy.

The question, then, is not whether to do a marrow transplant but when. Transplantation of younger patients with ANL in first remission seems to offer the best hope of long-term survival. Transplantation of older patients, some 20% of whom may be alive in remission at 5 years after chemotherapy, might be deferred until relapse has occurred. Once relapse has occurred, whether or not a subsequent remission is induced, marrow transplantation offers the only hope of long-term remission and cure. A careful consideration of all these factors as well as prospective studies will be needed in order to determine the best treatment for a particular patient.

## Acknowledgements

The Seattle Marrow Transplant Team is composed of physicians and scientists of a wide range of disciplines, nursing and nursing support teams, technicians, dieticians, and an administrative and secretarial team. It is a pleasure to acknowledge their contribution to this work.

## References

1. Tsoi MS, Storb R, Dobbs S, Santos E, Thomas ED: Specific Suppressor Cells and Immune Response to host antigens in long term human allogeneic marrow recipients: Implications for the mechanisms of graft-host tolerance and chronic graft-vs-host disease. Transplant Proc 13: 237–240, 1981.
2. Santos GW, Tutschka PJ, Brookmeyer R, Saral R, Beschorner WE, Bias WB, Braine HG, Burns WH, Elfenbein GJ, Kaizer H, Mellits D, Sensenbrenner LL, Stuart RK, Yeager AM: Marrow Transplantation for Acute Non-Lymphocytic Leukaemia (ANL) following treatment with Busulphan (BU) and Cyclophosphamide (CY). N Engl J Med (in press, 1983).
3. Ramsay NKC, Kersey JH, Robinson LL, McGlave PB, Woods WG, Krivit W, Kim TH, Goldman AI, Nesbit ME Jr: A randomised study of the prevention of acute graft-vs-host disease. N Engl J Med 306: 392–297, 1982.

## General references for further reading

1. Buckner CD, Appelbaum FR, Thomas ED: Bone marrow and fetal liver, chap. 16. In: *Organ preservation for transplantation,* Karow AK Jr, Pegg DE (eds). Marcel Dekker, Inc, New York, 1981, pp 355–375.
2. Gale RP: Clinical trials of bone marrow transplantation in leukemia. In: *Biology of bone marrow transplantation,* Gale RP, Fox CF (eds). Academic Press, New York, 1980, pp 11–27.
3. Gale RP (ed): *Recent Advances in Bone Marrow Transplantation.* New York, Alan R. Liss (in press).
4. Meyers JD, Thomas ED: Infection complicating bone marrow transplantation, chap. 15. In: *Clinical approach to infection in the immunocompromised* host, Rubin RH, Young LS (eds). Plenum Press, New York, 1982, pp 507–551.
5. Storb R, Doney KC, Thomas ED, Appelbaum F, Buckner CD, Clift RA, Deeg HJ, Goodell BW, Hackman R, Hansen JA, Sanders J, Sullivan K, Weiden PL, Witherspoon RP: Marrow transplantation with or without donor buffy coat cells for 65 transfused aplastic anemia patients. *Blood* 59: 236–246, 1982.
6. Sullivan KM, Shulman HM, Storb R, Weiden PL, Witherspoon RP, McDonald GB, Schubert MM, Atkinson K, Thomas ED: Chronic graft-versus-host disease in 52 patients: Adverse natural course and successful treatment with combination immunosuppression. *Blood* 57: 267–276, 1981.
7. Thomas ED, Clift RA, Buckner CD for the Seattle Marrow Transplant Team: Marrow transplantation for patients with acute nonlymphoblastic leukemia who achieve a first remission. *Cancer Treat Rep* 66: 1463–1466, 1982.
8. Thomas ED, Storb R, Clift RA, Fefer A, Johnson FL, Neiman PE, Lerner KG, Glucksberg H, Buckner CD: Bone-marrow transplantation. *N Engl J Med* 292: 832–843, 895–902, 1975.

# 33. Renal auto-transplantation and extracorporeal renal surgery

GEORGE M. ABOUNA

## Introduction

The impact of and the experience gained in renal transplantation has resulted in the development of newer techniques to treat various vascular and urological conditions of the kidney which otherwise might have resulted in serious renal function impairment or even nephrectomy. Among the vascular problems which can be successfully managed by extracorporeal renal surgery and auto-transplantation are renal artery stenosis from atheroma, fibromuscular disease, aneurysms, narrowing of segmental branches of the renal artery and renal trauma involving the vascular pedicle (1–9). There are many urological conditions which are best treated by work bench surgery and autotransplantation such as high stricture or injury of the ureter, recurrent Staghorn calculi, renal tumours in solitary kidney and renal trauma (9–13).

Historically the first renal autotransplantation was carried out by Shackman for reno-vascular hypertension (1). Hardy was the first to report autotransplantation of the kidney for high ureteric injury (10). Woodruff coined the term work bench surgery (14). Later, *ex vivo* surgical repair followed by autotransplantation was carried out by Ota (2) and by Gelin (5). In a relatively recent review (15) a total of 80 cases of work-bench surgery and autotransplantation were reported in the English literature during the period 1963 to 1975. Since that time many investigators have used this procedure for vascular and urological renal problems employing various cooling techniques including hypothermic pulsatile perfusion (4, 7, 13). In these cases the incidence of successful outcome was reported to be 94% for vascular problems and 84% for urological conditions (15).

In Kuwait we have used the technique of extracorporeal hypothermic bench work surgery with transplantation in 10 patients with various urological and vascular renal problems and we review here our experience and results in these patients.

## Patients and methods

Since we have been interested in hypothermic renal surgery for sometime, we have used *in situ* cooling in cases of renal calculi which were only moderately large and where no previous surgery had been carried out. A combination of intra-arterial perfusion and surface cooling was used in 7 patients and the results were very satisfactory.

Later in our programme we were referred a group of 10 patients whose vascular or urological problems were too complex to be dealt with by *in situ* hypothermia. in 6 patients there were huge Staghorn calculi filling almost the entire pelvi-calyceal system which had been present for 3 to 11 years. In two patients these were bilateral and in four the Staghorn calculus had recurred after multiple previous pyelolithotomies or nephrolithotomies. In 1 patient with horse-shoe kidney there was cystic degeneration of part of the left side with hydronephrosis and multiple large calculi. In another patient a large Staghorn calculus had been growing in a single right kidney after left nephrectomy for calculus disease 6 years previously. There were two patients with vascular problems. One patient, a renal transplant donor, was found on investigation to have a large aneurysm in one of the main branches of intra-renal arteries with mild hypertension. Another patient had been unsuccessfully treated for severe hypertension was found to have stenosis and kinking of the renal artery with aneurysmal formation close to the hilum of the kidney (Table 1). All patients were evaluated according to a specific protocol which included full clinical assessment, renal function studies, biochemical and haematological profiles, renal isotope scans, I.V.P., urine culture and angiography. Full biochemical examinations were carried out for the investigation of hypercalcuria, hypercalcemia and hyperuricemia and other metabolic causes of renal calculi. One patient with cystinuria and cystinosis had been fully investigated for this abnormality and had received medical treatment with penicillamine together with repeated previous pyelolithotomies for recurrence of calculi. Three patients had multiple renal arteries. In all patients with previous renal calculus surgery, deformities of the drainage system were present and at operation they were found to have intense fibrosis locally which would have made any *in situ* surgery difficult and quite hazardous. Indeed one patient with bilateral renal calculi and previous surgery underwent pyelonephrolithotomy on one of his kidneys in another institution before his referral to us and he required several units of blood and almost lost his kidney during the procedure.

## Techniques

The kidney and the ipsi lateral iliac vessels are exposed through an S shaped extraperitoneal incision from loin to groin. Our technique of *in situ* hypothermia is carried out by a combination of surface cooling and intra-arterial perfusion

*Table 1.* Details of patients undergoing extracorporeal work bench surgery and transplantation.

| Patient No. | Age & sex | Date of operation | Diagnosis | Length of history | Previous surgery |
|---|---|---|---|---|---|
| 1 G.S. | 41 M | 19.11.80 | Cystinosis-recurrent bilateral Staghorn calculi | 10 years | Pyelolithotomy Ureterlithotomy |
| 2 I.I | 50 M | 14. 1.81 | Staghorn calculus left kidney (recurrent) | 4 years | |
| 3 H.H.S | 36 M | 1. 4.81 | Staghorn calculus left kidney (recurrent) | 3 years | Pyelolithotomy |
| 4 K.H.B. | 46 M | 27. 5.81 | Staghorn + multiple calculi right kidney | 4 years | |
| 5A.A.H | 62 M | 1. 9.81 | Bilateral massive. Staghorn calculi + renal impairment | 11 years | Nephrolithotomy |
| 6 M.A.H. | 53 M | 24. 9.81 | Recurrent Staghorn calculus left kidney | 8 years | Pyelolithotomy × 2 |
| 7 S.S | 55 | 18.10.81 | Staghorn calculus single left kidney | 6 years | Right nephrectomy for Staghorn calculus |
| 8 M.A.H | 28 M | 1. 2.82 | Congenital horse shoe kidney. Multiple calculi + cysts hydronephrosis | 5 years | |
| 9 N.A.H | 30 F | 6. 5.82 | Aneurysm of segmental branch left renal artery | Unknown | |
| 10 N.M | 28 M | 11.12.82 | Aneurysm of renal artery and reno-vascular hypertension | 8 years | |

using a 16 or 20 size intracath attached to a chilled heparinized Hartmann solution. On the left side a 16 intracath is introduced through the aortic wall close to the renal artery and is then inserted into the renal artery. The aorta is then gently occluded with an oblique clamp and cooling of the kidney begun. On the right side a curved 18 or 20 intracath is introduced directly into the renal artery very close to its origin and after clamping the proximal artery, cooling is begun as previously. Perfusion is carried out under manual pressure of 120 to 150 mm of mercury and continued until the kidney blanches, which usually takes 10 to 15 min in the *in situ* situation. After completion of the procedure the intracath is removed and bleeding at the entrance of the needle stopped, with one or two vascular sutures. In the extracorporeal work-bench surgery the renal vascular pedicle is isolated, clamped and divided and the kidney is delivered to the surface and placed in a basin containing ice slush. Intra-arterial cooling is carried out as above but using a large arterial cannula and Collins solution rather than Hartmann's solution is used. Usually within five minutes the kidney blanches out and is cooled to about 10° C. The ureter is mobilized sufficiently to allow the kidney to come to the surface. If the ureter is not divided a bulldog clamp is placed across its upper part to prevent retrograde arterial flow into the kidney and also the escape of calculi into the lower ureter during lithotomy. In cases of calculi the kidney with its contained stone is then radiographed directly, to identify the exact location and extent of the sone. A large pyelolithotomy is then made over the calculus and the stone is crushed gently and removed piecemeal. When the individual calyces are exposed, the stones are removed from within each calyx, with care not to injure the epithelium. The procedure is continued until all stones are removed and the calyceal system is then thoroughly flushed with saline to remove debris and sand. A head mounted light is used together with a magnifying loops which give an excellent view even of the minor calyces. The kidney is then re-radiographed and when it is confirmed that all calculi are removed the ureter is then flushed with a catheter to remove any calculi. Redundant tissue from the pelvis of the kidney is excised and the pyelolithotomy is closed with interrupted 4/0 or 5/0 dexon sutures. If the problem is a vascular one this is repaired using manifying

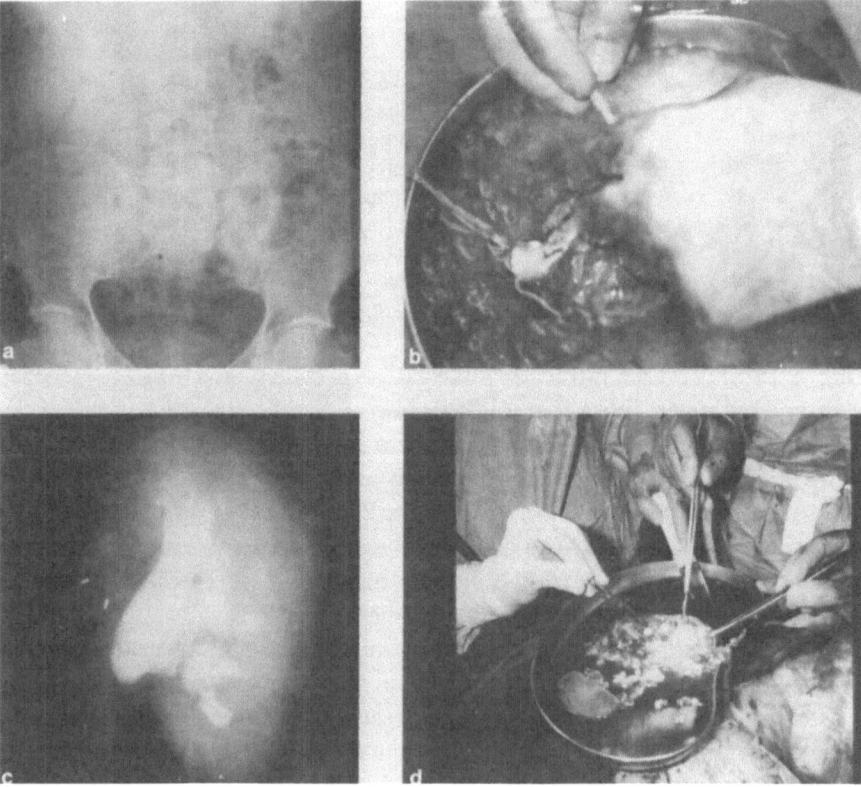

*Fig. 1.* Techniques of extracorporeal hypothermic renal surgery for complicated calculus disease: (a) Large recurrent staghorn calculus; (b) Kidney removed with intact ureter and cooled by perfusion; (c) Radiograph of extracorporeal kidney showing large branching calculus; (d) Stones being removed via long pyelotomy.

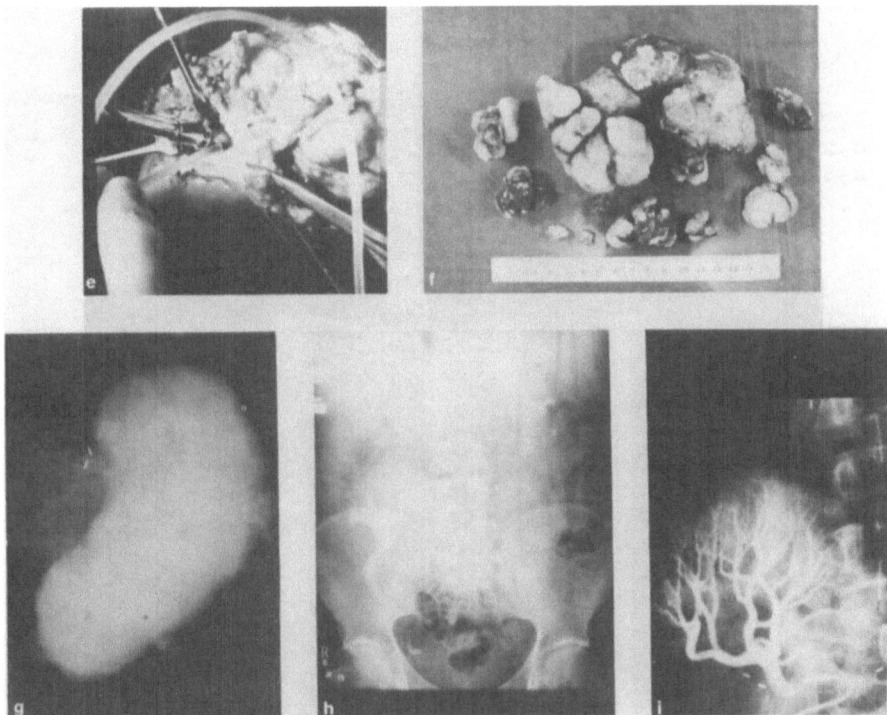

*Fig. 1.* (e) Deeper stones and debris removed and calyces flushed; (f) Crushed stones removed; (g) Radiograph of kidney now showing no calculi; (h) Kidney autotransplanted to ipsilateral fossa with normal IVP at one month; (i) Arteriogram of autotransplanted kidney showing normal perfusion.

loops while the kidney is in the ice solution. For aneurysms of the intra-renal artery 7/0 proline is used. (Figs. 1 and 2). At the conclusion of the procedure the kidney is replaced and it is autografted either orthotopically in its original prosition or in the ipsi-lateral iliac fossa employing the iliac arteries and the iliac vein for anastomosis with the renal vascular pedicle. When a single artery is present we prefer to use the hypogastric artery end to end with the renal artery but when multiple vessels are present we employ the main branches of the internal iliac artery and the external iliac artery as well. All vascular anastomoses at this level are carried out with 6/0 proline sutures. If the ureter has been divided a uretroneocystostomy is carried out after opening the bladder using an antireflux technique and employing a 4/0 or 5/0 dexon. The main wound then is closed in layers with closed drainage. Mannitol and high fluid intake is given from the time of surgery and continued for the first two to three postoperative days. If multiple vessels are present small dose heparin is continued for five days. Postoperative evaluation of the patient is carried out as already outlined above.

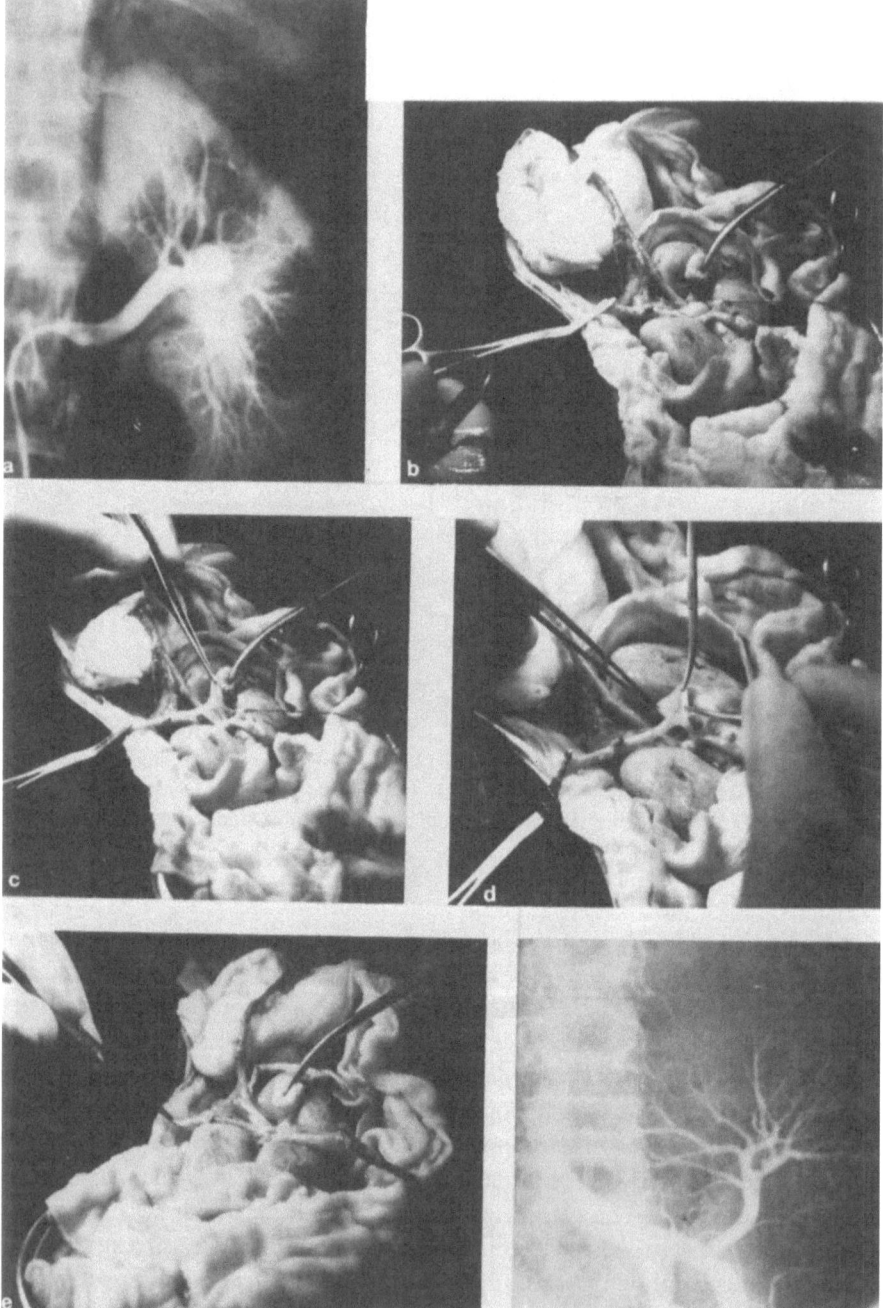

*Fig 2.* Technique of extracorporeal renal surgery and transplantation for intra renal artery aneurysm. (a) Renal angiogram shown site of aneurysm before operation; (b) Kidney removed and cooled by perfusion; (c) Aneurysm isolated; (d) Aneurysm being excised and intra renal artery repaired; (e) Intra renal arteries after excision of aneurysm; (f) Arteriogram of kidney after transplantation.

## Results

In all cases, excepting the allotransplant situation, the kidney was autografted to the ipsilateral side. In three cases (2 with calculus disease and one with renal artery stenosis and aneurysm) it was possible to regraft the kidney to its normal orthotopic position. In the remaining 7 patients the kidney was placed in the ipsilateral iliac fossa. The ureter was divided and shortened in one patient who had recurrent stones from cystinuria in the hope that this may facilitate passage of future stones into the bladder. In the remaining patients the ureter was not divided (Table 2). The weight of the stones removed in these patients varied from a 150 to 450 g. Indeed in one patient, case no. 6, the kidney was almost replaced by a solid branching marble which weighed 450 g and had to be broken up with difficulty before removal.

The ischemic time required to carry out the procedures varied from 52 to 106 min. The longest time required was in the difficult cases of recurrent Staghorn calculi. In all cases of calculus disease it was possible to obtain calculus free radiographs after the procedure. The immediate function was good in all cases except case no. 7 in whom A.T.N. developed in a single kidney which required two dialysis sessions before full function was restored. One patient, case no. 5, with two renal arteries developed thrombosis of one of the arteries after grafting with small drop in renal function but has remained free from calculi.

In the case of renal allograft with arterial aneurysm, excellent immediate function was obtained and normal anatomy was restored on angiography but

*Table 2.* Techniques and immediate results following extracorporeal renal surgery and transplantation.

| Patient no. | Renal arteries | Transplant site | Ureter | Total ischaemia minutes | Immediate operative X-ray | Immediate function |
|---|---|---|---|---|---|---|
| 1 | 1 | Ipsi lateral | Divided & re-implanted | 88 | No calculi | Good |
| 2 | 2 | Orthotopic position | Not divided | 96 | No calculi | Good |
| 3 | 1 | Ipsi lateral I.F. | Not divided | 85 | No calculi | Good |
| 4 | 1 | Ipsi lateral I.F. | Not divided | 72 | No calculi | Good |
| 5 | 2 | Ipsi lateral I.F. | Not divided | 104 | No calculi | Good |
| 6 | 1 | Ispi lateral I.F. | Not divided | 54 | No calculi | Good |
| 7 | 2 | Orthotopic position | Not divided | 92 | No calculi | A.T.N. (7 days) |
| 8 | 1 | L.I.F. | Not divided | 81 | No calculi | Good |
| 9 | 1 | Recipient L.I.F. | Divided & re-implanted | 106 | Normal angiogram | Good |
| 10 | 1 | Orthotopic | Not divided | 52 | Not done | Normal BP |

unfortunately the graft was rejected by a highly sensitized recipient one month after transplantation. In the patient with renovascular hypertension and arterial aneurysm, case no. 10, normal blood pressure was restored soon after operation. The complications seen in this series were two mild wound infections which responded to chemotherapy. Long term follow up of these patients for a period of 1 to 3 years has shown normal function and anatomy in all patients except case no. 1 and 2 who have developed recurrence of calculi and 18 and 24 months after the procedure.

### Discussion

There are numerous situations both vascular and urological in which the best and sometimes the only procedure which ensures cure and preservation of renal function is by extracorporeal work-bench surgery and auto-transplantation. This procedure is widely employed by many transplant, vascular and urological sur-geons with increasing success, particularly with the advent of successful tech-niques of hypothermic renal preservation (6, 8, 16 & DuBernard, personal communication). In the cases of Staghorn calculi there is debate regarding the indications for work-bench surgery versus hypothermic *in situ* procedure. There

*Table 3.* Renal function, complications and long-term result of extracorporeal renal surgery and transplantation.

| Patient no. | Patient survival | Complications | Serum creatinine MG% | | Comments current status |
| --- | --- | --- | --- | --- | --- |
| | | | Before operation | On discharge | |
| 1 | Alive | Nil | 0.8 | 0.6 | Recurrence at 24 months |
| 2 | Alive | Wound infection | 0.9 | 0.5 | Recurrence of stone at 18 months |
| 3 | Alive | Nil | 0.8 | 0.9 | Normal |
| 4 | Alive | Nil | 0.8 | 0.8 | Do |
| 5 | Alive | Thrombosis of one of 2 arteries | 1.6 | 2.0 | Do |
| 6 | Alive | Nil | 0.8 | 0.9 | Do |
| 7 | Alive | Temporary A.T.N. wound infection | 1.1 | 1.4 | Do |
| 8 | Alive | Wound infection | 0.8 | 0.7 | Do |
| 9 | Alive | Nil | Excellent initial function until rejection at 1 month | | Do |
| 10 | Alive | Nil | 0.9 BP 190/120 | 1.0 BP 140/80 | Do |

is no doubt that many cases of Staghorn calculi can be managed by *in situ* hypothermia alone. However, in our experience there are cases of recurrent calculi where the stone is so large and adherent that *in situ* removal becomes very difficult and hazardous to the kidney and even to the patient. In the Middle East where calculus disease is very common and late consultation with the surgeon is very common, such cases are not infrequent. Indeed many of our patients with calculus disease treated with extracorporeal procedure were referred by urological surgeons who had previously operated on these patients. The advantages of this procedure are: (a) ample time is available under hypothermia, to remove the stones carefully and unhurriedly; (b) the entire lithotomy can be carried out through a pyelotomy incision and without injury to the renal parenchyma; (c) complete removal of stones and debris is possible under direct vision and thus reducing the incidence of recurrence; (d) the whole procedure is done in a bloodless field with no blood loss and with accurate delineation of tissue margins. In the cases of vascular problems there is usually very little controversy since most of these problems can only be safely dealt with under extracorporeal and hypothermic conditions.

There was no mortality in this small series of patients and the immediate complications were few and minor. One patient developed acute tubular necrosis for a few days which required two dialysis sessions but recovered full renal function before discharge. Another patient aged 62 with double renal arteries thrombosed one of these vessels, resulting in minor deterioration of renal function. All the remaining patients had improved renal function on discharge. Long term follow-up has also been satisfactory although two patients developed recurrent stones. One of these is a patient suffering from the metabolic disease of cystinosis and recurrence was not unexpected. The patient with renal artery aneurysm and stenosis with severe hypertension, now has normal blood pressure and needs no medication. Various techniques have been reported for extracorporeal work-bench surgery and autotransplantation. Some surgeons have used trans-abdominal incision (5, 8, 13). Others have resorted to division of the ureter (4, 6, 9, 13). Some surgeons have used flank incision for nephrectomy and the kidney is transplanted through a second flank incision in one or the other iliac fossa (12–13). The technique which we have employed is simple and more direct. It is an extra peritoneal incision which extends from the loin to the groin and both nephrectomy and autotransplantation can be carried out without changing the operative circumstances of the patient. The ureter was divided in one patient on the theoretical assumption that this will facilitate passage of further calculi when they are formed as a consequence of his metabolic disease but we believe division of the ureter should not be carried out particularly in vascular cases since from experience in renal transplantation it has been shown that redundant ureter functions normally. Also the operation is shorter and avoids the possible complications of cystostomy and ureteroneo-cystostomy.

The method of preservation of the kidney in the extracorporeal position has also varied. Some surgeons have used hypothermic pulsatile perfusion (3, 6, 13) while many use simple cooling. In view of the fact that kidneys can be preserved for 48 h with Eurocollin's solution (16), in our opinion, it is much more simpler to use a simple cooling procedure than complicated perfusion machinery. The technique of autotransplantation has also been variable. Most surgeons prefer autotransplantation into the iliac fossa but it is possible to regraft the kidney back into its orthotopic position. This was performed in three of our patients in this series. If this is technically possible, in our opinion it should be performed since it saves time and unnecessary dissection but in most cases this is not easy technically and the ipsilateral iliac fossa should be used.

In conclusion we believe that extracorporeal work-bench surgery is a useful and effective technique for the treatment of patients with difficult urological and renal vascular problems. In cases of calculus disease, proper selection of patients is required and the procedure should be carried out only in those in whom the *in situ* cooling cannot be performed for technical reasons or for reasons of repeated recurrence resulting from incomplete removal of calculi at previous operations. Clearly this technique requires expertise in vascular and transplant surgery and it should not be practised by the occasional surgeon or urologist. Other aids to the success of this operation are to use magnifying loops, a good head mounted light and several delicate retractors.

### References

1. Shackman R, Dempster WJ: Surgical Kidney. Br Med J 2: 1724, 1963.
2. Ota K, Nori S, Awane Y, Ueno A: Ex Site Repair of the Renal artery for reno-vascular hypertension. Arch Surg 94: 395, 1971.
3. Belzer FO, Keaveny TV, Reed TW, Pryor JP: A new method of renal artery reconstruction. Surgery 68: 619, 1970.
4. McLoughlin MG, Williams GM: Renal Aneurysmictomy in the ex-vivo setting. J Urology 118: 15, 1977.
5. Gelin LE, Claes G, Gustafson A, Storm B: Total bloodlessness for extracorporeal Organ repair. Rev Surg 28: 395, 1971.
6. Corman JL, Anderson JT, Stables DP, Halgrimson CG, Poportzer M, Starzl TE: Ex-vivo Perfusion, arteriography and autotransplantation procedures for kidney salvage. Surg Gynec Obstet 137: 655, 1973.
7. Starr MG, Williams GM: Ispilateral extraperitoneal approach to renal autotransplantation. Surgery 94: 510, 1983.
8. Belzer FO, Salvatierra O, Palubinstras A, Stoney RJ: Ex-vivo renal artery reconstruction. Ann Surg 182: 456, 1975.
9. Lawson RK, Hodges CV, Potre TM: Nephrectomy, Microvascular Repair and Autotransplantation. Surg Forum 23: 539, 1972.
10. Hardy J: High uretral injuries management by autotransplantation. JAMA 124: 96, 1963.
11. Calne RY: Tumour in a single kidney-nephrectomy excision and autotransplantation. Lancet 2: 761, 1971.

12. Kearney GP, Mahoney EM, Demochouiski J: Radical nephrectomy, bench surgery and auto-transplantation in the potentially malignant renal mass. J Urol 116: 375, 1976.
13. Salvatierra O Jr, Olcott CV, Stoney RJ: Ex-vivo renal artery reconstruction using perfusion preservation. J Urol 119: 16, 1978.
14. Woodruff MFA, Doig A, Donald KW, Nolan B: Renal autotransplantation. Lancet 1: 433, 1966.
15. Kyriakides GK, Najarian JS: Renal Transplantation and Work-bench surgery. In: Vascular Surgery. Najarian JS, Delaney JP (eds). Symposia Specialists Inc, Miami, USA, 1978, p 395.
16. Abouna GM, Kumar AS, White AG, Daddah S, Omer OF, Samhan M, Kusma G, John P, Soubky AS, Abbas AR, Kremer G: Experience with imported human cadaveric kidneys having unusual problems and transplanted after 30–60 hours of preservation. Transplant Proceed 16: 61, 1984.

## 34. Hypothermic *in situ* perfusion and surface cooling in renal surgery

CH. CHAUSSY, F.J. MARX, W. STURM and A. SCHILLING

In the future it is unlikely that there will be any marked improvement in the operative technique of major stone surgery of the kidney. However, it seems worthwhile to avoid secondary damage of the organ due to this type of surgery. The main goal must be the preservation of kidney parenchyma and renal function.

It is common belief, that long lasting procedures for complete removing of Staghorn calculi or multiple concrements require a clamping of the renal vascular pedicle. Normothermic conditions limit the operation time to about 30 min ischemia time otherwise severe functional loss is to be expected. Complete removal of all concrements is essential to avoid recurrence and persistance of urinary tract infection and therefore techniques must be developed which allow one to exceed the restriction of time. For that purpose physical and biochemical operative conditioning of the kidney has been developed.

The aim of this paper is to present our experience with regional cooling of the kidney either by surface cooling or vascular *in situ* perfusion. A comparison of these two techniques should help to find out the advantages and disadvantages of each method.

Figure 1 shows our early results with 186 cases, who had undergone normothermic ischemia of the kidney for stone surgery. In more than 1/3 of the patients we had to operate for more than 30 min under warm ischemia. Nevertheless it was not possible to remove all the stones. A decrease of function and a high postoperative complication rate, including 10% secondary nephrectomies had to be accepted.

Because of these unsatisfactory results we were forced to review our strategy and look for alternative methods, which led to the development of hypothermic regional perfusion of the kidney, which we first published 10 years ago.

There are two procedures for cooling the kidneys. First surface cooling: After exposure of the kidney and clamping of the vascular pedicle the organ is wrapped in a plastic bag and covered with ice slush. The temperature was measured continuously with a probe. After approximately 20 min a temperature of 15° C is reached, when measured in the medulla. The ice is removed and surgery starts. In comparison to this universally applicable procedure, the hypothermic renal vas-

| | ISCHEMIA TIME | | |
| --- | --- | --- | --- |
| | 0 – 29 MIN. | 30 – 66 MIN. | TOTAL |
| INCOMPLETE REMOVAL OF STONES | 6 ( 4,7 %) | 17 (28,8 %) | 23 (12,4 %) |
| DELAY OF EXCRETION IN IVP | 23 (18,1 %) | 27 (45,8 %) | 50 (26,8 %) |
| SECONDARY NEPHRECTOMIES | 3 ( 2,4 %) | 6 (10,2 %) | 9 ( 4,8 %) |
| NUMBER OF PATIENTS | 128 | 58 | 186 |
| NUMBER OF COMPLICATIONS | 32 (25,2 %) | 50 (84,8 %) | 82 (44,0 %) |

*Fig. 1.* Clinical data of 186 patients undergoing stone surgery in normothermic ischemia (1960–1971).

cular perfusion is a more sophisticated technique, which needs certain mechanical applicances and a specially trained staff. A catheter is placed into the renal artery via a femoral arterial puncture. Ischemia is achieved either by closing a tourniquet around the renal artery and the inlying catheter or by using a double lumen balloon catheter and intraluminal balloon occlusion of the artery. Cooling is achieved by permanent perfusion with a solution consisting of 50% dextran 40, 50% saline and 2 500 i.U Heparin/l, which is cooled to 4° C. The perfusate is drained into the circulatory system via the renal vein. Usually after 10 min the correct temperature is reached and the renal vein is clamped (Fig. 2). In the last 4

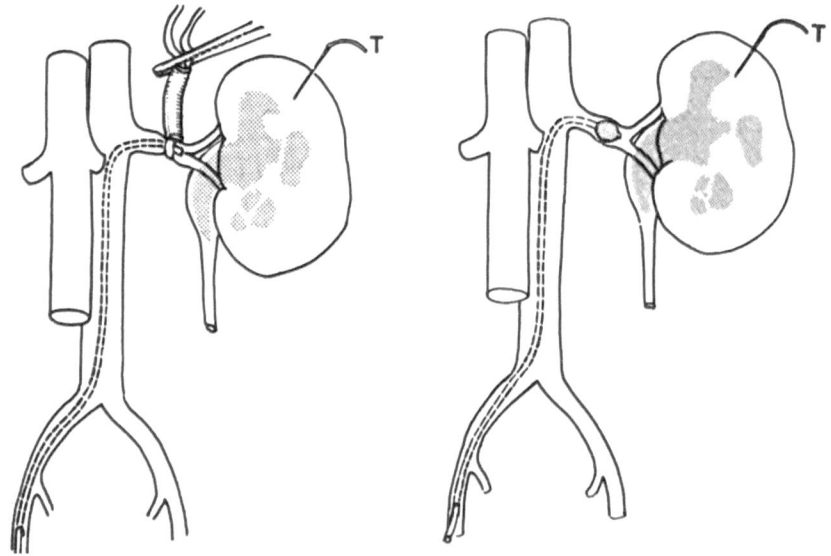

*Fig. 2.* Alternative techniques used for perfusion cooling: External occlusion by tourniquet, intraluminal occlusion using a balloon catheter.

years we were able to follow up 59 patients, who had undergone surgery of kidney stones under hypothermia (Fig. 3). Twentysix of these patients have had topical ice slush hypothermia, and 33, hypothermic renal perfusion.

Kidney function was measured by split radioisotope clearance studies using I 131 – Hippuran before, 1–2 weeks and 6–30 months after surgery.

As shown in Figure 3, it takes twice as long to cool the organ below 20° C with surface cooling than with perfusion. The interruption of renal circulation, given as cold ischemia in Figure 3, was not significantly different between the 2 methods. The average clamping time was 60 min with a range between 30 and 110 min.

The clinical data of the 59 cases, operated in hypothermia are given in Figure 4. As you can see, both groups are nearly identical with regard to age, sex, follow-up rate, surgery on residual kidneys or previous kidney surgery. The only difference between the two groups is that surface cooling was mostly done in cases with Staghorn calculi. The reason for this was clarified by analyzing the operation protocols. They gave evidence that in most cases we made the decision to use surface cooling before the intraoperative x-ray control showed remaining stones, which could only by removed with transrenal approach. At this time topical cooling was the only suitable technique to prolong the ischemic tolerance of the organ.

Figure 5 shows the complications found to be dependent on the technical procedure itself. Using the perfusion technique, with the exception of one case, all stones had been removed completely, where as using surface cooling, in 3 out of 26 cases concrements were found to be left. Severe complications were

|  | SURFACE COOLING | PERFUSION |
|---|---|---|
| TECHNIQUE | EMBEDDING OF THE KIDNEY WITH SLUSH ICE ↓ TEMPERATURE OF MEDULLA AFTER 20 - 25 MIN. < 20°C | PERFUSION OF RENAL ARTERY ↓ TEMPERATURE OF MEDULLA AFTER 10 MIN. < 20°C |
| LOWEST TEMPERATURE (MEDULLA) | $16,6 \pm 3,9$ °C | $18,4 \pm 4,2$ °C |
| COLD ISCHEMIA | $53 \pm 18$ MIN. (30 - 104) | $63 \pm 6$ MIN. (38 - 110) |
| n | 26 | 33 |

Fig. 3. Technical data during the different cooling procedures.

| | SURFACE COOLING | IN SITU PERFUSION |
|---|---|---|
| n | 26 (44,1 %) | 33 (55,9 %) |
| STAGHORN STONES | 19 | 30 |
| MULTIPLE STONES | 7 | 3 |
| RESIDUAL KIDNEY | 2 | 3 |
| KIDNEYS OPERATED BEFORE | 9 (34,6 %) | 11 (33,3 %) |

| | SURFACE COOLING | IN SITU PERFUSION |
|---|---|---|
| ♀ | 20 | 22 |
| ♂ | 6 | 11 |
| AGE | 48,9 ± 11,5 | 42,1 ± 15,5 |

| | SURFACE COOLING | IN SITU PERFUSION |
|---|---|---|
| FOLLOW UP AFTER 6 – 30 MONTH ($\bar{x}$ = 11,5) | 22 (84,6 %) | 28 (84,8 %) |

*Fig. 4.* Clinical data of 59 patients undergoing stone surgery in hypothermic ischemia.

| | SURFACE COOLING | PERFUSION |
|---|---|---|
| n | 26 | 33 |
| RESIDUAL CALCULI | 4 (15,4 %) | 1 (3,0 %) |
| SECONDARY NEPHRECTOMY | 0 | 4 (12,1 %) |
| | | 1 THROMBOSIS OF RENAL ARTERY<br>1 MASSIVE BLEEDING<br>2 UROSEPSIS |

*Fig. 5.* Complications of stone surgery using hypothermia *in situ* perfusion and surface cooling.

observed in the perfusion group, and we had to do secondary nephrectomies in 4 patients. But, as indicated at the bottom of the picture, this was only in cases of thrombosis, caused directly by the technical procedure.

When tested postoperatively within 1 or 2 weeks, a decrease of renal function was to be obtained after an average ischemia time of 60 min. This effect is demonstrated on the left side Figure 6, which shows a decrease down to 70% of initial values in both groups. There was no significant difference between the methods.

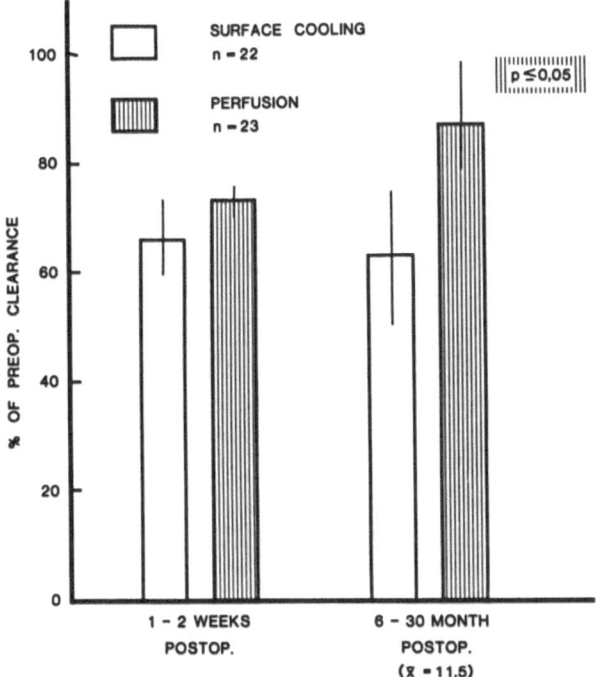

*Fig. 6.* Change of renal function (split radioisotope clearance studies using jodine-131 Hippuran) after surface and perfusion cooling.

However, a definite judgement of the efficiency in protecting renal function, can only be done by a longterm follow-up investigation. These results are shown on the right columns. These clearance studies were done after an average follow-up time of 11.5 months. At this time the renal function of the perfusion group showed a 90% recovery, reflecting a significant difference compared to the persistent loss of function in the group undergoing surface cooling. The function loss of 34% measured 2 weeks after surgery has to be accepted as permanent, as indicated by the longterm follow-up results. Since the perioperative adjunctive pharmacotherapy was identical in both groups the differences are certainly due to the different cooling methods.

Figure 7 shows the auxiliary therapy which we used in these patients. The most important was the preoperative sodium loading, which causes a significant decrease of plasma renin activity, as proved by our animal experiments. Nearly every patient was given saline in the preoperative period but the intraoperative injection of Procaine into the renal artery before and after clamping is reserved to the cases undergoing hypothermic renal perfusion. This should achieve blocking of the vascular spasm, induced by hypothermia, but this can only be done after discussion with the anaesthetist. The application of diuretics, of the osmotic or furosemid type induces an improvement of the washout of metabolic substances. Obviously with an infected kidney the preoperative management should include

302

the application of appropriate antibiotics, nephrotoxic agents like amino-glycosides should be restricted to cases without any alternative (Fig. 7).

The advantages and disadvantages of the perfusion and surface cooling techniques are summarised in Figure 8. Obviously in contrast to *in situ* perfusion, cooling with ice slush is easily applicable at any time and does not need special technical equipment. An additional advantage is the fact that surface cooling can be used for kidneys with multiple arteries.

One of the main drawbacks of surface cooling is non-homogeneous temperature profiles, leading in some cases to cortical necrosis. Figure 9, based on our experimental data, illustrates the different behaviour of an externally cooled or a perfused kidney. After 10 min of cooling the perfused kidney reached 20°C homogeneously, whereas in the surface cooled kidney differences of temperature between cortex and medulla of upto 10°C were found. As mentioned earlier it needs an extra 10 min to decrease the medullary temperature under 20°C. In our

---

1. PREOPERATIVE SODIUM LOADING

2. BOLUS INJECTION OF 3 ml 1 % PROCAINE

3. FORCED DIURESIS AFTER ISCHEMIA WITH MANNITOL

4. AVOIDING OF NEPHROTOXIC ANTIBIOTICS

---

*Fig. 7.* Perioperative adjunctive therapy in stone surgery under hypothermic ischemia.

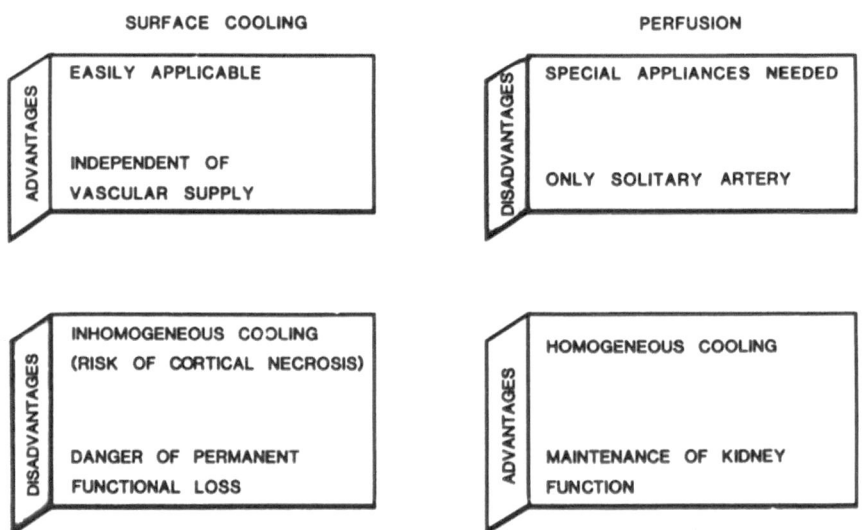

*Fig. 8.* Advantages and disadvantages of surface cooling and *in situ* perfusion.

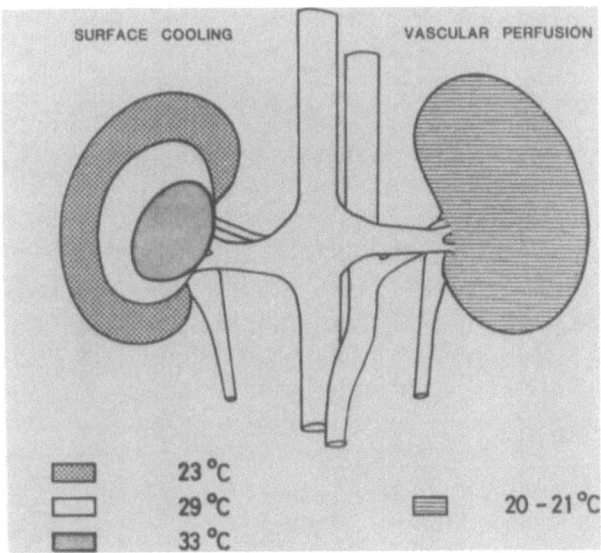

*Fig. 9.* Temperature profile after 10 min of surface and perfusion cooling (experimental data).

opinion the persistance of relatively high temperatures in the medulla may account for the permanent loss of kidney function, which could be demonstrated in our clinical study. The better functional results should justify the use of *in situ* perfusion. Inspite of the sophisticated technique and a certain danager of vascular complications the better results of *in situ* perfusion should lead us to favour this method.

## References

1. Chaussy CH, Eisenberger F, Riedl P: Langzeitfunktionsuntersuchungen nach hypothermer Perfusion und Oberflachenkuhlung der Niere bei schwierigen Eingriffen am Nierenparenchym. Verh Ber Dtsch Ges Urol 28: 368, 1977.
2. Eisenberger F, Chaussy CH, Klein U, Pfeifer KJ, Pielsticker K, Rothe R, Hammer C, Heinze HG: Tierexperimentelle Untersuchungen zur in situ Perfusion und Kuhlung der Niere. Urologe A 12: 268, 1973.
3. Marberger M, Eisenberger F: Regional Hypothermia of the Kidney. Surface or transarterial perfusion cooling? A functional study. J Urol 124: 179, 1980.
4. Riedmuller H, Thuroff J, Alken P, Hohenfellner R: Doppler and b mode ultrasound for a vascular nephrotomy. J Urol 130: 224, 1983.

# 35. Extracorporeal shock wave lithotripsy: a new aspect in the treatment of kidney stones

CHRISTIAN CHAUSSY, EGBERT SCHMIDT and DIETER JOCHAM

Until now, surgical removal of renal concrements has been the first choice of therapy, although the search for noninvasive treatment of nephrolithiasis has been going on for 50 years.

Chemotherapy of renal concrements is restricted to treatment of uric acid calculi only, while physical methods like ultrasound-lithotripsy or electro-hydraulic waves are applicable only in the lower urinary tract and require direct contact between energy source and concrement.

The aim of this paper is, to report about our experiences with high energy shock waves as applied to biological systems and expecially to discuss our results of the extracorporeal contact-free destruction of renal calculi in experimental animals and patients.

The principles of this procedure is extracorporeal generation and administration of shock waves focused at the renal concrements as a target. The shock waves are generated by underwater high-voltage condenser spark-discharge of 1 $\mu$sec duration (Fig. 1).

The spark electrodes are localized in the geometrical focus of an ellipsoidal reflector. High-voltage discharge causes an explosive evaporation of the surrounding water, which in turn leads to the generation of shock waves through the surrounding fluid due to the sudden expansion.

Because the shock wave source is localized in the focus of an ellipsoid, the waves, that means all the energy generated, are reflected from the surrounding wall and collected again. This 2nd focus is the area of highest energy density and the target area where concrements must be localized for destruction. The theoretical basis of this new procedure is summarised in Figure 2.

The shock waves, entering the body, spread homogenously through soft tissue because conductivity of soft tissue is very similar to that of water. However, at the borderline between normal tissue and concrement, the shock wave, which is partially reflected, produces high pressure gradients leading to tear and shear forces, destroying the concrement in zone A.

The penetrating part of the wave is again reflected at the opposite part of the concrement, where it is subjected to change in phase. Therefore again high tension forces are built up, which destroy the part of the concrement in zone B,

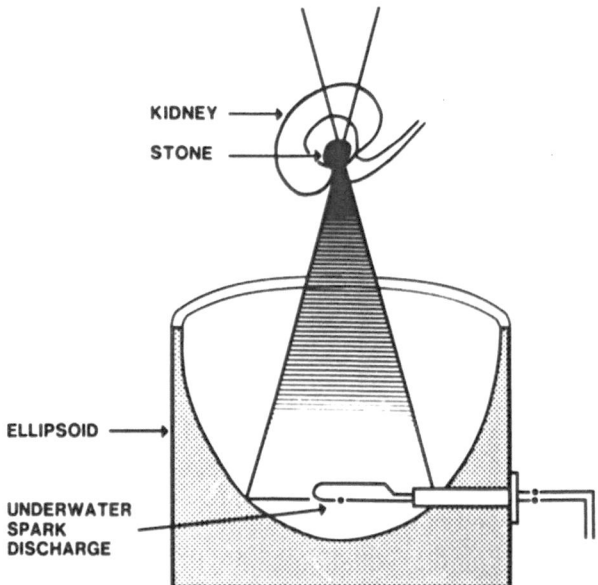

*Fig. 1.* Schematic representation of pressure transmission of shock wave exposure. The density of the screen compares with the approximate pressure density of the transmitting pressure as it moves through the tissue.

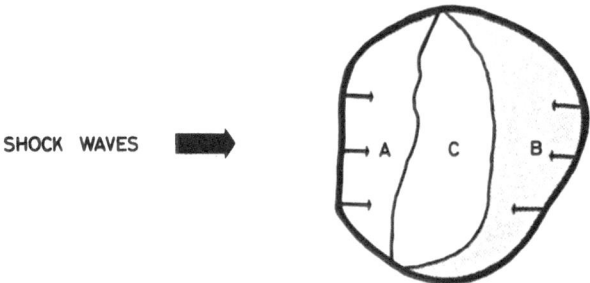

*Fig. 2.* Schematic description of stone destruction.

while zone C must be exposed again. When a technically and experimentally reliable solution of this concept became available, we were interested to investigate two points under *in vitro* and *in vivo* conditions, which are most important in this context.

The questions were:

1. Does the available energy suffice to destroy kidney stones?
2. To what extent do shock waves induce damage to the surrounding normal tissue?

In *in vitro* experiments, human kidney stones were exposed to shock waves. A typical result of this experiment is shown in Figure 3.

On the left, there is an oxalate-stone, approximately 1.5 cm in diameter, before shock wave exposure, and on the right, the result of shock wave application.

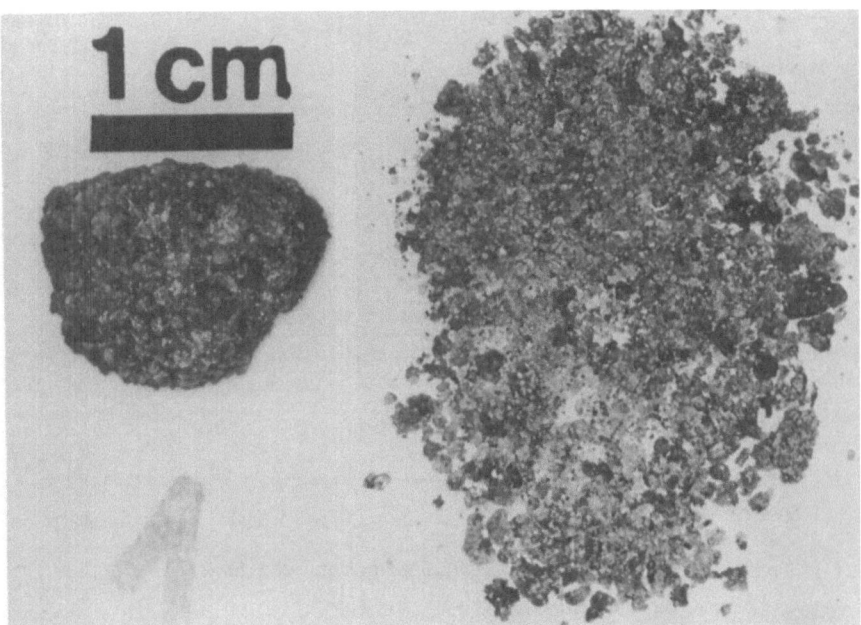

*Fig. 3. In vitro* kidney stone destruction of a calcium oxalate stone. Number of exposures: 500.

The same effect can be obtained with concrements of different chemical components. These series of investigations showed that calculi of different chemical structure can be destroyed by shock waves.

The question to what extent exposure to shock waves causes tissue damage was tested in red blood cells. Figure 4 shows the concentration of plasma hemoglobin in 10 ml of human blood exposed to shock waves, which illustrates the hemolytic effect of exposure. There is a linear correlation between hemolysis and the number of exposures but only up to 400 mg %.

Employing mixed lymphocyte culture, the question studied was whether and how nucleated cells are damaged by shock waves particularly so far as proliferation activity is concerned. The proliferation of these cells was measured prior to and after exposure to shock waves, as shown in Figure 5, demonstrating a typical experiment.

Evidently, there is no significant change in cell count after exposure. Furthermore no significant reduction of proliferation could be detected, both after nonspecific mitogen stimulation with PHA, and after stimulation with LD-different irradiated responder cells, which are marked with a cross in this diagram.

The first *in vivo* experiments were performed in rats. We subjected anaestesized rats to shock waves, exposing the abdominal region. No pathological changes were observed 24 h, or two weeks later. In contrast to these findings, tissue damage should be expected in organs such as the lung because of the marked difference in accoustic impedance. Exposure to lung tissue led to exten-

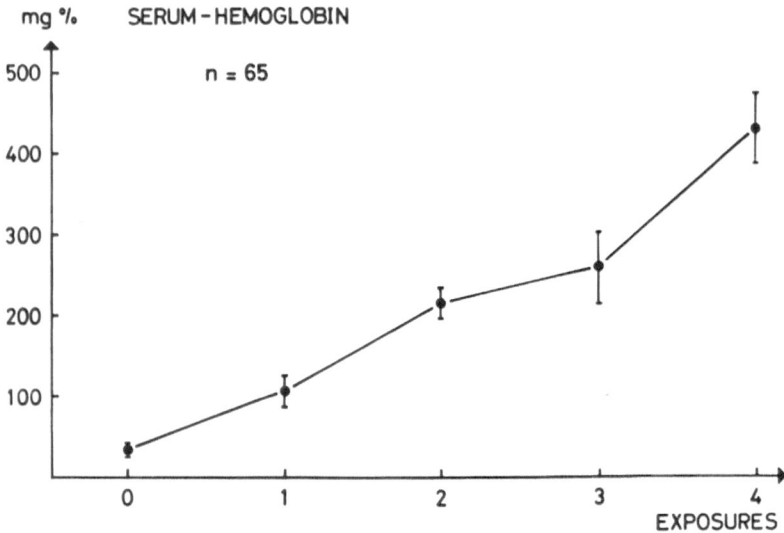

*Fig. 4.* Behaviour of serum-hemoglobin concentration after repeated shock wave exposures.

| MLC 88 | UNTREATED CELLS | | TREATED CELLS | |
|---|---|---|---|---|
| | cpm | Ratio | cpm | Ratio |
| A + Ax | 2 708 | | 2 030 | |
| A + Bx | 87 849 | 32, 4 | 57 325 | 28, 2 |
| B + Bx | 2 515 | | 2 815 | |
| B + Ax | 102 274 | 40, 6 | 142 317 | 50, 2 |
| A Cont. | 1 553 | | 1 250 | |
| A + PHA - P | 369 149 | 237 | 278 720 | 222 |
| B Cont. | 1 506 | | 1 225 | |
| B + PHA - P | 382 314 | 253 | 367 775 | 300 |

*Fig. 5.* Example of the stimulation study in the lymphocyte culture before and after shock wave exposure. Also given are the impulses per minute (cpm) and the quotient which is given from cpm (experimental) to cpm (untreated cells). Irradiated cells are marked with an x.

sive damage of the alveolar tissue, and consequently resulted in death of the experimental animal. This area, however, is easily protected, employing air containing material such as styropor or by exact focussing outside the lung.

Based on these results, the next step was the development of an experimental model of renal concrement destruction under *in vivo* conditions. The problem was to induce renal concrements in experimental animals.

A solution was the implantation of human kidney stones into the renal pelvis of dogs. This was actually a two step procedure with the first step (Fig. 6) to induce hydronephrosis by ureter ligation. After the renal pelvis had dilated sufficiently,

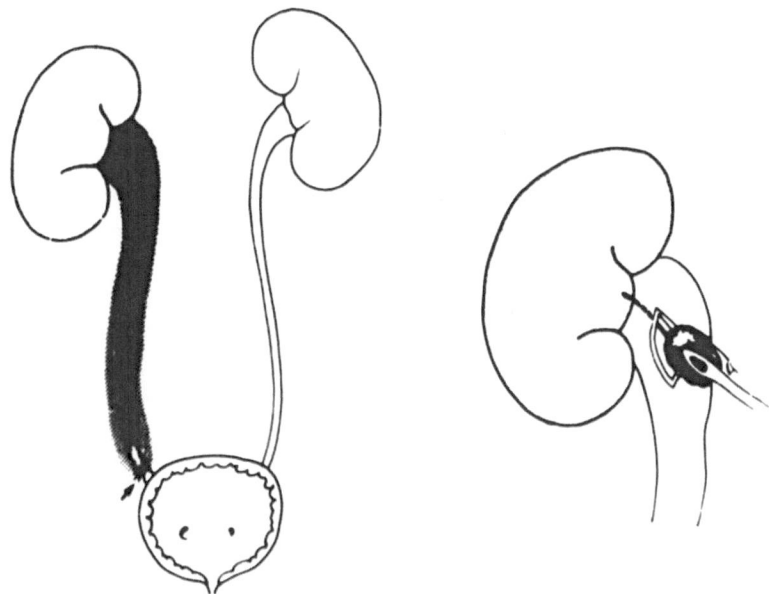

*Fig. 6.* Experimental procedure for the implantation of human kidney stones in the renal pelvic calyx system of the dog.

the concrement was implanted. In a 2nd surgical step the ureter was reanastomosed to the bladder (Fig. 7).

For shock wave exposure, the anaesthesized dogs were placed into a heated water bath containing the spark discharge electrodes at the bottom. As previously mentioned, the method requires the renal concrements to be positioned with utmost precision in the 2nd focus, the target focus, of the ellipsoidal reflector. For that purpose, an integrated 2-dimensional x-ray scanning system was used. The intersect of the x-ray beams is used for target focus and the calculus (within the animal,) is moved over the ellipsoid, until the stone is visualized in both crosshairs of the x-ray conversion system (Fig. 8).

After initial experiments of shock wave exposure using ultrasound for localization, which was unsatisfactory, we conducted experiments employing the described x-ray scanning system. In 22 out of 25 dogs, the implanted concrements were destroyed to such a degree that they were discharged spontaneously. Figure 9. shows an x-ray of one of these experiments. On the left side, there is the implanted concrement before shock wave treatment. The x-ray 1 h after treatment shows the crushed concrements covering the walls of the renal pelvis; and, on the right, there is no concrement left, 7 days after treatment.

After successful conclusion of the experimental investigation the application of shock wave lithotripsy in patients seemed to be justified. For this purpose it was necessary to design a new lithotripter, which satisfied the clinical requirement. Before coming to the clinical results it is important to emphasize that the principle

310

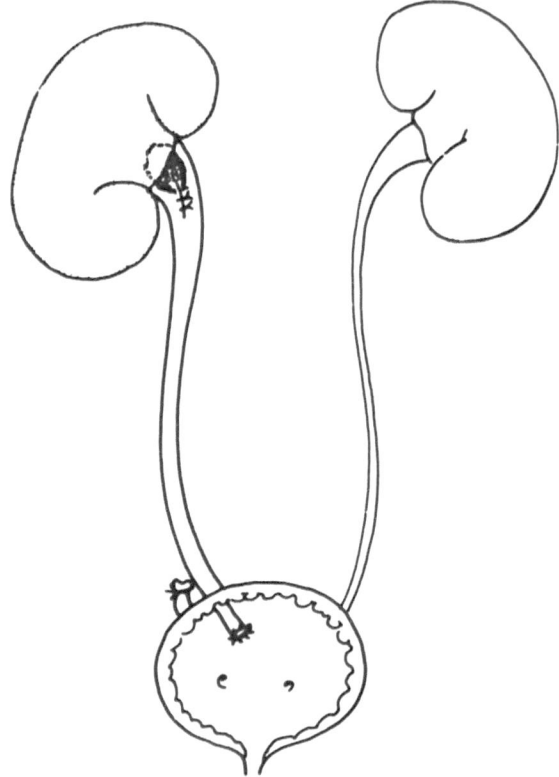

*Fig. 7.* Situation after the stone implantation and ureteroneocystostomy.

of the technique is based on shockwaves and not, as is often believed, ultrasound. The differences become clearer, when the time pressure distribution of super-sonic and shock waves are compared (Fig. 10). While supersonic waves are characterized by a sinusoidal pressure impulse, a shock wave only consists of a single pressure impulse with a steep wave front and a slow fall in the typical case. Rise and decay are characteristic quantities for shock wave pulse and depend on shock wave generation and the speed of propagation. The pressure of the shock wave we use, increases to a maximum of approximately 600 bars in less than 10 nano sec (1 nano-sec = $10^{-9}$ sec).

The way we arrange the shock wave source is explained in Figure 11. The shock wave is produced by an underwater spark discharge in the first focal point of an ellipsoidal reflector. The shock wave spreads out homogenously and is focused in the second focal point, after being reflected from the wall of the ellipsoid.

The calculus has to be positioned in the area of highest energy density. By means of a positioning device, the patients is moved over the shock wave source, so that the kidney stone is centered in the crosshairs of the two x-ray pattern

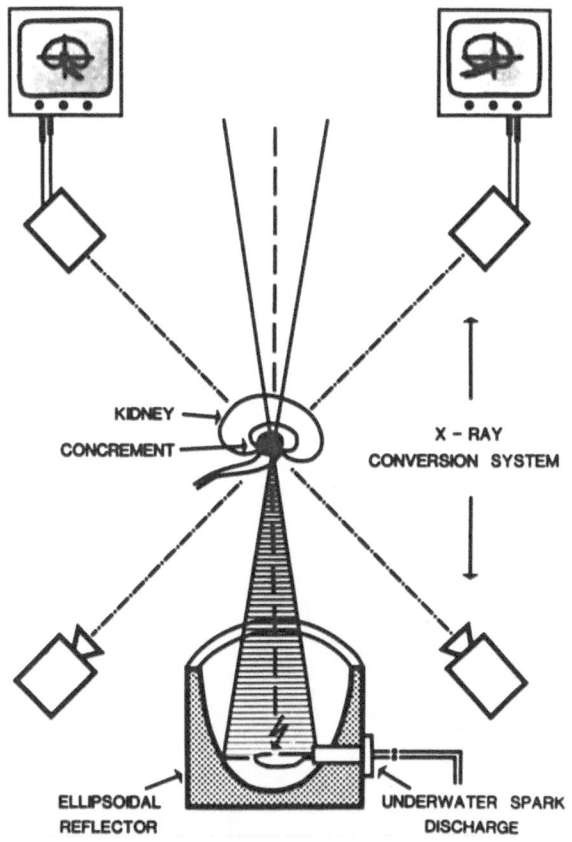

*Fig. 8.* Schematic arrangement of the shock wave lithotripter with ellipsoid, electrodes, X-ray tubes, and image intensifier systems.

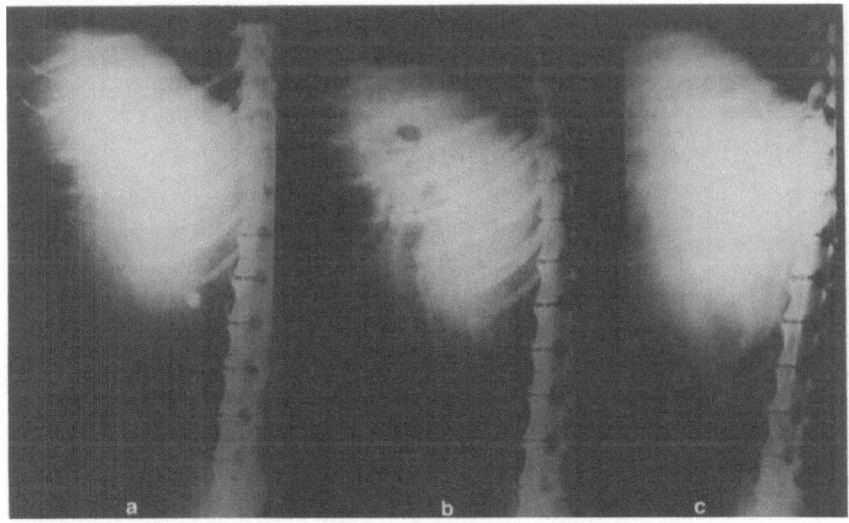

*Fig. 9.* X-ray monitoring (a) before; (b) immediately after; and (c) 7 days after shock wave exposure.

312

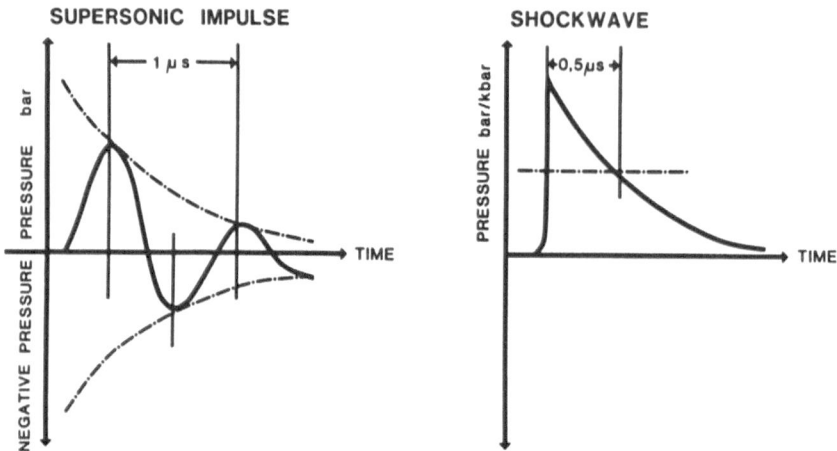

SUPERSONIC IMPULSE

SHOCKWAVE

Fig. 10. Comparison of the pressure vs. time diagrams for ultrasound and a shock wave.

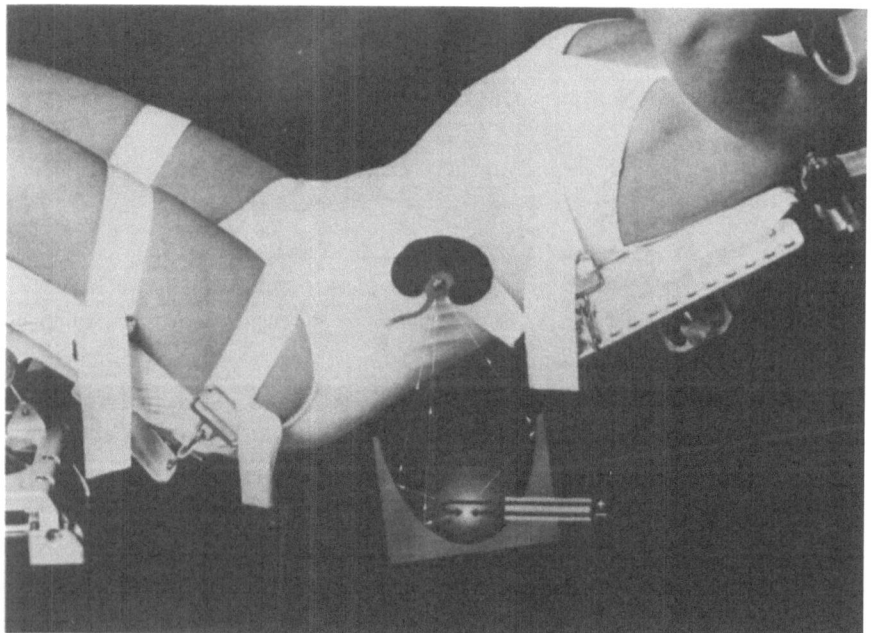

Fig. 11. Schematic drawing of the ellipsoid and the positioned patient.

conversion system (Fig. 12). The apparatus which we use for patient treatment is shown in Figure 13. The x-ray system is shown on both sides of the bath top, the fluoroscopic screen for stone localization and the operator console.

Since February 1980 514 patients with renal stones have been treated by the shock wave technique. Each patient is treated with 500–1000 single shock wave exposures, each with a duration of 0.5 μsec. The complete procedure, which

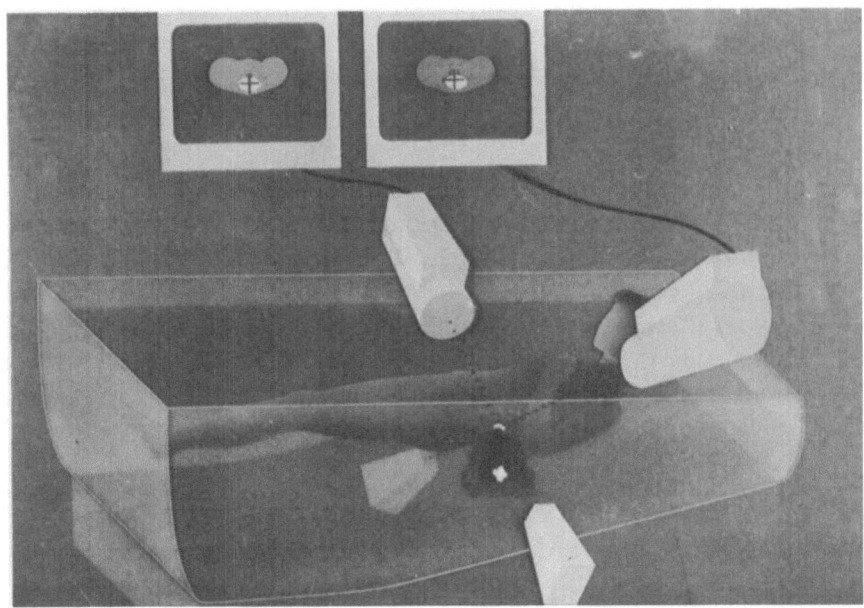

*Fig. 12.* Arrangement of the localization system at the waterbath.

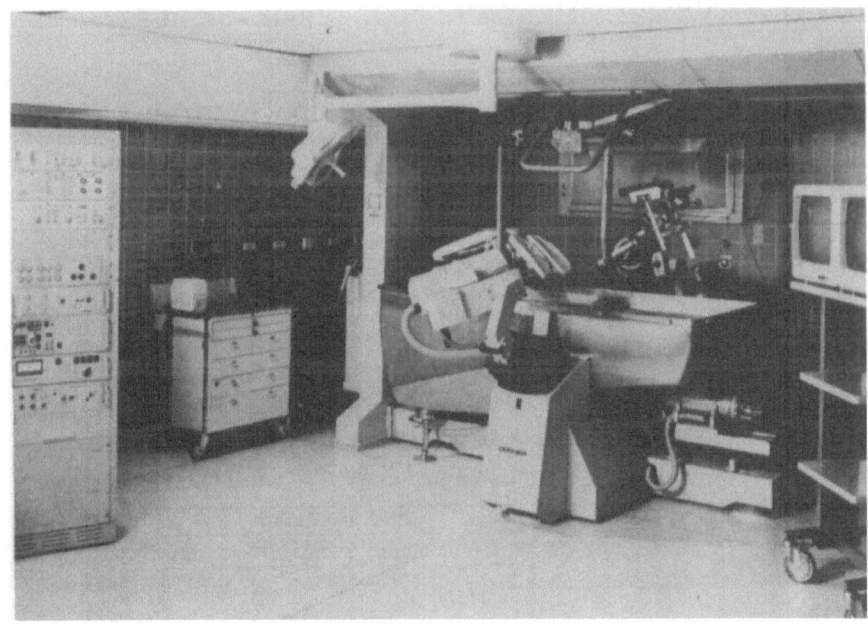

*Fig. 13.* Lithotripter for clinical use.

includes periodic repositioning of the patient, takes approximately 45 min (Fig. 14).

Follow-up radiographs made 3 months after treatment demonstrate, that 90% of the patients were stone-free. In 9.3% of the patients residual stone fragments were identified at the 3 month follow-up. Only 2 patients, that means 0.7% required operative treatment, because of obstruction caused by stone fragments (Fig. 15). Split isotopic studies made before and after treatment demonstrated no differences in kidney function post treatment. Approximately 20% of the patients had trouble with colic as the fragments passed. In Figure 16 a–c one example of an x-ray follow-up after shock wave treatment is shown. Initially we followed very strict conditions for the acceptance to shock wave treatment. These first contraindications are listed in Figure 17. However, as we gained experience we were able to eliminate some of these first criteria of exclusion.

|  | n |
|---|---|
| PATIENTS  TREATED | 514 |
| SHOCK WAVE  TREATMENTS | 576 |
| SHOCK WAVE  EXPOSURES PER  TREATMENT | 350 – 1850 |
| TIME  OF  TREATMENT APPR.  45  MINUTES | |

*Fig. 14.* Analysis of treatments.

| free of stones | 90,0 % |
|---|---|
| residual stones | 9,3 % |
| surgery | 0,7 % |

IODINE $_{131}$ – HIPPURAN STUDIES

| before treatment | after treatment | |
|---|---|---|
| | 3 – 6  month | 12 – 18 month |
| 100 % | 106 % | 110 % |

*Fig. 15.* Results of extracorporeal shock wave treatment.

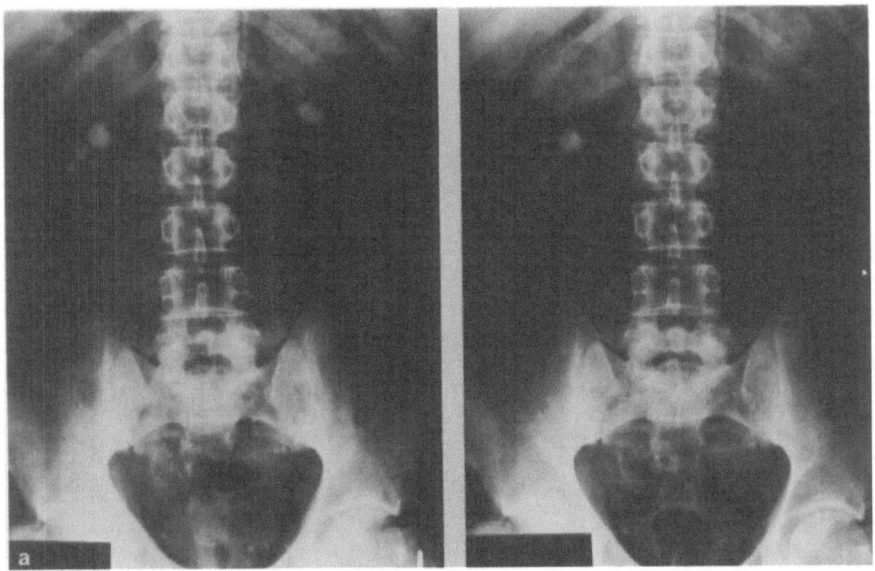

*Fig. 16a.* Kidney stone on both sides – Situation after the first treatment on the left side.

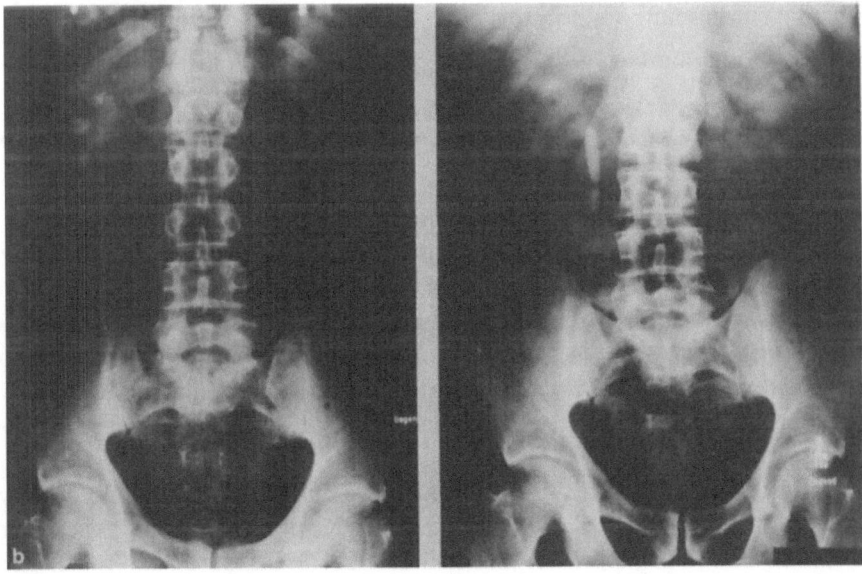

*Fig. 16b.* Left side stone-free and follow-up study after treatment on the right side.

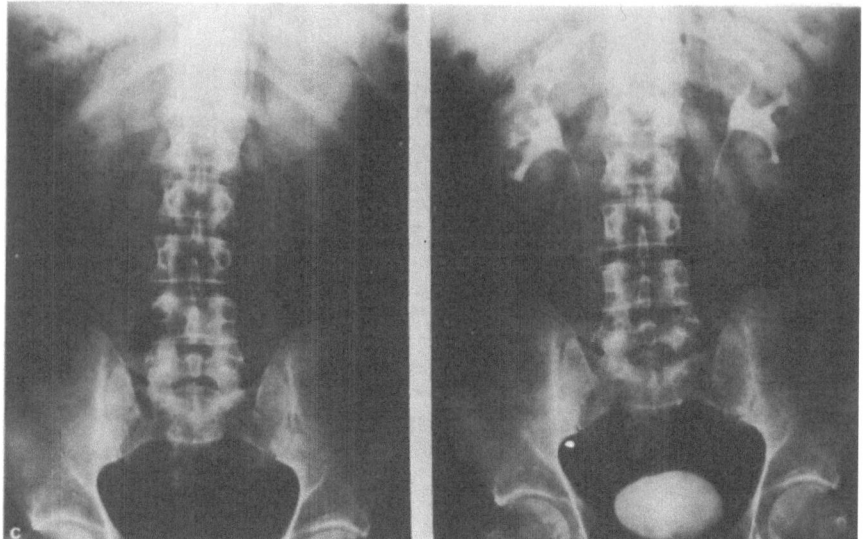

*Fig. 16c.* Stone-free collecting system on both sides and undisturbed discharge conditions in the IVP.

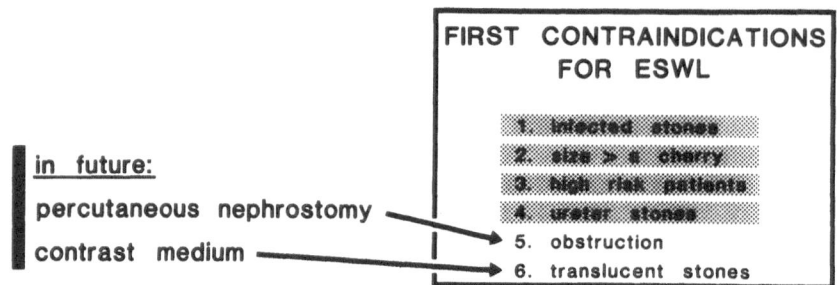

*Fig. 17.* Still existing contraindications for ESWL.

*Infected stones.* Transitory obstruction during debris discharge may in the case of urinary obstruction cause pyelonephritis as well as damage of the parenchyma with subsequent urosepsis. Therefore we excluded infected stones in the beginning. However, antibiotic pretreatment has proven to prevent this complication in 27 infected patients, so infected stones are no longer regarded as a contraindication. Furthermore in complicated infections a percutaneous nephrostomy can be done to support undisturbed urinary flow.

*Size of the stone.* Since the transport even of the smallest particles theoretically is a quantitative problem, we accepted for the early applications only concrements of smaller size. As experience was gained, the discharge of the concrements created fewer problems than anticipated. For that reason we accept stones up to partial Staghorn calculi at the moment.

*High risk patients.* In the beginning we did not accept high risk patients, because we needed a clear appraisal of possible side effects of shock wave therapy. The addition of complications of a serious internal disease could have made the true appraisal of the shock wave effect impossible. After having treated 150 patients without any side effects, we slowly began to treat high risk patients.

*Ureter stones.* In the beginning we had to operate on 2 patients, suffering for a long time from ureter stones, after a non-effective shock wave treatment. In these cases, we found at surgery, that the stones were totally fractured, but embedded in the wall of the ureter and therefore could not disintegrate in parts. Treatment of another 8 patients with ureter stones, was more successful. Here the stone had passed into the upper ureter only a short time before treatment. In all cases we could destroy the stones, so that the particles passed spontaneously within a few days.

*Obstruction and radio-translucent stones.* At the present time, obstruction below the stone and not caused by the stone, and an insufficient contrast density of the stone still represent containdications for extracorporeal shock wave therapy. For this problem, it is planned, however, to extend the application by means of percutaneous nephrostomy, to allow the localization of stones with little or no contrast using a contrast medium.

In conclusion as the indications for shock wave treatment have been expanded, a high success rate continues to be obtained. It can be concluded, that non invasive treatment of patients with kidney stones by high energy shock waves is efficient. In an expanding range of indications shock wave treatment of renal calculi can replace surgical removal.

### References

1. Chaussy CH, Eisenberger F, Wanner K, Forssmann B, Hepp W, Schmiedt E, Brendel W: The use of shock waves for the destruction of renal calculi without direct contact. Urological Research 4: 175, 1976.
2. Chaussy CH, Schmiedt E, Forssmann B, Brendel W: Contact free renal stone destruction by means of shock waves. Europ Surg Res 11: 36, 1979.
3. Chaussy CH, Schmiedt E, Brendel W: Instrumentelle Harnsteinentfernung. In: Urolithiasis 2. W Vah-lensieck (Hrsg). Springer Verlag, Berlin – Heidelberg – New York, 1979.
4. Chaussy CH, Brendel W, Schmiedt E: Extracorporeally induced destruction of kidney stones by shock waves. Lancet, Dec 13: 1265–1268, 1980.
5. Chaussy CH (ed): Extracorporeal shock wave lithotripsy – New aspects in the treatment of kidney stone disease. Karger, Basel, 1982.
6. Chaussy CH, Schmiedt E, Jocham D, Brendel W, Forssmann B, Walther V: First clinical experiences with extracorporeally induced destruction of kidney stones by shock waves. J Urol 127: 417–420, 1982.
7. Chaussy CH, Schmiedt E, Jocham D: Nonsurgical treatment in renal calculi with shock waves. In: Stones – Clinical Management of Urolithiasis. RA Roth, B Finlayson (eds): Wailliams & Wilkins, Baltimore – London.

# Index

Acute tubular necrosis (ATN) 81
Antilymphocyte globulin (ALG) 41, 42, 49–56, 58, 61–77, 87, 196, 201, 226, 234, 235
Antibodies to vascular endothelial cells (VEC) 16–20
Antithymocyte globulin (ATG) 4, 32, 156, 243, 250, 253, 258
Azathioprine 39, 41, 42, 57–60, 91, 156, 159, 177, 195, 210, 226, 234, 244, 250, 253, 262

Biliary atresia 263, 264
Blood transfusion and transplantation 23–35, 43, 44, 158
  Composition of the transfusate 26, 27
  Donor specific transfusion 158–159
  HLA matched blood 28–30
  Mechanism of the transfusion effect 33–35
  Numbers of transfusions 24–26
  Timing of transfusion 30, 31
Bone marrow transplantation 269–283
  Autologous marrow 275, 276
  Buffy coat supplementation 271
  Graft versus host disease 278, 279
  Graft versus leukaemia effect 281, 282
  Granulocyte transfusions 280
  Indications for non-malignant disease 270, 271
  Indications for malignant disease 271–275
  Infections 280, 281
  Interstitial pneumonia 280, 281
  Irradiation 273, 277
  Marrow transplant versus chemotherapy 282
  Marrow treatment 279, 280
  Partially matched grafts 276, 277
  Recipient preparation 270
  Recurrent leukaemia 277

Cardiac transplantation 239–245
  Donor selection 101, 240
  Heterotopic transplantation 243
  Immunosuppression 253–259
  Operation 242
  Recipient selection 241, 242
Centre effect 10–12, 203

320

Chronic granulocytic leukaemia 274
Cyclophosphamide 41, 156, 270, 279
Cyclosporine 44–46, 57–60, 87, 88, 90, 100, 157, 173, 174, 195, 204, 206, 209, 219, 222, 226, 228–230, 234, 235, 244, 247, 249, 255, 257, 258, 261, 266, 273, 274, 279
    Nephrotoxicity 59, 81, 82, 157, 226, 241, 274
Cytomegalovirus 280, 281

Diabetes 215, 225
    Diabetic nephropathy reversal 206
    Renal transplantation diabetics 173–175
DNCB skin reactivity 1, 33
Donor age for renal transplantation 115–121
Donor specific blood transfusion 158, 159

Edothelial monocyte antigens (EM) 18, 19
    Graft rejection 18, 19

Fine needle aspiration biopsy (FNAB) 79–95
    Bone marrow transplantation 82
Fungal infection in renal transplantation 177–182

Graft irradiation 156
Graft rejection 15, 16, 39, 49–55, 79–95, 156, 178, 211, 239, 250, 253, 254, 258
Graft survival 42, 43, 49
    HLA A and B antigens 7–13, 15, 196, 197, 210, 222, 269, 270, 276
    HLA DR. 2, 5, 222, 269
    MLR 7–12, 155, 158, 159, 163, 196
Graft versus host disease 278, 279

Haemodialysis in Kuwait 187–191
Heart and lung transplantation 247–252
    Donor selection 101, 248, 249
    Operation 249
    Post-operative management 249, 250
    Recipient selection 248
Hepatitis B 201, 206
High and low responders 1, 2, 4, 33
High dose steroids 90, 91
HLA identical living donors and rejection 18, 19
HLA A and B and graft survival – see under 'Graft Survival'
HLA DR and graft survival – see under 'Graft Survival'
HLA DRW 6  1–4

Immunosuppression 39–47
    see also, Antilymphocyte globulin; antithymocyte globulin; azathioprine; cyclophosphamide; cyclosphorine; high dose steroids, methotrexate, methylprednisone; prednisone
    Complications of 59, 201, 204, 255–258
    for Cardiac transplantation 253–259
Interferon 264, 277, 280
Islet cell transplantation 215–244
    Immunogenicity of 221
    Registry of 220

Kidney antigenicity 17
Kidney preservation *in situ* 107–114
Kidney and pancreas simultaneous transplantation 217, 225, 228, 236

*Listeria monocytogenes* 198, 206
Liver transplantation 88–90, 261–267
    Biliary atresia 263–264
    Demand for 261, 262
    Donors 100
    Indications for 263
    Non-heparin bypass 266, 267
    Rejection 262
    Results 266, 267
Living donors for renal transplantation 155, 163–171, 189, 193, 196, 209–213

Methotrexate 270, 273, 279
Methylprednisone 92, 93, 210
Mixed lymphocyte reaction (MLR) 7–13
    Graft survival – see 'Graft survival'
    Rejection episodes 8, 11, 12
Monoclonal antibodies
    to Lymphocyte subsets 34, 157, 158, 278, 279
    Tumours 276

Organ preservation
    Kidney 123–130, 131–139, 155, 219
    Normothermic perfusion 131–139
    Pancreas preservation 222
Organ procurement 97–106
    Donor maintenance 101, 102
    Donor operation 102–104
    Heart/heart/lung donors 101, 240
    Kidney donors 100, 107, 107–114, 154, 155
    Liver donors 100
    Pancreas donors 101
    Transportation 105

Paediatric renal transplantation 200, 204
Pancreas transplantation 215–224, 225–231, 233–238
    Pancreas preservation 222
    Pancreas registry 216
Peritoneal dialysis in Kuwait 187–191
Placental eluates 69
Plasmaphoresis 157
Prednisone 39, 41, 42, 87, 156, 175, 195, 244, 254

Renal autotransplantation 285–295
    Indications for 285–286
    Techniques 286–289
Renal diseases
    In Kuwait 189

322

In Turkey 209
Renal replacement therapy in Kuwait 187–191
Renal surgery
    Hypothermic *in situ* perfusion and surface cooling techniques 297–303
Renal transplantation
    Current status 153–161
    Indications for 153
    Immunological contraindications 154–156
    In diabetics 173–175
    In Kuwait 189, 193–208
    Results 158, 159
    In Turkey 209–213

Sensitized patients 23
Sexual dysfunction in transplanted patients 183–186
Splenectomy 57, 156, 212, 213
Suppressor cells 34, 35, 73

Thoracic duct drainage 44, 61–77
Tolerance 41

Vascular access 141–145, 147–151
    Bovine heterografts 147–151
    Brescia cimino fistula 147–151
    Goretex grafts 147–151
    Upper arm A-V fistula 141–145
Vascular endothelial cell antigens (VEC) 15
    On monocytes 17, 19, 20